Problem-Oriented
Medical Diagnosis

Problem-Oriented
Medical Diagnosis

EDITOR   H. Harold Friedman, M.D.

Clinical Professor of Medicine, University of Colorado School of
Medicine; Attending Physician and Director, Heart Station, General
Rose Memorial Hospital; Attending Physician, Saint Joseph
Hospital, Denver

**Consulting
Editor**   Solomon Papper, M.D.

Distinguished Professor of Medicine, University of Oklahoma College
of Medicine; Distinguished Physician, Oklahoma City Veterans
Administration Hospital, Oklahoma City

Contributing Authors

Robert G. Chapman, M.D.
S. Robert Contiguglia, M.D.
Paul M. Cox, M.D.
Lane D. Craddock, M.D.
Sidney Duman, M.D.
William C. Earley, M.D.
Barry W. Frank, M.D.
H. Harold Friedman, M.D.
Stanley Ginsburg, M.D.
Gilbert Hermann, M.D.
Walter A. Huttner, M.D.
Robert C. Jacobs, M.D.
Herbert Kaplan, M.D.
Harvey B. Karsh, M.D.
A. J. Kauvar, M.D.
Melvyn H. Klein, M.D.

Henry M. Lewis, M.D.
Jeffrey L. Mishell, M.D.
Kenneth H. Neldner, M.D.
Jerome S. Nosanchuk, M.D.
Solomon Papper, M.D.
Stanley B. Reich, M.D.
John C. Riley, M.D.
Alan D. Rothberg, M.D.
John H. Saiki, M.D.
Janet E. Schemmel, M.D.
Marvin I. Schwarz, M.D.
David Shander, M.D.
N. Balfour Slonim, M.D., Ph.D.
Charley J. Smyth, M.D.
Joseph C. Tyor, M.D.
Phillip S. Wolf, M.D.

Little, Brown and Company
Boston

To our parents   To the memory of
Morris and Sarah Friedman

and to
Max and Lillian Papper

Preface

The goal of medical practice is the solution of the varied problems presented by the patient. To accomplish this purpose, it is necessary to identify the patient's problems, investigate them by suitable means, arrive at a diagnosis, determine the prognosis, and institute proper treatment.

Problem identification begins with a complete history and physical examination. From the information thus obtained, it is possible to select appropriate laboratory procedures that may assist in establishing a diagnosis. Many physicians also order routinely a battery of laboratory tests for screening purposes. The findings on the history, physical examinations, and laboratory investigations provide the essential data on which the diagnosis, prognosis, and management of the patient are based.

The method of recording the medical history is a subject of much controversy today. The question of whether the traditional, chronological narrative form or the problem-oriented (Weed) system should be employed for history-taking is still being debated. However, it is hardly debatable that one of the physician's major responsibilities is to discover all the patient's problems. Such problems may present themselves as symptoms, signs, abnormal laboratory findings, or clinical diagnosis.

The purpose of this book is to provide a practical approach to many of the problems encountered in the everyday practice of adult medicine. The subjects selected for discussion were chosen because they occur frequently or because they are clinically important. It is obvious that, in a field as vast as internal medicine, a great deal of selectivity had to be exercised to keep the size of the book within reasonable limits. We recognize that some readers may disagree with our choice of subjects.

The problem list (the sections within the chapters) is composed of presenting symptoms, physical signs, selected laboratory and radiologic findings of abnormalities, and a few disease entities and symptom complexes. To deal with these problems, we have chosen academically oriented physicians who are primarily engaged in the care of patients. It is hoped that their work will give this manual the imprimatur of both authenticity and practicality.

This book is intended for the medical student, the intern, the family practice or internal medicine resident, and the private practitioner whether he be a family physician or a general internist. It is not intended for the subspecialist in internal medicine.

Most textbooks of medicine are organized about diseases rather than patients, and properly so. However, because of that frame of reference, such books do not provide the methodology for proceeding from symptoms, signs, or abnormal laboratory findings to the diagnosis of disease. This text, by providing the diagnostic approach to presenting problems, should help to bridge the gap. It is thus intended to supplement, not to replace, conventional textbooks of medicine.

The format of the book deserves brief mention. It is written primarily in outline form for clarity and conciseness but also tries to provide a reasonable degree of comprehensiveness. Because individual contributors were permitted some latitude in dealing with the topics assigned to them, the presentations of the various problems are not uniform throughout the book. Most of the authors, however, have used the following basic format: definition of the entity, consideration of its etiology and significant clinical features, and, finally, presentation of a practical diagnostic approach to the problem. Brief interpretations of the relevant laboratory tests are also given. Discussions of pathophysiology, prognosis, and treatment have been omitted, however, not only because they are not within the scope of the book but also because this information is readily available from other sources. For similar reasons a bibliography is not included.

We express our thanks to those who did most of the typing of the manuscript: Cricket Beach, Fran Weinstein, Cathy Roberts, Esther Kandt, and especially Diane Yacovetta.

In the preparation of the book, we have had the generous support of the Administrative Staff and the Board of Trustees of General Rose Memorial Hospital in Denver.

H. H. F.
S. P.

Contents

Contributing Authors

Robert G. Chapman, M.D.
Associate Professor of Medicine, University of Colorado School of Medicine;.
Attending Hematologist, University of Colorado Medical Center, Denver

S. Robert Contiguglia, M.D.
Clinical Instructor in Medicine, University of Colorado School of Medicine;
Co-Director, Division of Renal Medicine and Dialysis, General Rose Memorial
Hospital, Denver

Paul M. Cox, M.D.
Associate Director, Division of Pulmonary Medicine, Maine Medical Center,
Portland

Lane D. Craddock, M.D.
Assistant Clinical Professor of Medicine, University of Colorado School of Medicine;
Attending Physician and Director, Division of Cardiology, General Rose Memorial
Hospital, Denver

Sidney Duman, M.D.
Assistant Clinical Professor of Medicine (Neurology), University of Colorado
School of Medicine; Attending Physician, General Rose Memorial Hospital and
Saint Joseph Hospital, Denver

William Charles Earley, M.D.
Assistant Clinical Professor of Radiology, University of Colorado School of
Medicine; Head, Division of Nuclear Medicine, General Rose Memorial Hospital,
Denver

Barry W. Frank, M.D.
Associate Clinical Professor of Medicine, University of Colorado School of
Medicine; Attending Physician, General Rose Memorial Hospital and Saint Joseph
Hospital, Denver

H. Harold Friedman, M.D.
Clinical Professor of Medicine, University of Colorado School of
Medicine; Attending Physician and Director, Heart Station, General
Rose Memorial Hospital; Attending Physician, Saint Joseph
Hospital, Denver

Stanley Ginsburg, M.D.
Clinical Instructor in Medicine (Neurology), University of Colorado School of
Medicine; Attending Physician, General Rose Memorial Hospital and Saint Joseph
Hospital, Denver

Gilbert Hermann, M.D.
Associate Clinical Professor of Surgery, University of Colorado School of Medicine;
Attending Surgeon, General Rose Memorial Hospital, Denver

Walter A. Huttner, M.D.
Associate Clinical Professor of Medicine, University of Colorado School of
Medicine; Attending Physician and Chief, Division of Endocrinology, General
Rose Memorial Hospital, Denver

Robert C. Jacobs, M.D.
Clinical Instructor in Medicine, University of Colorado School of Medicine;
Attending Physician, General Rose Memorial Hospital, Denver

Herbert Kaplan, M.D.
Assistant Clinical Professor of Medicine, University of Colorado School of
Medicine; Attending Physician, General Rose Memorial Hospital, Denver

Harvey B. Karsh, M.D.
Assistant Clinical Professor of Medicine, University of Colorado School of
Medicine; Attending Physician, General Rose Memorial Hospital, Denver

A. J. Kauvar, M.D.
Associate Clinical Professor of Medicine, University of Colorado School of
Medicine; Davis Distinguished Research Fellow, Eleanor Roosevelt Cancer
Institute; Attending Physician and Chief, Division of Gastroenterology, General
Rose Memorial Hospital, Denver

Melvyn H. Klein, M.D.
Clinical Instructor in Medicine, University of Colorado School of Medicine;
Co-Director, Division of Renal Medicine and Dialysis, General Rose Memorial
Hospital, Denver

Henry M. Lewis, M.D.
Associate Clinical Professor of Medicine (Dermatology), University of Colorado
School of Medicine; Attending Physician, General Rose Memorial Hospital;
Consulting Physician, Fitzsimons General Hospital, Denver

Jeffrey L. Mishell, M.D.
Clinical Instructor in Medicine, University of Colorado School of Medicine;
Co-Director, Division of Renal Medicine and Dialysis, General Rose Memorial
Hospital, Denver

Kenneth H. Neldner, M.D.
Associate Clinical Professor of Medicine (Dermatology), University of Colorado
School of Medicine; Associate Attending Physician, General Rose Memorial
Hospital, Denver

Jerome S. Nosanchuk, M.D.
Assistant Professor of Pathology, University of Colorado School of Medicine;
Pathologist, General Rose Memorial Hospital, Denver

Solomon Papper, M.D.
Distinguished Professor of Medicine, University of Oklahoma School of Medicine;
Distinguished Physician, Oklahoma City Veterans Administration Hospital,
Oklahoma City

Stanley B. Reich, M.D.
Professor of Clinical Radiology, University of Colorado School of Medicine;
Chairman, Department of Radiology, General Rose Memorial Hospital, Denver

John C. Riley, M.D.
Clinical Assistant Professor of Radiology, University of Colorado School of
Medicine; Radiologist, General Rose Memorial Hospital, Denver

Alan D. Rothberg, M.D.
Clinical Instructor in Radiology, University of Colorado School of Medicine;
Radiologist, General Rose Memorial Hospital, Denver

John H. Saiki, M.D.
Associate Professor of Medicine, University of New Mexico School of Medicine;
Hematology-Oncology Section, Department of Medicine, Bernalillo County
Medical Center, Albuquerque

Janet E. Schemmel, M.D.
Associate Clinical Professor of Medicine, University of Colorado School of
Medicine; Chief of Medicine, Saint Joseph Hospital; Attending Physician,
General Rose Hospital, Denver

Marvin I. Schwarz, M.D.
Assistant Professor of Medicine, University of Colorado School of Medicine;
Chief, Pulmonary Division, Denver Veterans Administration Hospital, Denver

David Shander, M.D.
Clinical Instructor in Medicine, University of Colorado School of Medicine;
Associate Director, Division of Cardiology, General Rose Memorial Hospital,
Denver

N. Balfour Slonim, M.D., Ph.D.
Director, Cardiopulmonary Diagnostic Laboratory; Associate Attending Physician,
General Rose Memorial Hospital, Denver

Charley J. Smyth, M.D.
Professor of Medicine and Head, Rheumatic Disease Division, University of
Colorado School of Medicine, Denver

Joseph C. Tyor, M.D.
Associate Clinical Professor of Medicine, University of Colorado School of
Medicine; Attending Physician, General Rose Memorial Hospital, Denver

Phillip S. Wolf, M.D.
Assistant Clinical Professor of Medicine, University of Colorado School of
Medicine; Vice-Chairman, Department of Medicine, and Associate Director,
Division of Cardiology, General Rose Memorial Hospital, Denver

1.

General Problems

Clubbing

Solomon Papper

DEFINITION

Clubbing is a condition characterized by bulbous enlargement of the distal phalanges of the fingers and toes. Hypertrophic osteoarthropathy is a more advanced stage of clubbing associated with periosteal proliferation of the long bones, often with arthralgia or joint swelling.

CLINICAL FEATURES

1. The earliest evidence of clubbing is thickening of the nail bed, manifested by increased ballotability of the nail in its bed and a reduction in the angle made by the nail and the dorsum of the distal phalanx. (The normal angle is about 15°.) Later there may be warmth and redness and sometimes tenderness of the skin of the distal phalanges. Sometimes the patient has a burning sensation in the affected areas, but pain is uncommon. Exaggeration of the curvature of the nail is not clubbing but a normal variant.

2. When the periosteum of the long bones is involved, there may be pain near the joints as well as redness, warmth, and tenderness.

3. The joints adjacent to long bone involvement may be swollen.

4. Early the x-rays are normal. Later there is flaring of the ungual process and demineralization. The long bones may reveal periosteal thickening, especially near the joints.

1

DIFFERENTIAL DIAGNOSIS

In some patients joint symptoms predominate and may be confused with arthritis. When there is superficial warmth, redness, and tenderness about the ankle, thrombophlebitis or cellulitis may be considered.

ASSOCIATED CONDITIONS

1. Clubbing may be hereditary and not associated with any disease state.

2. Pulmonary disease.
  a. Bronchogenic carcinoma (rare with metastatic lung tumor).
  b. Pleural neoplasms.
  c. Chronic infections other than tuberculosis (e.g., bronchiectasis, abscess, empyema).
  d. Emphysema with cor pulmonale.
  e. Mediastinal lesions.

3. Cardiac disorders.
  a. Cyanotic congenital heart disease.
  b. Infective endocarditis.
  c. Pulmonary arteriovenous fistula.

4. Chronic liver disease: cirrhosis.

5. Gastrointestinal disorders.
  a. Ulcerative colitis.
  b. Granulomatous colitis.
  c. Regional enteritis.
  d. Neoplasms.
  e. Steatorrhea of unknown cause.

6. Hyperthyroidism.

7. Unilateral clubbing is usually due to local vascular disease (e.g., anomalies of the aortic arch, aortic or subclavian aneurysm, pulmonary hypertension with persistent patency of the ductus arteriosus).

DIAGNOSTIC APPROACH TO BILATERAL CLUBBING
History

A family history of clubbing and long duration of clubbing without evidence of associated illness suggest that it is of the hereditary type. Specific history information related to associated illnesses should be sought: cough, dyspnea, cigarette smoking, cyanosis, fever, jaundice, alcoholism, diarrhea, and tremulousness.

Physical Examination

Specific points related to associated illness should be sought: wheezes, rales, supraclavicular nodes, murmurs, jaundice, vascular spiders, palmar erythema, enlarged liver, abdominal mass (regional enteritis), thyromegaly, and thyroid eye signs.

Laboratory Studies

1. CBC.
2. Urinalysis.
3. Chest films.
4. Electrocardiogram.
5. Liver function tests.
6. T_4 and T_3 resin uptake.
7. Stools for occult blood.
8. Sigmoidoscopy, barium enema, and upper GI and small bowel study if the history suggests gastrointestinal disease or if stools are positive for blood.

Edema

Solomon Papper

DEFINITION

Edema is an increase in the volume of interstitial fluid, i.e., the extravascular portion of the extracellular compartment. The plasma volume may or may not be increased.

DIAGNOSIS

There may be a considerable increase in the interstitial fluid volume before it is clinically appreciated. The symptoms and signs of edema are unexplained weight gain, tightness of a ring or shoe, puffiness of the face, swollen extremities, enlarged abdominal girth, and persistence of indentation of the skin following pressure.

ETIOLOGY

Localized Edema

This term usually refers to edema produced by regional obstruction to venous or lymphatic flow, or both. It is usually limited to one or two limbs. Examples include unilateral lower extremity edema due to deep venous thrombosis and unilateral lymphedema due to pelvic neoplasm. The term is also sometimes used to refer to patches of "vascular" edema seen in allergic states.

Hydrothorax and ascites may be localized phenomena or occur in any generalized edematous state. When such an association is not evident, or if the effusions do not respond to treatment, the involved serous cavity should be tapped and the fluid examined by appropriate means (see Differential Diagnosis of Pleural Effusion, Chapter 4, and Abdominal Distention and Ascites, Chapter 5).

Generalized Edema

The more common causes of generalized edema are listed below.

1. Congestive heart failure.
   a. *Symptoms.* A history of heart disease can usually be obtained. Exertional dyspnea, orthopnea, paroxysmal nocturnal dyspnea, fatigue, weakness, and swelling of the lower extremities are common.
   b. *Signs.* Physical examination usually reveals distended jugular veins, cardiomegaly, bibasilar rales, hepatomegaly, and dependent edema.
   c. *Laboratory findings.* The hemogram is usually normal. Urinalysis may disclose proteinuria (trace to 2+). Mild azotemia due to renal hypoperfusion is not unusual.

2. Pericardial disease.
   a. Chronic constrictive pericarditis.
      (1) *Symptoms.* The major symptoms are dyspnea, fatigue, weakness, abdominal distention, and edema.
      (2) *Signs.* The classic findings are markedly elevated venous pressure, often with a deep Y trough and Kussmaul's sign; pulsus paradoxus; a quiet precordium; slight to moderate cardiac enlargement; and absence of significant murmurs.
   b. Pericarditis with effusion.
      (1) *Symptoms.* Chest pain is common but may not be present. Dyspnea, orthopnea, and cough are frequent complaints.
      (2) *Signs.* The area of cardiac dullness is increased. The apical impulse may be impalpable or if present may be located well within the lateral border of cardiac dullness. A pericardial friction rub is often but not always present. When cardiac tamponade occurs, there may be elevated venous pressure, decreased blood pressure with a narrow pulse pressure, pulsus paradoxus, ascites, and edema.
   c. *Laboratory findings.* Chest films and an electrocardiogram are helpful in the diagnosis of pericardial disease. Echocardiography and other procedures may be useful in the diagnosis of pericardial effusion. Hemodynamic studies are important in the evaluation of chronic constrictive pericarditis (see Table 3-15, p. 119).

3. Liver disease.
   a. *Symptoms.* A history of alcoholism and jaundice may be obtained. Weakness, fatigability, anorexia, and weight loss are common.
   b. *Signs.* Physical examination usually reveals evidence of liver disease: jaundice, spider nevi, palmar erythema, hepatomegaly, sometimes splenomegaly, parotid swelling, gynecomastia, testicular atrophy, and clubbing. Although lower extremity edema is not uncommon, the edema may be limited to the peritoneal cavity (ascites).
   c. *Laboratory findings.* An elevated serum bilirubin, abnormal liver function tests, and reduced serum albumin are typical. Urinalysis may reveal proteinuria (0 to 1+).

4. Hypoalbuminemic states.
   a. Nephrotic syndrome.
      (1) *Symptoms.* The history may or may not reveal evidence of renal disease or a systemic illness that can produce the nephrotic syndrome (e.g., diabetes mellitus, systemic lupus erythematosus). Constitutional symptoms may be present but are nonspecific.
      (2) *Laboratory findings.* Urinalysis shows marked proteinuria (>3.5 gm in 24 hours) and lipiduria. Hypoalbuminemia, hyperlipemia, and hypercholesterolemia are typically present.
   b. Protein-losing enteropathy.
      (1) *Symptoms.* This is a rare disorder that may occur in association with chronic inflammatory enterocolonopathies, Menetrier's disease, gastric carcinoma, etc. The symptoms are those of the underlying disease.
      (2) *Signs.* There are no specific signs.
      (3) *Laboratory findings.* Decreased serum albumin and a normal urinalysis are typical.
   c. Malnutrition. Malnutrition associated with severe protein deficiency may result in edema.

5. Miscellaneous causes.
   a. Acute nephritic syndrome. This disorder is characterized by oliguria, proteinuria, hematuria, red blood cell casts, hypertension, and edema. Acute poststreptococcal glomerulonephritis is the most common cause of the acute nephritic syndrome.
   b. Idiopathic cyclic edema. This perplexing disorder of unknown cause occurs predominantly in premenopausal women. Large daily fluctuations in body weight are characteristic. The edema is most prominent while the patient is upright and ambulatory and tends to disappear with recumbency.
   c. Myxedema. Patients with hypothyroidism often have puffiness below the eyes and in the pretibial region. At the latter site it may be firm and nonpitting.

   d. Trichinosis. This disease, commonly associated with the ingestion of raw or improperly cooked pork, has as symptoms and signs
   muscle aches, fever, periorbital edema, and eosinophilia.
   e. Hemiplegia. Unilateral edema in the paralyzed extremity or extremities is a common finding in stroke victims.

DIAGNOSTIC APPROACH

   1. As a first step it is essential to determine whether the edema is localized
   or generalized. This can usually be accomplished by careful attention
   to the history and physical examination. Once localized edema and
   its causes have been excluded, it can be assumed that the edema is
   generalized.

   2. The three most common causes of generalized edema are congestive
   heart failure, liver disease, and the nephrotic syndrome. The diagnosis
   is usually apparent on clinical grounds in the first two conditions, while
   heavy proteinuria suggests the third.
   a. Congestive heart failure and cardiac tamponade sometimes present
   a problem in differential diagnosis. The presence of an apical impulse that is displaced downward and to the left and a gallop
   rhythm are strong evidence in favor of congestive heart failure
   rather than cardiac tamponade. It is also worth noting that congestive heart failure is so frequently associated with cardiomegaly
   that a normal cardiac silhouette almost excludes the diagnosis.
   b. Liver disease as the cause of edema is usually evident from the
   physical examination. Abnormal liver function tests support the
   diagnosis.

   3. When generalized edema is found not to be due to cardiovascular or
   hepatic disease or to the nephrotic syndrome, consideration must be
   given to other, less frequent causes.

   4. Routine studies in patients with edema should include the following:
   a. CBC.
   b. Urinalysis.
   c. Biochemical screening (e.g., SMA-12), including T_4 and T_3 resin
   uptake, serum albumin and total protein, serum cholesterol, and
   liver function tests.
   d. Chest films.
   e. Electrocardiogram.

   5. Urinary findings of heavy proteinuria, hematuria, cylindruria, and
   formed elements in the sediment are generally indicative of renal
   parenchymal disease (see Renal and Urinary Tract Disorders, Chapter 7).

6. Moderate to heavy proteinuria, with or without hypoalbuminemia, suggests the nephrotic syndrome. Additional studies are necessary to determine its etiology.

7. Hypoalbuminemia without proteinuria requires investigation for malnutrition or protein-losing enteropathy, provided liver disease is excluded.

8. The diagnosis of idiopathic cyclic edema is based on an appropriate clinical setting and the exclusion of other causes.

Fatigue

H. Harold Friedman

Fatigue is one of the most common symptoms for which patients seek medical attention.

DEFINITION

Fatigue is a sense of weariness, described by patients variously as exhaustion, tiredness, lack of pep and energy, loss of ambition or interest, low vitality, or a feeling of being "all in." It is often accompanied by a subjective sensation of weakness and a strong desire to rest or sleep.

ETIOLOGY

Fatigue is normal when it is the end result of a full day's work or sustained physical activity. It may also be a consequence of a period of prolonged emotional stress or mental strain. In these circumstances, the cause of the fatigue is usually evident to the patient, and he rarely seeks advice because of it. Chronic fatigue, however, is not a normal state. Although chronic fatigue may be due to a physical ailment, it is most often psychogenic in origin. Table 1-1 lists the more common causes of chronic fatigue.

DIAGNOSTIC APPROACH
History

1. Much can be learned from the history of a patient with fatigue. Because fatigue is most commonly psychic in origin and the result of anxiety, anger, or chronic conflict, a careful inquiry into the emotional state of the patient and his life situation is warranted. Depressive reactions, also a common cause of fatigue, are often associated with weakness, anorexia, weight loss, apathy, insomnia, withdrawal, lack

TABLE 1-1.   Causes of Chronic Fatigue

A. Fatigue of psychogenic origin (80% of cases)
  1. Anxiety states
  2. Depression
B. Fatigue of physical origin (20% of cases)
  1. Infectious disease
    a. Febrile states
    b. Tuberculosis
  2. Metabolic disorders
    a. Diabetes mellitus
    b. Hypothyroidism
    c. Hyperparathyroidism
    d. Hypopituitarism
    e. Addison's disease
  3. Blood dyscrasias
    a. Anemia
    b. Lymphoma and leukemia
  4. Renal disease
    a. Acute renal failure
    b. Chronic renal failure
  5. Liver disease
    a. Acute hepatitis
    b. Chronic hepatitis and cirrhosis
  6. Chronic pulmonary disease
  7. Chronic cardiovascular disease
  8. Neoplastic diseases
  9. Neuromuscular diseases (see Weakness of Neuromuscular Origin, Chapter 10)

of a desire to go on, and self-depreciation. The presence of such symptoms should alert the physician to the possibility of serious depression with its attendant risk of suicide. Therapy should be instituted promptly, even before diagnostic studies are completed.

  2. Clues to the etiology of fatigue may be found in the analysis of the symptom itself.
    a. Patients with psychic fatigue are typically tired when they go to bed and just as tired when they wake up in the morning. As a general rule the fatigue appears to lessen during the day. Many patients complain that they are "always tired" and that no amount of rest or sleep seems to improve their weariness or give them strength. Inquiry will often disclose that there is considerable variation in the patient's fatigue: at one time he feels exhausted, and at another time—sometimes only a few minutes later—he is full of energy and capable of any task confronting him. Motivation appears to be a large factor in the patient's ability to cope with the situations of everyday life. Headaches and other pains, as well as subjective weakness, commonly accompany the fatigue.
    b. Fatigue due to physical illness, on the other hand, is relieved by decreased activity and by rest and sleep. The patient probably awakens refreshed in the morning, but less than ordinary activity causes fatigue.

c. Denial or minimization of fatigue in a patient who looks tired or is described as being weak or tired by his family usually implies organic disease rather than a psychological disturbance.

Physical Examination

1. Fatigue per se is not associated with any specific physical findings.

2. The patient who is pale, wan, and sickly in appearance, who looks tired and worn, and whose face sags and body slumps should be suspected of having organic illness.

3. The facial expression of the depressed patient, once seen, is rarely forgotten.

4. Most physical ailments that cause fatigue can be diagnosed by clinical observation alone.

Diagnostic Work-up

1. The major purpose of the diagnostic work-up is to exclude organic disease. To this end, the following procedures are recommended:

   a. CBC.
   b. Sedimentation rate.
   c. Urinalysis.
   d. Biochemical screening (e.g., SMA-12).
   e. Thyroid function tests (e.g., T_4 and T_3 resin uptake).
   f. Two-hour postprandial glucose or glucose tolerance test.
   g. Chest films.
   h. Electrocardiogram.

2. If the initial work-up is negative in a patient who is apparently well except for fatigue, usually organic disease can be excluded and no further work-up is necessary. The patient should be kept under observation until systemic illness can reasonably be excluded. Patients with fatigue of physical origin sooner or later develop other symptoms or signs. Should these occur, further investigation is then warranted.

Fever of Unknown Origin

H. Harold Friedman

DEFINITION

Fever of unknown origin (FUO) is defined as continuous fever of at least 3 weeks' duration with daily temperature elevation above 101°F and re-

maining undiagnosed after 1 week of intensive study in the hospital (Petersdorf and Wallace), or as temperature greater than 100.5°F persisting for
at least 3 weeks in patients in whom the history, physical examination,
blood count, urinalysis, and chest films fail to indicate the diagnosis (Sheon
and Van Ommen). Regardless of which of these criteria is employed, the
diagnostic approach to FUO must be individualized for each patient. No
hard and fast rules can be set, because each patient with cryptic fever
presents a unique problem in diagnosis. The requirement of fever of 3
weeks' duration for the diagnosis of FUO is most important because it
eliminates from consideration most viral and bacterial infections as well as
other self-limited diseases associated with fever.

ETIOLOGY

Most patients with FUO do not have rare diseases but usually suffer from
common disorders that are difficult to diagnose because they present
atypically. Most reported series of FUO reveal that infections comprise
about 40 percent of cases; neoplasms (primary or metastatic), 20 percent;
connective tissue diseases, 20 percent; and miscellaneous disorders, 10 percent. In approximately 10 percent of cases, the cause is unknown, but
long-term follow-up studies in this group have shown that most patients
had benign disorders that were simply undiagnosable at the time of the
initial investigation. Table 1-2 lists most of the diagnostic entities encountered by Pertersdorf and Wallace in several hundred patients with FUO.

DIAGNOSTIC CLUES

The type of fever curve, whether intermittent, remittent, or continuous, is
of little or no help in the diagnosis of FUO.

Infections

1. *Tuberculosis* is the most common infectious disease responsible for
   FUO. It may be disseminated without radiologic evidence of pulmonary involvement, and the tuberculin test may be negative. Fun-
   duscopic examination may provide the first suggestion of this disease
   if choroid tubercles are demonstrable. However, the diagnosis is usually made by smear and culture of gastric aspirates or by demonstrating
   tubercles in biopsies of the liver, lymph nodes, bone marrow, or pericardium. Sometimes only a therapeutic trial with antituberculotic
   drugs will establish the correct diagnosis.

2. *Infective endocarditis* may present initially as FUO, particularly if the
   patient has received antibiotics in the early stages of the disease. *Atrial
   myxoma* may mimic endocarditis when it presents with fever, a heart
   murmur, and embolic phenomena. Angiocardiography and echocardiography will help distinguish between the two.

TABLE 1-2. Common Disease Entities Responsible for Fever of Unknown Origin

I. Neoplastic diseases
  A. Tumors of reticuloendothelial system
    1. Leukemia
    2. Lymphoma, Hodgkin's disease
    3. Multiple myeloma (rare)
  B. Metastatic tumors
    1. From gastrointestinal tract
    2. From lung, kidney, bone
    3. Melanoma
  C. Solid localized tumors
    1. Kidney
    2. Liver
    3. Lung
    4. Pancreas
    5. Atrial myxoma
II. Infections
  A. Granulomatous infections
    1. Tuberculosis
    2. Coccidioidomycosis
    3. Histoplasmosis
    4. Actinomycosis
    5. Nocardiosis
  B. Pyogenic infections
    1. Right upper quadrant infections
      a. Cholangitis
      b. Cholecystitis (stone)
      c. Liver abscess
      d. Subphrenic abscess
      e. Subhepatic abscess
      f. Lesser sac abscess
    2. Abscesses secondary to bowel diseases
      a. Diverticulitis
      b. Appendicitis
    3. Pelvic inflammatory disease
    4. Renal infections
      a. Pyelonephritis (rare)
      b. Perinephric abscess
      c. Intrarenal abscess
      d. Ureteral obstruction with infection
  C. Subacute bacterial endocarditis

II. Infections (continued)
  D. Other bacteremias
    1. Meningococcemia
    2. Gonococcemia
    3. Vibriosis
    4. Listeriosis
    5. Brucellosis
  E. Miscellaneous
    1. Malaria
    2. Infectious mononucleosis
    3. Cytomegalovirus disease
    4. Coxsackie B diseases
    5. Amebiasis
    6. Leptospirosis
    7. Trichinosis
    8. Q fever
III. Connective tissue diseases
  A. Rheumatic fever
  B. Disseminated lupus erythematosus
  C. Rheumatoid arthritis
  D. Giant cell arteritis (temporal arteritis, polymyalgia rheumatica)
  E. Rare
    1. Scleroderma
    2. Dermatomyositis
    3. Polyarteritis nodosa
IV. Unclassified
  A. Drug fever
  B. Multiple pulmonary emboli
  C. Thyroiditis
  D. Sarcoidosis
  E. Hemolytic anemia
  F. Cryptic trauma
  G. Regional enteritis
  H. Granulomatous hepatitis
V. Psychogenic fevers
  A. Habitual hyperthermia
  B. Factitious fever
VI. Periodic fevers
  A. Familial Mediterranean fever
  B. Etiocholanolone fever
VII. Undiagnosed fever of unknown origin

Source: R. G. Petersdorf and I. F. Wallace, Fever of unknown origin. In J. A. Barondess (Ed.), *Diagnostic Approaches to Presenting Syndromes.* Baltimore: Williams & Wilkins, 1971. P. 305.

3. *Urinary tract infections* rarely cause FUO unless associated with intrarenal or perinephric abscess or obstructive uropathy. Rare organisms causing FUO are diagnosed primarily by blood cultures.

4. *Liver abscess and subphrenic abscess* may present initially as FUO without localized findings. Radioisotope scanning of the liver and combined scanning of the lung and liver are useful, safe procedures in diagnosing these entities. Arteriography may also be helpful in some situations.

Neoplasms

Most patients with cancer have fever at some time during the course of their illness. The fever may be related to concomitant infection, localized obstruction by the tumor, surgery and postoperative complications, or the neoplasm itself. The diagnosis is most often established by biopsy of the bone marrow, liver, lymph nodes, or tumor masses. Neoplasms that are most frequently associated with fever are *hypernephromas, lymphomas,* and *metastatic tumors* of the liver. Carcinoma of the stomach, colon, or pancreas, and aleukemic leukemia are examples of other malignancies that may cause fever.

Connective Tissue Diseases

It is not unusual for rheumatic fever, systemic lupus erythematosus, rheumatoid arthritis (particularly the juvenile variety), and polymyalgia rheumatica (temporal arteritis, giant cell arteritis) to present as FUO. On the other hand, scleroderma, dermatomyositis, and polyarteritis nodosa rarely present in this manner. The clinical history, physical findings, and laboratory tests are more important than biopsy in establishing the diagnosis of connective tissue disease. One exception is temporal artery biopsy, which may establish the diagnosis of polymyalgia rheumatica.

Miscellaneous Causes

1. Drugs are an important cause of FUO. A careful inquiry must be made in every case of FUO to determine whether the patient is taking any medications, because elimination of the offending agent may solve the problem and eliminate the need for extensive work-up.

2. Multiple pulmonary emboli may cause FUO. Lung scans and pulmonary angiography will usually establish the diagnosis.

3. Regional enteritis, granulomatous disease of the colon, and ulcerative colitis may present as FUO in the absence of abdominal complaints.

DIAGNOSTIC APPROACH

1. Check the *history.*

   a. If other members of the family have been affected or are affected by a similar illness, exposure to a common etiologic agent may be involved or the disease may have a hereditary basis (e.g., familial Mediterranean fever).

b. A past history of episodic illnesses over a period of years involving multiple organ systems suggests the possibility of connective tissue disease.

c. The occupation of the patient may provide a clue to the cause of FUO. For example, a veterinarian, a butcher, or one engaged in animal husbandry may be suffering from a disease of animal origin.

d. Inquiry about travel abroad is important because the geographic locale in which the patient has been may lead to a search for illnesses endemic in that area rather than those commonly found in the United States. For example, among United States military personnel in Vietnam, the causes of FUO have included such diseases as dengue, malaria, Chikungunya, scrub typhus, and enteric diseases.

2. Rule out *habitual hyperthermia*. This usually occurs in young, psychoneurotic women, and is characterized by afternoon temperatures between 100° and 100.5°F, vague complaints, vasomotor instability, and a normal sedimentation rate. Removal of the patient from her stressful life situation or the administration of tranquilizers, or both, will result in the disappearance of the fever.

3. Rule out *factitious fever* (malingering). Clues to the diagnosis are the failure of the temperature curve to follow the normal diurnal cycle, excessively high temperatures (106° or 107°F, which is rare in adults), normal pulse and respiratory rates at the time of fever, and rapid defervescence unaccompanied by diaphoresis. If malingering is suspected, all temperatures should be taken by a nurse with a carefully checked thermometer, and the patient should be carefully observed throughout the procedure.

4. Perform careful and repeated complete *physical examinations*.

a. Pay particular attention to the eyes, since ocular manifestations of systemic disease may provide the first clue to the diagnosis of obscure fever. An ophthalmologist may be of great help in interpreting ocular findings.

b. Examine carefully for lymphadenopathy, particularly in the area about the clavicles.

c. Listen for bruits, which may provide evidence for malignant vascular tumors.

d. Check for sternal and bony tenderness, which may suggest myeloproliferative disease or metastatic tumor.

e. Check the navel, since intraabdominal neoplasms may metastasize early to the navel, where their presence is readily detectable by palpation. Moreover, such metastases are easily biopsied under local anesthesia.

f. Examine the skin for nodules that likewise may represent the earliest manifestation of metastatic malignancy.

g. Rectal examination and proctosigmoidoscopy are indicated in all patients with FUO.

5. Depending on circumstances, perform most or all of the following *laboratory tests.* It may be necessary to do these tests serially. Surgical procedures, with the exception of easily performed biopsies, should be considered only after routine studies have failed to reveal the source of FUO.

  a. Routine laboratory tests.

  (1) CBC.

  (2) Sedimentation rate.

  (3) Urinalysis, and urine culture and sensitivity studies.

  (4) Stools for ova, parasites, occult blood, culture and sensitivity studies.

  (5) Blood cultures: Take at least five at 4-hour intervals; repeat single cultures on the second and third days. All specimens should be cultured aerobically and anaerobically and retained for several weeks.

  b. Serologic tests.

  (1) Febrile agglutinins (rarely of help).

  (2) ASO titer to help in the diagnosis of rheumatic fever.

  (3) LE preparation × 3.

  (4) RA test or its equivalent.

  (5) Serum for ANA.

  (6) Mono test and heterophil agglutination.

  c. Blood chemistries.

  (1) Biochemical screening, including serum levels of calcium, phosphorus, alkaline phosphatase, bilirubin, BUN or creatinine, SGOT, LDH, GGPT, glucose, and T_4.

  (2) Serum protein electrophoresis and immunoglobulins.

  d. Miscellaneous tests.

  (1) Bone marrow core biopsy (not aspiration alone) and culture.

  (2) Gastric aspirate for acid-fast smear and culture.

  e. Skin tests. Tuberculin, histoplasmin, coccidoidin, and possibly others, depending upon the circumstances.

  f. Radiographic procedures.

  (1) Chest films.

  (2) Intravenous pyelogram.

  (3) Barium enema and upper GI series, including small bowel study.

  (4) Bone films to detect infection or neoplastic disease.

  g. Radioisotope scanning procedures.

  (1) Lung scan to detect pulmonary embolism.

  (2) Liver scan to detect hepatic lesions.

  (3) Bone scans to detect neoplastic disease.

h. Tissue examination.

   (1) Biopsy of lymph nodes or readily accessible tumor masses.

   (2) Needle biopsy of the liver often will reveal the diagnosis if there is hepatic involvement.

   (3) Consider biopsy of the skin and skeletal muscle in suspected connective tissue disease. Usually this procedure is not very helpful.

   (4) Biopsy of the temporal artery in suspected polymyalgia rheumatica, which may establish the diagnosis.

i. Angiographic studies.

   (1) Lymphangiography to detect lymphomas.

   (2) Celiac aortography to detect hepatic, renal, and pancreatic tumors.

   (3) Angiocardiography to detect atrial myxoma.

   (4) Pulmonary angiography to detect pulmonary embolism.

j. Surgical procedures.

   (1) Peritoneoscopy may be useful in detecting tuberculous peritonitis, peritoneal carcinomatosis, cholecystitis, and pelvic inflammatory disease.

   (2) Exploratory laparotomy should not be done in FUO unless all noninvasive techniques have been exhausted and only if the clinical picture, roentgenographic studies, or laboratory findings point to the abdomen as the source of the fever.

   (3) Exploratory thoracotomy with biopsy may be useful in the presence of unidentified pulmonary disease. Needle biopsy of the lung is less useful.

k. Therapeutic trials. Therapeutic trials should be employed only as a last resort and only if they are reasonably specific. Shotgun mixtures of antibiotics, steroids, and other drugs are to be condemned since they usually solve nothing, confuse the clinical picture, and are not without hazard. Examples of more or less specific therapeutic trials include antituberculotic drugs for suspected tuberculosis, aspirin for rheumatic fever, heparin and anticoagulant therapy for pulmonary emboli, steroids for polymyalgia rheumatica, rheumatoid arthritis, or systemic lupus erythematosus, and penicillin and streptomycin for suspected bacterial endocarditis.

Unexplained Weight Loss

Harvey B. Karsh

Weight loss is often an early manifestation of many acute or chronic illnesses. It may occur in a broad spectrum of conditions, including endocrine or metabolic diseases, drug intoxications, neoplastic processes, and psychiatric disorders.

HISTORY

Special attention should be focused on the following:

1. Documentation that weight loss has actually occurred.

2. An increased or decreased appetite.

3. The composition of the diet and the eating habits of the patient.

4. The presence of any gastrointestinal symptoms, regardless of how vague they might be.

5. A complete social and psychiatric history to elicit sources of anxiety, fear, depression, or special situational problems.

WEIGHT LOSS WITH INCREASED APPETITE

Weight loss in spite of an increased appetite suggests the possibility of diabetes or hyperthyroidism.

CONDITIONS ASSOCIATED WITH ACCELERATED METABOLISM AND WEIGHT LOSS

1. Neoplasms.   Unexplained weight loss in middle-aged or elderly persons should suggest the possibility of occult malignancy. Neoplasms produce weight loss by increasing the metabolic processes of the host even in the absence of complicating anatomic, endocrine, or metabolic abnormalities.

2. Fever.   Infections, neoplasms, cerebrovascular accidents, and metabolic disorders may be accompanied by fever. Since the basal metabolic rate increases by 7 percent with each degree of temperature rise, fever by itself can cause weight loss. Moreover, the anorexia, dehydration, and increased protein catabolism that commonly accompany any febrile illness may also contribute to the weight loss. Fever of unknown origin is discussed in the preceding section.

3. Congestive heart failure.

4. Chronic infections.

5. Excessive physical activity.

6. Periods of rapid growth.

CONDITIONS PRIMARILY ASSOCIATED WITH ANOREXIA OR DECREASED FOOD INTAKE

Psychogenic Disorders

1. Anxiety and depression are among the most common causes of weight loss. The importance of psychological and emotional problems as causes of weight loss should not be underestimated. Depression, anxiety, hysteria, or serious psychosis may cause an unnoticed but nevertheless significant decrease in food intake. Correct diagnosis requires a thorough psychiatric and social history.

2. Anorexia nervosa.

    a. *Definition.* Anorexia nervosa is a psychogenic disorder characterized by loss of appetite and refusal to eat. It occurs predominantly in young women between 11 and 35 years of age.

    b. *Signs and symptoms.*

        (1) Weight loss, varying from 10 to 50 percent of the premorbid weight.

        (2) Spontaneous or deliberate vomiting is a common occurrence.

        (3) Overactivity is usual and is out of proportion to the degree of cachexia.

        (4) Diarrhea may result from laxative abuse.

        (5) Although the patient may sleep poorly, he awakens refreshed (unlike the depressed individual, who is always tired).

        (6) Acrocyanosis is often observed.

        (7) Pubic and axillary hair growth is normal.

        (8) Bradycardia and hypotension occur commonly.

        (9) Because of malnutrition, gonadal function is diminished. Decreased urinary estrogens, absence of cornified cells on vaginal smears, and low urinary gonadotropins are common findings. Urinary 17-ketosteroids may also be decreased. However, the plasma cortisol levels are normal, a finding which helps to differentiate anorexia nervosa from panhypopituitarism. Thyroid function is also normal.

Dietary Causes

With few exceptions, malnutrition is rare in the United States. However, the possibility of nutritional deficiencies should be considered in drug addicts, alcoholics, poor people, elderly people (particularly those living alone), and food faddists. Physicians, in the treatment of certain diseases by special diets, may sometimes inadvertently prescribe nutritionally deficient diets and thereby initiate or perpetuate weight loss.

Affections of the Mouth and Pharynx

1. Mechanical. Ill-fitting dentures or a lack of dentures may so interfere with mastication that the quantity and quality of the food eaten is substandard.

2. Neurologic lesions. Neurologic disorders that affect the ability to chew or swallow food can result in an insufficient caloric intake and weight loss. Included in this group of diseases are such conditions as muscular dystrophy, strokes, amyotrophic lateral sclerosis, brainstem lesions, and syringomyelia.

3. Painful oral lesions.
   a. Nutritional diseases, including vitamin deficiencies.
   b. Painful lesions of the oropharynx due to connective tissue or other diseases.
   c. Candidiasis which is often associated with the use of antibiotics.
   d. Gingivitis due to diphenylhydantoin or other drugs.
   e. Heavy-metal intoxication.

Drug Effects

Drugs may cause weight loss as a by-product of their actions. Thus, digitalis and the amphetamines may cause anorexia. Drugs may induce anorexia, nausea, and vomiting by a direct effect on the gastrointestinal mucosa. Laxative abuse may result in malassimilation of necessary nutriments. Finally, some drugs may produce nutritional deficiencies, which in turn can cause anorexia, decreased food intake, and weight loss.

Anorexia and Weight Loss as Symptoms

Anorexia and weight loss may be early or prominent symptoms in the following disorders.
1. Infectious diseases (e.g., tuberculosis).
2. Metabolic disorders.
   a. Hypopituitarism.
   b. Hyperthyroidism.
   c. Addison's disease.
3. Blood dyscrasias.
   a. Pernicious and other anemias.
   b. Lymphoma and leukemia.
4. Renal disease.
5. Liver disease.
   a. Acute hepatitis.
   b. Chronic hepatitis and cirrhosis.
6. Malabsorptive states (see Diarrhea, Chapter 5).
7. Malignancy.
   a. Carcinoma of the stomach.
   b. Carcinoma of the pancreas.
   c. Carcinoma of the colon.
   d. Other neoplasms.

DIAGNOSTIC APPROACH

1. It is manifestly impossible to investigate every possible cause of unexplained weight loss. Clues to the diagnostic approach should be sought in the history and physical examination.

2. When no obvious cause for weight loss can be discovered and when psychogenic disorders can be excluded, the initial work-up should include, as a minimum, the following tests:
   a. CBC.
   b. Sedimentation rate.
   c. Urinalysis.
   d. Biochemical screening (e.g., SMA-12), serum electrolytes, and T_4 and T_3 resin uptake.
   e. Two-hour postprandial glucose or glucose tolerance test.
   f. Stools for occult blood, ova, and parasites.
   g. Chest films.

3. If the initial studies are unrevealing, further investigation is warranted in any patient who continues to lose weight without an adequate explanation. Consideration should be given to at least some of the following tests or procedures:
   a. Skin tests (e.g., tuberculin, histoplasmin).
   b. Serologic tests (syphilis, RA, LE, and ANA).
   c. Serum protein electrophoresis and immunoglobulins.
   d. X-ray studies (intravenous pyelography, complete GI series, bone survey).
   e. Tests to rule out endocrinopathies (e.g., Addison's disease, hypopituitarism).
   f. Tissue biopsy (bone marrow, liver, skin, and muscle).
   g. Radioisotope scanning procedures.
   h. Angiographic studies.

4. Patients with unexplained weight loss should be kept under observation until systemic illness can be excluded. If the weight loss is due to physical causes, other symptoms and signs almost invariably develop over a period of time. As these occur, additional diagnostic studies should be undertaken.

2.

Dermatologic Problems

Pruritus

Kenneth H. Neldner

Itching sensations can be elicited only from a physical or chemical stimulation of cutaneous nerve receptors, located primarily in the region of the epidermal-dermal junction and around hair follicles. The stimuli may come from internal or external sources. It is currently believed that pain, temperature, and touch are all subserved by the same unmyelinated free nerve net as it terminates in the skin. Minimal stimulation of these fibers is believed to cause itching while more intense stimulation of the same fibers induces pain.

Histamine, kallikrein, and various endopeptidases (papain, trypsin, cathepsins, erythrocyte proteases, and lysosomal enzymes) are known chemical mediators of pruritus, but by unknown mechanisms. In its broadest sense, itching may be viewed as a uniform response to a wide variety of physical or chemical stimuli.

ETIOLOGY

There are four general reasons why people itch. These are discussed below in order of frequency.

Itching Associated with a Visible Cutaneous Eruption

A discussion of itching skin rashes encompasses essentially the entire field of dermatology, since virtually any skin lesion may itch. This is beyond the purpose and scope of this text. Therefore, only the major categories and types of dermatoses that most commonly produce itching are summarized in Table 2-1.

TABLE 2-1.   The Most Common Itching Dermatologic Disorders

A. Papulosquamous skin diseases
1. Eczema (atopic, nummular, dyshydrotic)
2. Lichen planus
3. Seborrheic dermatitis
4. Psoriasis
5. Pityriasis rosea
B. Vesicobullous diseases
1. Dermatitis herpetiformis
2. Erythema multiforme
C. Allergic reactions
1. Contact dermatitis
2. Systemic drug eruptions
3. Urticaria
4. Photoallergy
D. Infestations
1. Bites (lice, fleas, scabies, bedbugs, mosquitoes, chiggers)
2. Nematodes (creeping eruption, onchocerciasis)
E. Infection
1. Bacterial (impetigo, folliculitis)
2. Viral (exanthem, herpes simplex, varicella)
3. Fungal (tinea capitis, tinea corporis, tinea pedis, *Candida*)
F. Environmental causes
1. Wool, fiber glass, pollen, dust
2. Miliaria (prickly heat)
3. Sunburn
G. Miscellaneous conditions
1. Purpura simplex
2. Phototoxic reactions
3. Urticaria pigmentosa
4. Ichthyosis
5. Juvenile rheumatoid arthritis
6. Primary cutaneous amyloidosis

Itching Secondary to an Internal Disorder and without a Visible Skin Rash

Itching without an associated skin rash is more difficult to evaluate. It must first be determined whether the patient has genuine pruritus or whether his symptoms are neurologic or psychosomatic in nature. A careful history and physical examination will usually establish the presence of any existing neurologic defect. Psychosomatic problems are more difficult to assess. The major categories of internal disorders associated with itching are summarized in Table 2-2.

The most common cause for itching in the patient without a rash is simple dryness of the skin, followed in order of frequency by obstructive biliary disease and lymphoma, particularly Hodgkin's disease and mycosis fungoides. Diagnostic work-up should therefore concentrate initially on these areas and then proceed to less common possibilities, as the situation dictates.

1. Increasing *dryness* of the skin with age is common and may be considered a normal physiologic consequence of aging. It varies in sever-

TABLE 2-2. The Most Common Internal Conditions Associated with Pruritus

---

A. Dry skin
B. Metabolic and endocrine causes
   1. Obstructive biliary disease
      a. Extrahepatic
         (1) Common duct stones
         (2) Common duct stricture
         (3) Carcinoma of bile duct or pancreas
      b. Intrahepatic
         (1) Biliary cirrhosis
         (2) Carcinoma of liver
         (3) Drug-induced cholestasis
         (4) Viral hepatitis
   2. Uremia
   3. Thyroid disease
   4. Hyperparathyroidism
   5. Diabetes mellitus
   6. Gout
C. Malignancy
   1. Lymphoma (Hodgkin's disease, mycosis fungoides, leukemia)
   2. Carcinoma
   3. Carcinoid
D. Parasitosis
   1. Hookworm
   2. Pinworm
E. Drug reactions
   1. Opium derivatives
   2. Histamine liberators
F. Miscellaneous causes
   1. Polycythemia vera
   2. Pregnancy

---

ity from person to person. It is generally aggravated in the winter, especially in those geographic areas where prolonged heating decreases the humidity in the living and sleeping quarters. Dry skin pruritus is also called senile pruritus, pruritus hiemalis, or asteatosis.

2. Pruritus associated with *liver disease* nearly always implies the presence of an obstructive condition, since pruritus occurs seldom with jaundice secondary to hemolytic anemia and only rarely in infectious hepatitis. The constituent of bile responsible for itching has not been identified with certainty, but it is generally accepted that elevated circulating levels of bile acids (cholic, desoxycholic, and chenodesoxycholic acids) with deposition in the skin are the cause for itching. It is difficult to measure bile acids themselves; there is a general, but not absolute, correlation with serum conjugated bilirubin level, bromsulphalein retention, serum alkaline phosphatase, and SGOT levels. Intrahepatic obstruction (cholestasis) may be induced by medications such as chlorpromazine, testosterone, and erythromycin estolate.

3. *Uremia* is a more common cause of itching in chronic renal disease than in acute nephropathy. The slow development of uremia seems to correlate better with pruritus than do absolute levels of azotemia. Most patients with chronic renal disease have marked relief of itching following hemodialysis, but some do not, suggesting that factors other than azotemia itself may be involved.

4. *Hypothyroidism* is commonly associated with generalized pruritus and is most likely related to the dry skin that characterizes this disease. Hyperthyroidism is seldom associated with itching, but itching does occur in rare instances in the absence of any observable cutaneous reaction other than temperature change secondary to increased circulation.

5. *Hyperparathyroidism* secondary to renal disease is the most common parathyroid disorder producing pruritus. Relief of itching with return of the elevated serum calcium and phosphorus levels to normal following parathyroidectomy suggests that increased blood and tissue levels of calcium may be the pruritogenic stimulus, but the etiologic factors are not completely clear since not all hypercalcemic disorders are accompanied by pruritus.

6. *Diabetes mellitus* is actually a rare cause of itching—certainly less than "common knowledge" would have it. The increased susceptibility of diabetics to cutaneous bacterial and yeast infection with secondary pruritus is a more common cause for itching than is the diabetes per se.

7. *Gout* is a rare cause of itching. When present, it is presumed to be due to elevated blood and tissue levels of uric acid.

8. Of all the *malignancies* known to induce pruritus, Hodgkin's disease is the most common, and itching may be the first symptom in as many as 25 to 30 percent of the cases. Mycosis fungoides may also be preceded by itching in areas where characteristic skin lesions subsequently develop. Chronic leukemia is less commonly pruritic; if itching is present, it is somewhat more common in lymphatic leukemia than in the granulocytic types. Carcinoma of any organ may produce itching, but this is most frequently associated with involvement of the stomach, pancreas, bowel, bronchi, esophagus, ovaries, and prostate gland. The carcinoid syndrome is characterized by flushing of the skin, but pruritus is rare.

9. Intestinal *parasitosis* with hookworm (*Ancylostoma duodenale* or *Necator americanus*) may produce generalized pruritus. The constitutional phase of the disease is preceded by evanescent skin lesions ("ground itch"), usually on the feet, at the sites where the *Ancylostoma* larvae penetrate the skin. Pinworm (*Enterobius vermicularis*) infestation is a common cause of pruritus ani, especially in children.

10. Subclinical *drug reactions* that do not result in urticaria or other rashes may be responsible for itching. It is particularly common in opium or heroin addicts and may occur in patients receiving morphine, codeine, or other histamine-liberating drugs, such as aspirin and polymyxin B.

11. Mild, generalized pruritus is a frequent complaint during *pregnancy* and, in some patients, is very severe and distressing. Approximately 65 percent of pregnant women have mild to moderate elevations of serum bilirubin (0.75 to 3.0 mg/100 ml) during the last trimester, with a rapid return to normal after parturition. The degree of itching generally parallels the serum bilirubin level. If the pruritus does not disappear in the immediate postpartum period, underlying liver disease should be suspected.

12. *Polycythemia vera* is frequently associated with itching. Here, the itching is unique in that it is markedly aggravated after a hot bath.

Psychosomatic Pruritus

1. Neurotic excoriations (factitial dermatitis). The patient presents with multiple, dug out, superficial ulcerations of the skin and complains of severe, intractable pruritus. Most individuals freely admit to deep scratching and relate the intensity of the itching to nervous tension. Some are more evasive and deny that they had anything to do with the obviously self-induced lesions; situations of this type generally indicate a more severe underlying neurosis.

2. Psychotic states. The usual complaint is that "bugs" or parasites are crawling in the skin, producing intense pruritus. *Delusions of parasitosis* and *acarophobia* are the terms applied to this condition. Deep, self-inflicted excoriations and ulcerations are the rule. This is one of the most intractable and incurable forms of pruritus. The patient will readily report that "bugs" are in his skin but will adamantly refuse to accept any evidence or explanation to the contrary. Psychiatric treatment has been disappointing.

Neurologic and Circulatory Disturbances

Any neurologic disease with manifestations of cutaneous paresthesias, hypoesthesia, or hyperesthesia may produce sensations in these areas that the patient interprets as pruritus. Neurologic examination will in most instances quickly establish the presence or absence of such a neurologic defect. Neurologic disease of this type is actually a rare cause of itching. Circulatory disturbances secondary to cardiovascular disease are also uncommon causes for itching. When itching is present, the lower extremities are most frequently involved, with the pruritus secondary to ischemic changes.

DIAGNOSTIC APPROACH

1. Those patients with obvious skin lesions should be clinically and, if necessary, histologically evaluated in order to establish a diagnosis. A trained observer should be able to diagnose most dermatologic disorders with a high degree of accuracy. Patients with urticaria present special problems because of the diverse nature of the possible etiologic factors. Urticaria is therefore considered separately (see the next section).

2. Pruritus without an associated cutaneous reaction presents the most challenging diagnostic problem. The initial history and physical examination should specifically include an evaluation for possible low-grade jaundice and generalized dryness of the skin.

TABLE 2-3. Procedures for Evaluating Pruritus of Undetermined Etiology

1. Hematologic studies
    a. Complete blood count
    b. Sedimentation rate
    c. Esosinophil count
2. Gastrointestinal work-up
    a. Liver profile
    b. Cholecystography
    c. Serum amylase
    d. Stool for ova and parasites
    e. Liver biopsy
3. Endocrine evaluation
    a. Blood sugar and glucose tolerance tests
    b. Thyroid function studies
    c. Serum calcium and phosphorus
4. Genitourinary studies
    a. Urinalysis
    b. Blood urea nitrogen
    c. Serum creatinine
    d. Creatinine clearance
    e. Intravenous pyelogram
5. Evaluation for malignancy
    a. Lymph node biopsy
    b. Chest x-ray
    c. Bone marrow biopsy
    d. Upper GI examination
    e. Barium enema
    f. Proctosigmoidoscopy
    g. Mammograms
    h. Papanicolaou test
    i. Skull x-rays
    j. Pelvic x-rays
    k. Serum acid phosphatase
6. Miscellaneous studies
    a. Psychiatric evaluation
    b. Pregnancy test
    c. Blood and urine toxicology

3. The diagnostic work-up then proceeds according to the results of the history and physical examination. In some instances, the clinical findings alone will establish a diagnosis with certainty and no laboratory studies will be necessary. At other times, extensive laboratory evaluation will be required. The procedures that may be indicated are listed in Table 2-3. This list is neither complete enough to cover all possible exigencies nor is it to be considered routine work-up for each and every case of pruritus of undetermined etiology. Each significant symptom or sign should be evaluated with an appropriate laboratory test, based on the best clinical judgment of the examining physician.

Urticaria
Henry M. Lewis

DEFINITION

Urticaria may be defined as transient wheal formation with erythema and pruritus. When extensive, the process is termed *angio-edema*. The diagnosis is usually made by the patient. Because of its evanescent nature, many will not seek medical assistance unless urticaria is severe or persistent. Diagnosis is merely a prelude to a rational, systematic investigation of potential causal agents. It has been estimated that these agents cannot be found in 25 to 90 percent of chronic cases. Nevertheless, a rational breakdown of urticarial agents, with emphasis on their relative importance, helps to orient the quest for the causative agent or agents.

ETIOLOGY

Yeast Hypersensitivity

In 26 percent of patients with chronic urticaria, *Candida albicans* sensitivity may be an important factor, and there are cross reactions between this organism and food and inhalant yeasts. Exacerbations of urticaria by intentional feeding of food yeast tends to establish this as a causal agent, and a positive prick test result for yeast antigen is confirmatory. The diagnosis of yeast hypersensitivity should be considered established if the drinking of a bottle of beer severely exacerbates the urticaria.

Ingestants

1. *Foods.* Acute urticaria from ingestion of strawberries, nuts, chocolate, or shellfish is a frequent diagnosis in office practice. Often urticariogenic foods may be eaten with impunity after a full meal even if their preprandial ingestion, particularly with alcohol, induces urticaria. Chronic urticaria due to foods may be diagnosed by food diaries and questionnaires. Skin tests are of no value. The yeast-fungus group—cottonseed, soybean, egg, corn, wheat, and milk—may be causative. Purgation, followed by a 3-day rice diet, while the patient is hospitalized, is the simplest way to rule out food allergy.

2. *Drugs.* Patients with known penicillin sensitivities should avoid all dairy products if their lesions persist unreasonably; the clue may lie in trace quantities of penicillin. Other antibiotics derived from yeasts or molds may produce lesions in yeast-sensitive individuals. Aspirin sensitivity usually develops after middle age and is often associated with asthma. Other salicylates apparently do not produce urticaria. Quinidine, sodium dehydrocholate, hydralazine, opium derivatives, and thiamine may incite hives.

3. *Chemicals.* Of the ubiquitous food additives, preservatives (especially sodium benzoate and its congeners) have been responsible for many cases of persistent urticaria. Also, synthetic food colors have been cited for their hive-producing capability, and there have been instances of urticaria induced by the fluoride in drinking water.

Emotional Factors

Although the role of anxiety states in the production of urticaria is difficult to assess, experience suggests that emotional upsets often trigger exacerbations. Patients readily volunteer this information without leading interrogation. The time interval between emotional stress and the appearance of urticaria appears to be only a few minutes. Transient flushing of the anterior chest in young women during states of embarrassment, a phenomenon familiar to physicians, is probably a form of subclinical urticaria.

Cholinergic Urticaria

Exercise, heat, or emotional stress may produce the pathognomonic lesions of cholinergic urticaria. These are 1- to 2-mm wheals surrounded by large red flares. Sometimes these lesions are accompanied by other parasympathetic manifestations, such as abdominal cramps, syncope, headache, sweating, and salivation. The palms and soles are characteristically exempt from this disorder. Lesions may occur when the body temperature is increased 0.2° to 1.0°F. To test for cholinergic urticaria, simply soak an extremity in 100°F water; symptoms will be produced in 30 minutes. The methacholine (Mecholyl) skin test is diagnostic; but although this procedure is simple, it is unreliable.

Physical Agents

1. *Cold.* Cold urticaria may occur with or without the presence of cryoglobulin. The disorder is noncryoglobulinemic and idiopathic in a majority of patients, although the ice cube test gives a positive result in both the cryoglobulinemic and noncryoglobulinemic forms. One tests for this disorder by leaving an ice cube on the volar surface of the forearm for a full 5 minutes; an additional 10 minutes should elapse before the test is read. A negative reaction is simple erythema.

Whealing without purpura indicates the more common idiopathic form, and whealing with purpura indicates cryoglobulinemia. Patients with cold urticaria must be cautioned against sudden immersion in cold water.

2. *Heat.* The development of large wheals on exposure to heat constitutes the exceedingly rare, noncholinergic type of heat urticaria. To demonstrate it, immerse a hand in 100.5°F water for 5 minutes. Immediate flushing on withdrawal is followed in 5 minutes by a wheal at the site of exposure.

3. *Sunlight.* Sunlight of all wavelengths may rarely produce urticaria on exposed areas. Erythema followed by wheal formation may appear within a few minutes after exposure. Investigative measures should include determination of specific action spectra in order that suitable sunscreening preparations may be prescribed.

4. *Trauma.*
   a. *Immediate dermographism* is simply an accentuation of the normal triple-response phenomenon. In dermographic individuals, a firm stroke on the back with the edge of a tongue blade produces a red line in 15 seconds, an axon reflex flare in 45 seconds, and a wheal in 1 to 3 minutes. A therapeutic response to hydroxyzine is considered diagnostic of this disorder.
   b. *Delayed dermographism* is a rare abnormality that appears 3 to 6 hours after firm stroking as deep, wide, urticarial plaques that persist for hours and are accompanied by burning and tenderness.
   c. *Pressure urticaria*, distinct from dermographism, is also rare. Following application of intense pressure, affected individuals demonstrate poorly defined erythematous plaques after a latent period of several hours.

Endogenous Agents

1. *Infection.* Closed-space infections, i.e., chronic cholecystitis, prostatitis, sinusitis, tonsillitis, and especially apical tooth abscesses, may produce urticaria by liberation of bacterial antigen. Some authors have attributed more than 20 percent of chronic cases of urticaria to these sources. A therapeutic trial of an antibiotic or chemotherapeutic agent may be indicated if such lesions are demonstrable or suspected, but complete clearing of the urticarial lesions should not be anticipated. Urticaria as a prodrome to or occurring during the latent phase of viral hepatitis has recently received much-deserved attention. The hepatitis may be of serum, infectious, or mononucleosis origin.

2. *Infestation.* Urticaria is sometimes related to infestations, such as amebiasis, giardiasis, strongyloidiasis, ascariasis, uncinariasis, and trichinosis. When the causative agent has been identified by appropriate laboratory methods, therapeutic trials with specific agents should be undertaken.

3. *Endocrinopathies.* Three endocrine disorders (hyperthyroidism, hypothyroidism, and diabetes) may be associated with urticaria, but the precise mechanisms remain unclear.

4. *Systemic disorders.* Bizarre circinate or polycyclic lesions should make one suspicious of visceral carcinoma. Urticaria may be found in patients with systemic lupus erythematosus, juvenile rheumatoid arthritis, necrotizing angiitis, Hodgkin's disease, chronic myelogenous leukemia, polycythemia vera, and leukemoid reactions. Severe pruritus is one of the hallmarks of Hodgkin's disease. In mast cell disease (urticaria pigmentosa), rubbing the cutaneous lesions causes immediate mast cell degranulation and a typical histamine wheal.

Injectants

Injection of noxious agents by bees and mosquitoes is usually self-evident, but mite, flea, and bedbug bites may easily escape detection. Scabies is particularly difficult to diagnose in the presence of good personal hygiene. Of the injectable drugs, penicillin is the most common cause of urticaria, serum sickness reactions, and angio-edema. Vaccines and sera may produce similar reactions. Opiates are the most common cause of hospital-onset urticaria.

Inhalants

Patients with pollen urticaria usually have associated respiratory allergies. Formaldehyde urticaria may follow inhalation of tobacco smoke. The host of other potential causative inhalant agents includes animal danders, orrisroot, house dust, castor bean dust, flour, feathers, yeasts and molds, acroleins from frying fat, cottonseed, aerosols, and menthol.

Contactants

Nettles and the nettling hairs of certain caterpillars may produce wheals limited to contact sites, but these are seldom a diagnostic problem.

DIAGNOSTIC APPROACH

1. Have the patient drink one bottle of beer on an empty stomach. A severe exacerbation of urticaria is virtually diagnostic of yeast sensitivity.

2. Check carefully for a history of drug or insect bites.

3. Determine whether flare-ups follow heat, exercise, emotional stress, or exposure to sunlight. If necessary, perform the ice cube test for cold urticaria and the hot water soak or methacholine test for cholinergic urticaria.

4. Look for dermographism. If there is doubt, a therapeutic response to hydroxyzine is diagnostic.

5. Investigate for infestations and closed-space infections.

6. After purgation, try a 3-day rice diet or starvation to rule out food allergy.

7. If further work-up is indicated, the patient should be referred to an allergist or dermatologist.

3.

Cardiovascular Problems

Chest Pain

Phillip S. Wolf

Chest pain may have its origin in the heart; in the lungs or other organs of the chest; in the musculoskeletal structures of the thorax, neck, or shoulders; or in the upper abdominal viscera. The history, with particular attention to a detailed description of the pain and any associated symptoms, often provides most if not all of the essential information needed for a correct diagnosis. It is convenient for clinical purposes to classify chest pain into two categories: (1) recurrent, often paroxysmal, pain, which is mild or moderate in intensity, and (2) severe, prolonged pain, which is commonly associated with clinical evidence of acute, serious illness.

RECURRENT CHEST PAIN

Angina pectoris is the most important but not the most frequent cause of recurrent chest pain. Musculoskeletal disorders, as a group, are responsible for more cases of chest pain than is any other disease entity. They account for most errors in the diagnosis of angina pectoris, although they may coexist with this condition. By meticulous attention to the history and examination of the chest wall, especially by palpation, it is often possible to resolve the diagnostic difficulties.

Angina Pectoris

Atherosclerotic narrowing of one or more coronary arteries is the most common cause of angina pectoris. Other causes of angina include severe aortic stenosis, pulmonary hypertension, and primary myocardial disease. However, on rare occasions, typical angina may occur in the absence of

33

apparent heart disease or demonstrable abnormality of the coronary arteries. It is worth stressing that angina is uncommon in men below 35 years of age and in premenopausal women unless they have diabetes, hypertension, or hyperlipidemia.

Characteristics of Anginal Pain

1. Anginal pain is "visceral," meaning that it is poorly localized and squeezing, oppressive, burning, or heavy in quality.

2. It is of brief duration, usually lasting from 2 to 10 minutes, only rarely longer or shorter.

3. It is usually moderate in intensity.

4. The pain is typically retrosternal, but it may occur in other locations. Even then, at least a portion of the pain is usually beneath the sternum. The pain may be referred to the precordium, neck, lower jaws, shoulders, arms, back, and epigastrium. Radiation to the left shoulder and arm is especially common.

5. The pain is precipitated by effort or emotional stress, or both. It is most likely to occur after meals, on exposure to cold air or wind, and while walking uphill or climbing stairs. The pain often increases with recumbency. A key question to ask is "Do you get discomfort behind your breastbone if you walk rapidly in cold air?"

6. Anginal pain can usually be excluded under the following circumstances:
   a. If it can be localized with one finger.
   b. If it consistently lasts less than 30 seconds or longer than 30 minutes.
   c. If the pain is sticking, jabbing, or throbbing.
   d. If it occurs exclusively at rest with two exceptions: (1) angina preceding myocardial infarction, and (2) a variant form of angina, described by Prinzmetal, that is characterized by pain at rest but not with exertion.
   e. If the intensity of the pain is consistently severe.

Coexistence of Angina with Pain of Different Origin

1. Anginal pain may coexist with chest pain due to musculoskeletal disease. When this occurs, a history of a second type of chest discomfort, different in character from anginal pain, may be elicited. The finding of tenderness on palpation of the chest wall confirms the musculoskeletal origin of this additional pain.

2. Preexisting disease of the neck, arms, shoulders, thorax, or upper abdomen may so condition the nervous system that if angina pectoris develops subsequently, ischemic pain may erroneously be perceived as arising from these structures. This explanation probably accounts for at least some cases of angina that present atypically.

3. Some patients with long-standing chronic coronary artery disease, especially after open-heart surgery, may develop chronic burning precordial pain that is associated with tenderness of the anterior thoracic wall. This condition, whose etiology is unknown, has been termed *cardiac causalgia.*

4. In a majority of patients the diagnosis of angina can be established from the history alone. When doubt exists or diagnosis is difficult, the procedures listed below may be helpful.

Diagnostic Approach
1. Physical examination. Examination of the heart seldom provides the information needed for an unequivocal diagnosis of angina pectoris. However, the physical findings listed below provide supportive evidence for the diagnosis of angina, especially if they occur during an episode of pain.
   a. An audible or palpable fourth heart sound.
   b. A rise in blood pressure or pulse rate, or both.
   c. The appearance of the murmur of mitral regurgitation due to papillary muscle dysfunction.
   d. A palpable dyskinetic area or bulge at or around the cardiac apex.
   e. Paradoxical splitting of the second heart sound.
   f. Relief of pain by carotid sinus massage (the Levine test). The relief of pain appears to be related to slowing of the heart rate produced by carotid sinus pressure. In performing the test, to avoid influencing the patient's interpretation of the result, the physician should ask him whether the maneuver has made the pain worse. A reply that the pain was not made worse but was relieved constitutes evidence in favor of the diagnosis of angina.

2. Use of nitroglycerin. Sublingual nitroglycerin relieves anginal pain in 3 minutes or less in a large majority of cases, provided the tablets are potent (capable of inducing headache and flushing or producing a burning sensation under the tongue). Failure of nitroglycerin tablets (especially if taken at 3- to 5-minute intervals) to relieve chest pain indicates either that the pain is not anginal or, if it is anginal, that it may represent an episode of coronary insufficiency or myocardial infarction. On the other hand, a statement by a patient that his pain diminishes 10 minutes or more after nitroglycerin is evidence against, rather than for, the diagnosis of angina.

3. Electrocardiographic changes.
   a. No electrocardiographic changes are pathognomonic of angina pectoris. In fact, the resting ECG is frequently normal in patients with angina.
   b. During anginal attacks, ST-segment depression is the most commonly noted abnormality. However, this finding is nonspecific.
   c. Exercise testing increases the accuracy of the electrocardiographic diagnosis if the ECG is recorded both during and after exercise.

The presence of at least 1 mm of flat or downsloping ST-segment depression that is 0.08 to 0.12 second in duration is the major criterion of a positive result. Exercise testing may be performed by climbing stairs, walking a treadmill, or pumping a stationary bicycle.

   d. Exercise testing may be misleading in women under the age of 40 years. In this group, the incidence of coronary artery disease is remarkably low, but false-positive ST-segment depression is not uncommon.

4. Selective coronary arteriography. Coronary arteriography is currently the most accurate method for diagnosing coronary artery disease during life and determining its severity. The procedure is not without hazard, but the risk is low in competent hands. As a general rule, the symptomatology of ischemic heart disease correlates exceedingly well with arteriographic evidence of occlusive disease. However, the diagnostic value of arteriography decreases with advancing age, since some degree of arterial narrowing is present in a very high percentage of men above the age of 50 years. The mere presence of partially obstructive vessels in a person of this age does not establish that the lesions are causally related to chest pain. However, absence of arterial narrowing, with rare exceptions, is a most important finding in excluding angina as a cause of chest pain.

Musculoskeletal Pain

1. The musculoskeletal structures of the neck, shoulders, and thorax are the most common sources of chest pain.

2. Anterior or posterior chest pain, or both, may result from involvement of the nerve roots of the cervical and upper thoracic spine by osteoarthritis, disc disease, or deformities. The radicular nature of the pain and the presence of a posterior component to the pain help to differentiate it from angina. The pain tends to occur at night. It may be precipitated by fatigue, incorrect posture, and movement of the involved segments but not movement of the body as a whole. It may also intensify with coughing or sneezing. The discomfort is usually dull and aching in character but is often punctuated by brief sharp twinges of pain. The pain may last for hours at a time. Relief is often obtained by rest, analgesics, postural exercises, and local heat.

3. Costochondral and chondrosternal pain or swelling, or both (Tietze's syndrome), may simulate angina. The pain is usually well localized, but it may radiate across the chest and over to the arms. Tenderness to palpation over the involved articulations, especially with reproduction of the pain, is the clue to the diagnosis.

4. Fleeting, jabbing, lancinating, or sticking pains are common in many normal individuals. They are easily differentiated from angina by their brevity and character and by the lack of any relationship to effort or emotional excitement. The etiology of these pains is unknown.

5. The thoracic outlet syndromes (e.g., the scalenus anterior, costoclavicular, hyperabduction, cervical rib syndromes) may cause chest pain. Symptoms depend on whether neural or vascular structures are compressed at the thoracic outlet. Nerve compression is more frequent; pain and paresthesias are the leading symptoms. Demonstrable weakness is infrequent. Vascular compression is less common and is associated with more diffuse pain, coldness, weakness, and easy fatigue of the upper extremity. Signs of venous obstruction or thrombosis may be present. Arm and head movements may reproduce the discomfort and pain. It is often difficult to evaluate the effects of various maneuvers because they may produce signs of neurovascular compression in some normal persons. Decreased ulnar nerve conduction is currently considered the most reliable objective method for demonstrating thoracic outlet compression. Angiography may be indicated in those cases presenting with symptoms of vascular obstruction.

6. Disorders of the shoulder may produce pain that is referred to the chest. Although the pain may increase with effort, careful analysis usually reveals that aggravation of the discomfort is related specifically to shoulder movement and not to body motion. Local tenderness, pain on passive movements, and limitation of motion are commonly present.

7. Fibrositis involving the muscles of the chest wall may cause myalgia. Localized tenderness and relief with local analgesic injections are clues to the diagnosis.

8. Less common and usually obvious causes of pain in the chest are rib fractures, tumors or infections of the ribs, herpes zoster, and superficial phlebitis of the thoracic wall or breast.

Other Causes of Recurrent Chest Pain

1. The chest discomfort of angina may be mimicked by anxiety states. The discomfort may take various forms: (a) intermittent sharp, knife-like pains, (b) persistent precordial aching unrelated to effort, and (c) tight sensations in the chest. Sighing respirations and symptoms due to hyperventilation are commonly associated. A statement that "the pain is coming from my heart" is almost a giveaway for the diagnosis of psychogenic pain.

2. Pain due to reflux esophagitis, with or without hiatal hernia, may closely simulate anginal pain. The discomfort is substernal and may radiate to the left arm or lower jaw. It may be precipitated by overeating, excessive alcohol intake, or consumption of highly seasoned foods. The pain is often nocturnal and is most often triggered by recumbency. It may be relieved by assuming an upright position and by the ingestion of antacids. Cineradiographic studies of the barium-filled esophagus and esophageal motility studies provide substantiating evidence for this diagnosis.

3. Pulmonary hypertensive pain may resemble angina in that it is pre-cipitated by effort. The association of moderate or severe dyspnea and evidence of pulmonary hypertension are clues to the diagnosis. The response to nitroglycerin is not as clear-cut as it is in angina pectoris.

PROLONGED CHEST PAIN

Patients presenting with severe, protracted chest pain may have serious un-derlying disease, such as myocardial infarction, dissecting hematoma (aneu-rysm) of the aorta, pulmonary embolism, and pericarditis. Therefore, im-mediate hospitalization of such patients for diagnosis and therapy is almost always indicated.

Acute Myocardial Infarction

Characteristics of Pain in Myocardial Infarction

1. The pain in acute myocardial infarction is typically crushing, pressing, burning, aching, or vise-like in quality. Although it may be mild or moderate in severity, it is more commonly quite severe.

2. If the patient has had angina previously, inquiry often discloses that the frequency and severity of the anginal pain were greater during the period preceding the acute attack.

3. The duration of the pain is variable. It may last from half an hour to several hours or longer.

4. The pain is typically retrosternal but may be in the precordium or in other locations. Radiation of the pain to the anterior thorax, lower jaws, neck, shoulders, and arms is common. There is a tendency for it to be transmitted to the left shoulder and arm.

5. Symptoms of dyspnea, a cold sweat, and "indigestion" commonly ac-company the pain.

6. In some instances, myocardial infarction is painless, but more often there are symptoms that the patient has overlooked or has attributed to "gas" or other nonspecific gastrointestinal complaints.

Physical Findings

1. The patient may appear cold, diaphoretic, pale, cyanotic, and in obvious distress from the pain. Cardiogenic shock may be present in severe cases.

2. Physical signs of myocardial ischemia may be noted (see Angina Pec-toris, p. 35).

3. Signs of congestive heart failure without peripheral edema may be noted on physical examination or in the chest roentgenogram.

4. An evanescent pericardial friction rub is not an uncommon finding.

5. Disorders of the heartbeat occur in almost all cases. Ventricular premature contractions are the most common type of rhythm disturbance, but all types of arrhythmias, including conduction defects, may be seen.

Diagnostic Approach

1. The diagnosis of acute myocardial infarction is based primarily on objective evidence. Characteristic changes in the ECG and in serum enzyme activity, together with the clinical picture, establish the diagnosis.

2. The electrocardiographic diagnosis of myocardial infarction can be established with certainty in an appropriate clinical setting when abnormality of the initial 0.04 second of the QRS complex (abnormal Q, QS, or R waves) is combined with characteristic ST-segment changes or typical T-wave abnormalities, or both. Unfortunately, ECG abnormalities that are usually considered diagnostic of myocardial infarction may sometimes occur in conditions such as left or right ventricular hypertrophy, cardiomyopathy, myocarditis, tumor of the heart, obstructive pulmonary emphysema, acute cor pulmonale, ventricular preexcitation, and left anterior fascicular block, and thus may lead to an erroneous diagnosis. It is also important to realize that the ECG may be normal or may show only nonspecific abnormalities in myocardial infarction. Serial changes in the ECG may be significant, especially if the initial ECG is normal. It cannot be emphasized too strongly that a normal initial tracing does not necessarily rule out infarction.

3. Elevated serum levels of enzymes released from necrotic cardiac muscle support the diagnosis of myocardial infarction. The magnitude of the enzyme elevations corresponds roughly to the size of the infarct. The three enzymes commonly used in diagnosis are creatinine phosphokinase (CPK), serum glutamic oxaloacetic transaminase (SGOT), and lactic dehydrogenase (LDH). However, elevated levels of these enzymes may result from causes other than myocardial infarction, and it is important to be aware of this possibility. Determination of LDH isoenzymes is sometimes useful when differential diagnosis is a problem or when serum levels of LDH are normal. The CPK level is the first to rise (2 to 6 hours after myocardial infarction); next, the SGOT level; and last, the LDH concentration. Serum LDH levels ordinarily remain elevated longer (up to 10 days) than the other enzymes. A rise and fall in serum enzyme levels, a progressive fall in serum levels (when the patient is first seen 48 hours or longer after the onset), or elevated hydroxybutyric dehydrogenase (HBD) levels suggest myocardial necrosis. A rise and fall within the normal range may be the only change with minor myocardial injury. An elevated CPK level is virtually diagnostic of myocardial necrosis in the absence of muscle trauma, surgery, muscle disease, cerebral infarction, hypothyroidism, and recent cardioversion, provided intramuscular medications have not been administered. The last statement is important

because it is not widely appreciated that almost any type of intramuscular injection can cause a significant rise in serum CPK levels.
Therefore, such injections should be avoided in all patients in whom
the diagnosis of myocardial infarction is uncertain until the problem
has been resolved.

4. Fever, leukocytosis, and an elevated sedimentation rate are nonspecific
abnormalities commonly associated with myocardial infarction. However, a persistently normal sedimentation rate suggests that infarction
has not occurred.

5. The differential diagnosis between myocardial infarction and acute
pericarditis is discussed later in this section (see p. 44).

6. Patients with prolonged bouts of angina-like pain unaccompanied by
signs of myocardial necrosis are considered to have a condition variously called acute coronary insufficiency, preinfarction angina, the
intermediate coronary syndrome, or unstable angina. Such episodes
frequently precede the occurrence of myocardial infarction.

Dissecting Hematoma (Aneurysm) of the Aorta

Dissecting hematomas occur most frequently in hypertensive males between
40 and 70 years of age.

Characteristics of Pain in Dissecting Hematoma

1. The pain, which is inordinately severe and often unbearable, is usually described by the patient as having a sharp, tearing, or ripping
quality. Large, repeated doses of narcotics are often needed to relieve
the pain.

2. The location of the pain correlates with the site of intimal rupture.
When the tear is above the aortic valve, the pain is located in the
anterior chest; when the rupture is distal to the left subclavian artery,
the pain is referred to the back. The pain may radiate along the pathway of aortic dissection.

Physical Findings

Usually the patient appears to be very sick but does not show signs of shock
unless rupture through the aortic wall takes place. Dissection of the aorta
may spread and occlude major arteries, resulting in characteristic findings:

1. Carotid or vertebral occlusion may lead to syncope, coma, hemiplegia,
or blindness.

2. Interference with circulation to the arms or legs may cause vascular
insufficiency of the involved limb, with loss of arterial pulsations.

3. Renal artery occlusion may cause acute hypertension and oliguria.

4. Mesenteric artery occlusion may produce infarction of the bowel, with abdominal pain and ileus.

5. Dissection at the base of the aortic root may extend into the aortic ring and cause acute aortic regurgitation.

6. Coronary artery occlusion, which occurs occasionally, may lead to myocardial infarction.

7. External rupture of the aorta into the pericardial sac usually results in cardiac tamponade and death. External rupture into other sites, such as the mediastinum, peritoneum, or retroperitoneum, may occur, and likewise may terminate life.

Diagnostic Approach

1. The diagnosis of dissecting hematoma is often suggested by the clinical picture, provided it is considered in the differential diagnosis of severe chest pain.

2. The chest roentgenogram usually reveals widening of the aortic shadow in the mediastinum. Progressive widening of this structure in serial films is strongly suggestive of the diagnosis.

3. Aortography is the most precise method for diagnosing aortic dissection. Under ideal circumstances, the points of entry and exit of the dissection can be seen in the films. The location and extent of the dissection may help in deciding between surgical and pharmacologic management. The initial decision to perform aortography should be postponed until the diagnosis of myocardial infarction has been excluded. As a general rule, no harm is done to the patient with aortic dissection who is treated palliatively, but serious harm can come to the patient with myocardial infarction who is submitted to aortography.

4. The ECG usually shows nonspecific abnormalities. Evidence of myocardial infarction indicates involvement of the coronary arteries by the disease process.

Pulmonary Embolism

Chest Pain in Pulmonary Embolism

1. Chest pain is absent in the majority of patients with pulmonary embolism. When present, the pain is pleuritic or retrosternal.

2. Pleuritic pain is characteristic of pulmonary infarction and is seen in about one-fourth of the patients with embolism. Accompanying features include hemoptysis, a pleural friction rub, and a pulmonary infiltrate or pleural effusion.

3. With extensive embolism, severe substernal discomfort may occur, mimicking acute myocardial infarction. Signs of pulmonary hypertension and right ventricular failure are generally present.

Diagnostic Approach

1. The diagnosis of pulmonary embolism is usually suggested by the clinical setting in which it occurs. Embolism should be suspected whenever dyspnea develops acutely in patients who have been immobilized or bedridden for long periods of time because of surgery, trauma, hip fracture, congestive heart failure, or malignancy. The susceptibility to thromboembolic phenomena is apparently also increased in women taking oral contraceptives.

2. Chest roentgenograms reveal signs of infarction in only a minority of instances (15 percent). With extensive embolism, localized areas of decreased vascularity, a subtle finding, may be observed.

3. The ECG is of relatively little diagnostic value in a majority of instances of embolism. Signs supporting pulmonary embolism may be present in 15 to 20 percent of cases.

4. Arterial blood gases often reveal some degree of hypoxemia and are of supportive value in the diagnosis of embolism.

5. Lung scanning is the diagnostic method of choice and should be performed in any patient with suspected embolism. Further details may be found in the section Acute Pulmonary Radiographic Abnormalities, Chapter 4.

6. Pulmonary angiography is an accurate method for disclosing the presence of embolism, but because special techniques are required, angiography is less readily available than scanning. The procedure should be reserved for instances in which the information to be obtained is vital to proper diagnosis and treatment. Angiography may be indicated under the following circumstances: (a) when massive embolism is believed to be present and pulmonary embolectomy is contemplated. It is then essential to verify the diagnosis by angiography lest a seriously ill patient be subjected to unnecessary thoracotomy. (b) When a high suspicion of embolism exists and conventional studies fail to provide a diagnosis. (c) When the use of anticoagulants or other forms of therapy hinges on an accurate diagnosis.

Acute Pericarditis

Nearly all patients with acute pericarditis have chest pain. Since only the lower portion of the external surface of the parietal pericardium is pain-sensitive, much of the pain is presumably due to inflammation of the adjoining diaphragmatic pleura.

Pain in Acute Pericarditis

1. Three types of pain may occur in acute pericarditis:

   a. Pleuritic pain is the most common type.

   b. Steady, severe retrosternal pain of sudden onset, simulating that of myocardial infarction, may occur.

c. The rarest type is pain at the cardiac apex felt synchronously with each heartbeat.

2. Characteristics of pericardial pain:

   a. The pain is commonly sharp. It is normally increased by breathing deeply, rotating the trunk, swallowing, or yawning—maneuvers that have no effect on the pain of myocardial infarction. It is often worse in recumbency and is sometimes relieved by sitting up and leaning forward.

   b. The pain is most commonly located in the precordial region and may radiate to the neck or to the left shoulder and arm.

Diagnosis of Acute Pericarditis

1. The pericardial friction rub. On examination, the most important finding is the presence of a pericardial friction rub over the precordium. The rub is often very transient, but it may persist and may even last for weeks. Classically, it has a superficial quality and is grating or scratchy in character. It may have systolic, diastolic, and presystolic components. It is accentuated by deep breathing and may be heard only in certain body positions (e.g., with the patient sitting and leaning forward). Pericardial rubs are often quite changeable in character from minute to minute or hour to hour. When confined to either systole or diastole, a rub may be confused with a cardiac murmur. Repeated observation usually makes the distinction clear, since the friction rub either assumes a to-and-fro character or disappears.

2. Pericardial effusion. Acute pericarditis is often accompanied by pericardial effusion. The physical signs depend upon the amount of fluid and, in the case of tamponade, on the rapidity of its accumulation. Signs of pericardial effusion include an increased area of cardiac dullness and muffling of the heart sounds. Signs of tamponade include decreased systolic pressure with a narrow pulse pressure, tachycardia, pulsus paradoxus, and inspiratory elevation of the jugular venous pressure. Several techniques are available to demonstrate the presence of pericardial effusion, including:

   a. Radioisotope scanning of the cardiac blood pool.

   b. Angiocardiography.

   c. Injection of CO_2 into the right atrium by a catheter.

   d. Echocardiography, which appears to be the simplest, safest, and most accurate method of diagnosis.

3. Electrocardiographic changes. The electrocardiographic diagnosis of acute pericarditis is based primarily on the presence of sequential changes in the ST segments and T waves in multiple leads. The QRS abnormalities of myocardial infarction are absent. Low-voltage and electrical alternans may occur when effusions are large. The cardiac rhythm is usually a sinus tachycardia, but atrial arrhythmias occur commonly.

4. Differential diagnosis of acute pericarditis and myocardial infarction. Because of the similarity in pain and, occasionally, in the ECG findings, it may be difficult to differentiate between acute pericarditis and myocardial infarction. The following points may be helpful:

   a. The presence of a pleuritic component to the pain favors pericarditis.

   b. The development of pathologic Q waves in the ECG occurs only with myocardial infarction.

   c. ST-segment abnormalities are more widespread in pericarditis than in infarction. When elevated, the ST segments may be concave upward in pericarditis, whereas convex changes are more consistent with infarction. Reciprocal ST changes are usually absent in the limb leads in pericarditis but are commonly present in infarction. In pericarditis, the T waves are usually not inverted until the ST segment is iso-electric; in infarction, they begin to invert while the ST segment is still elevated.

   d. Serum enzyme elevations are absent or minimal in acute pericarditis.

   e. A pericardial friction rub may occur in either condition but is far less likely in infarction. The rub is more persistent in pericarditis.

   f. Large pericardial effusions occur only in pericarditis.

Other Causes of Prolonged Chest Pain

Pneumothorax, mediastinal emphysema, acute pancreatitis, acute cholecystitis, peptic disease, and perforated ulcer may sometimes cause severe chest pain. Usually, local symptoms, signs, radiographic studies, and laboratory findings provide the information needed for correct diagnosis.

Venous Pressure

H. Harold Friedman

MEASUREMENT

1. The peripheral venous pressure is measured most accurately by manometry. However, an adequate approximation of the venous pressure for clinical purposes can be obtained by inspection of the jugular pulsations.

2. Although internal or external jugular pulsations may be used to estimate venous pressure, the former are preferred for this purpose.

3. Right-sided pulsations are preferred for measurement because left-sided ones may be falsely elevated by kinking of the left innominate vein.

4. The reference level for bedside evaluation of venous pressure is the sternal angle.

5. The height of the jugular pulsations varies with the position of the chest. For this reason, the patient should be examined in a position that is optimal for revealing the venous pulsations.

6. The vertical distance between the top of the venous column and the sternal angle represents the venous pressure.

7. The upper limits for normal venous pressure at various degrees of body elevation are:
   Recumbent, 2 cm.
   30°, 3 cm.
   45°, 4.5 cm.
   Upright, at the level of the suprasternal notch.

8. When the findings on inspection are equivocal, the 1-minute abdominal compression test (hepatojugular reflux) may unmask latent elevation of the venous pressure.
   a. The abdominal compression test is considered to give a positive result if abdominal pressure for 1 minute causes a rise of at least 1 cm in the level of venous pulsations.
   b. A positive response is usually indicative of right-sided heart failure.
   c. Pure left-sided heart failure usually elicits a normal or, at most, an equivocal response.
   d. False-positive results may occur in severe emphysema, superior vena cava obstruction below the azygos vein, hypervolemia, restrictive cardiomyopathy, pulmonary embolism, and increased sympathetic stimulation.

9. The maximum normal antecubital venous pressure, as determined by manometry, is 12 cm when the zero level is located 5 cm below the sternal angle, and 15 cm when the zero level is 10 cm from the back.

10. The central venous pressure (CVP) can be determined by the transvenous placement of a plastic catheter into the superior vena cava or right atrium. The CVP is an indicator of right ventricular filling pressure. When performed serially, CVP determinations are useful in following patients after cardiac or thoracic surgery or shock, and in monitoring those with complex fluid and electrolyte problems or serious cardiac disorders. The normal range for CVP is between 5 and 15 cm of water.

ABNORMALITIES OF VENOUS PRESSURE

1. Unilateral nonpulsatile distention of the neck veins usually is indicative of venous obstruction. Unilateral distention of the left jugular

veins, however, may be caused by compression of the left innominate vein, a condition that is clinically unimportant.

2. Bilateral nonpulsatile neck vein distention associated with venous collaterals in the upper thorax is strongly suggestive of superior vena cava obstruction in the absence of heart disease, hepatic congestion, or venous engorgement in the lower half of the body.

3. Bilateral pulsatile neck vein distention associated with generalized elevation of venous pressure is commonly found in the following conditions:

   a. Right-sided congestive heart failure from any cause.
   b. Pericardial effusion with tamponade.
   c. Chronic obstructive pulmonary disease.
   d. Bronchial asthma.
   e. Pleural effusion.
   f. Hyperkinetic circulatory states.
   g. Tricuspid stenosis.
   h. Tricuspid regurgitation.
   i. Central circulatory congestion due to noncardiac causes.

4. Inspiratory distention of the neck veins (Kussmaul's sign), formerly considered to be pathognomonic of chronic constrictive pericarditis or cardiac tamponade, may also occur in severe right ventricular failure and the restrictive cardiomyopathies.

5. Expiratory increase in venous pressure may occur in some cases of bronchial asthma and chronic obstructive pulmonary disease.

Jugular Venous Pulse
H. Harold Friedman

THE NORMAL JUGULAR VENOUS PULSE

The normal visible jugular venous pulse (see Fig. 3-1) consists of three positive waves (A, C, and V) and two negative waves (X and Y). The A wave is normally the tallest wave, exceeding both C and V waves in amplitude. The X wave is usually deeper than the Y wave. The heart sounds are preferable to the carotid pulse for timing the venous pulsations at the bedside.

The A Wave

The A wave is produced by right atrial contraction. It begins before S_1 and peaks just before or during this sound. If an S_4 is present, it coincides with the summit of the wave. It precedes the carotid pulse.

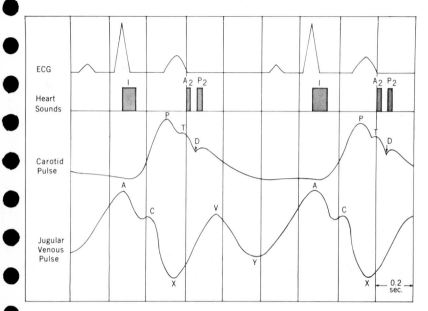

FIG. 3-1. Relationships between the electrocardiogram, heart sounds, arterial pulse, and jugular venous pulse. 1 = first heart sound; A_2 = aortic component of the second heart sound; P_2 = pulmonary component of the second sound; P = percussion wave; T = tidal wave; D = dicrotic notch; A, C, X, V, and Y = waves and troughs of the jugular venous pulse.

The C Wave

The C wave is probably produced by right ventricular systole and the bulging of the tricuspid valve into the right atrium. Impact of the carotid pulse against the jugular vein may contribute to its genesis. It begins at the end of S_1 and peaks shortly thereafter. It coincides with the upstroke of the carotid pulse.

The X Descent ("Systolic Collapse" of the Venous Pulse)

The X descent is produced by right atrial relaxation and downward displacement of the base of the heart. It begins with the downslope of the A wave and terminates in the X trough. Some authorities divide it into the X and X′ descents, the C wave separating the two. The X trough occurs about 0.10 second before S_2. The X descent occurs during the peak of the carotid pulse.

The V Wave

The V wave is produced by right atrial filling during right ventricular systole while the tricuspid valve is closed. It begins shortly before P_2 and peaks

0.06 to 0.08 second after this sound. The peak of the V wave occurs after the dicrotic notch of the carotid pulse.

The Y Descent ("Diastolic Collapse" of the Venous Pulse)

The Y descent is produced by the rapid flow of blood into the right ventricle after the opening of the tricuspid valve. It begins with the end of the V wave and ends with the Y trough. The Y trough occurs about 0.20 second after P_2. The Y descent comes long after the carotid pulse is felt.

ABNORMALITIES OF THE JUGULAR VENOUS PULSE

The types of abnormalities of the jugular venous pulsations and their causes are listed below.

The A Wave

1. Large or giant A waves are caused by increased resistance at the tricuspid valve or increased resistance to right ventricular filling in the following conditions:
   a. Tricuspid stenosis or atresia.
   b. Ebstein's anomaly.
   c. Pulmonary stenosis.
   d. Pulmonary hypertension.
      (1) Primary.
      (2) Eisenmenger's syndrome (uncommon).
      (3) Mitral stenosis.
      (4) Acute and chronic cor pulmonale.
      (5) Tricuspid regurgitation (nonrheumatic cases secondary to pulmonary hypertension).
   e. Cardiomyopathy.
   f. Idiopathic hypertrophic subaortic stenosis.
   g. Aortic stenosis (some cases).

2. Decreased A waves are seen in the presence of a markedly dilated right atrium.

3. Absent A waves are seen in atrial fibrillation and atrial flutter (A waves replaced by flutter waves).

4. Cannon A waves are produced by fusion of giant A waves with C or V waves.
   a. Regular cannon waves.
      (1) Atrioventricular (AV) junctional rhythm.
      (2) First-degree AV block (some cases).
      (3) 2:1 AV block.
      (4) Atrial tachycardia (some cases).

b. Irregular cannon waves.
  (1) Premature systoles.
    (a) Ventricular (frequently).
    (b) AV junctional (sometimes).
    (c) Atrial (rarely).
  (2) Complete AV dissociation.
    (a) Complete AV block.
    (b) AV junctional tachycardia (some cases).
    (c) Ventricular tachycardia (some cases).
  (3) Atrial flutter (difficult to detect).

The X Descent

The X descent is decreased in atrial fibrillation. It is partially or completely obliterated by a regurgitant wave (called the CV, S, or V wave) in tricuspid regurgitation. It may be deeper than the Y descent in some cases of chronic constrictive pericarditis.

The V Wave (Large V Wave)

1. Tricuspid regurgitation.
2. Right-sided heart failure.
3. Atrial septal defect (about 50 percent of cases).
4. Anomalous pulmonary venous drainage.

The Y Descent

1. A slow, shallow Y descent is seen in tricuspid stenosis.
2. A rapid, steep Y descent is seen in constrictive pericarditis and in severe right-sided heart failure.

Arterial Pulse
H. Harold Friedman

THE NORMAL ARTERIAL PULSE

Routine examination of the arteries should include palpation of the carotid, arm, and leg pulses. The normal carotid pulse (see Fig. 3-1, p. 47) consists of a brisk upstroke, a smooth dome-shaped summit, and a downstroke that is more gradual than the upstroke. The systolic percussion and tidal waves, as well as the dicrotic notch, are not normally palpable, but they can be recorded. Most pulse wave abnormalities are detected best in the carotid arteries.

ABNORMALITIES OF THE ARTERIAL PULSE

Hypokinetic Pulse (Weak Pulse, Pulsus Parvus)

A small pulse signifies a narrowed pulse pressure. It is usually produced by low cardiac output in association with increased peripheral resistance. The causes are listed in Table 3-1.

Hyperkinetic Pulse (Bounding Pulse)

A bounding pulse usually implies a widened pulse pressure. It is produced by varying combinations of increased stroke volume, increased cardiac output, and lowered peripheral resistance. The causes are listed in Table 3-2. A water-hammer pulse is an exaggerated type of bounding pulse. Corrigan's sign, as originally described, consists of visible abrupt distention and rapid collapse of the carotid pulse. It is therefore a sign detected by inspection, not by palpation. The sign is quite characteristic of aortic regurgitation.

Pulsus Parvus et Tardus

This is a pulse of low amplitude that rises slowly to a late summit. It is usually found in valvular aortic stenosis. Although it may occur with lesser frequency in subvalvular aortic stenosis due to a fibrous ring or diaphragm, it is not found in idiopathic hypertrophic subaortic stenosis. The anacrotic pulse, a variant of pulsus parvus et tardus, in which a notch is palpable on the upstroke of the pulse wave, is indicative of severe aortic stenosis.

Pulsus Bisferiens

Pulsus bisferiens is a twice-beating pulse in which both peaks occur during systole. The initial, or percussion, wave is brisk and forceful. The second,

TABLE 3-1.   Causes of Decreased Pulse Pressure*

A. Decreased cardiac output
   1. Congestive heart failure
   2. Shock
   3. Hypovolemia
   4. Acute myocardial infarction
   5. Cardiac tamponade
   6. Chronic constrictive pericarditis
   7. Cardiomyopathy and myocarditis
B. Peripheral vasoconstriction
   1. Shock
   2. Hypovolemia
C. Mechanical
   1. Valvular disease
     a. Aortic outflow obstruction
     b. Mitral stenosis or regurgitation, or both
   2. Aortic disease
     a. Coarctation of the aorta
     b. Aortic arch syndrome

* More than one mechanism may be operative.

TABLE 3-2.   Causes of Increased Pulse Pressure*

1. Decreased distensibility of the arterial system
   a. Atherosclerosis (most common)
   b. Hypertension
   c. Coarctation of the aorta
2. Increased stroke volume
   a. Normal
   b. Anxiety, exercise
   c. Complete heart block
   d. Aortic regurgitation
3. Increased cardiac output or decreased peripheral resistance, or both
   a. Fever
   b. Anemia
   c. Thyrotoxicosis
   d. Hyperkinetic heart syndrome
   e. Arteriovenous fistula
   f. Paget's disease
   g. Beriberi
   h. Cirrhosis of the liver

* More than one mechanism may be operative.

or tidal, wave is slower-rising and less prominent than the percussion wave. Pulsus bisferiens occurs most commonly in combined aortic stenosis and regurgitation, but it may occur in pure aortic regurgitation. Pulsus bisferiens is also characteristic of idiopathic hypertrophic subaortic stenosis.

Dicrotic Pulse

A dicrotic pulse is a double-peaked pulse in which the initial wave occurs during systole and the final (dicrotic) wave occurs during diastole. It occurs in some fevers, notably typhoid fever, and occasionally in mild or moderate aortic regurgitation.

Pulsus Alternans

Pulsus alternans is a condition in which the pulse waves during regular rhythm are alternately strong and weak. It may be detected by palpation but it is more accurately assessed by sphygmomanometry. To detect pulsus alternans, inflate the blood pressure cuff rapidly above the systolic pressure and then deflate it slowly until sounds are first audible. At this point, the beats are heard at one-half of the heart rate. When the cuff is deflated further, the rate doubles. There may be some variation in the intensity of the strong and weak beats. Pulsus alternans can be diagnosed only if the heart rate is regular. It is often accentuated when the patient is sitting or standing. Severe degrees may be palpable over the radial and other peripheral arteries.

Pulsus alternans is virtually diagnostic of left ventricular failure and is commonly associated with a ventricular (S_3) gallop rhythm. However, it may occasionally occur during or after paroxysmal tachycardia in an otherwise normal heart. Pulsus alternans must be differentiated from bigeminy produced by premature systoles. In pulsus alternans, the intervals between the strong and weak beats are equal. In extrasystolic bigeminy, weak ectopic beats occur prematurely and are followed by strong normal beats after pauses, resulting in ventricular cycles that are alternately short and long.

Pulsus Paradoxus

Pulsus paradoxus is a condition in which the inspiratory decline in systolic pressure exceeds 10 mm Hg (maximum normal value during quiet respiration). To detect pulsus paradoxus, inflate the cuff rapidly above the systolic pressure and then slowly deflate it. The difference between the systolic pressures at which sounds are just heard only during expiration and later during both expiration and inspiration is a measure of the magnitude (in mm Hg) of the paradoxical pulse. Deep inspiration may cause a 10- to 15-mm fluctuation in the systolic pressure of a normal person but does not cause the radial pulse to disappear. Hence, disappearance of the radial pulse on deep inspiration suggests significant pulsus paradoxus.

Classic pulsus paradoxus occurs in cardiac tamponade and constrictive pericarditis, but it may also be found in chronic obstructive airway disease and occasionally in cardiomyopathy or shock. Pulsus paradoxus due to constrictive pericarditis or cardiac tamponade is sometimes associated with an inspiratory increase in venous pressure (Kussmaul's sign), whereas pulsus paradoxus due to pulmonary disease usually shows an expiratory increase in venous pressure.

PULSE AND PRESSURE DIFFERENCES BETWEEN THE ARMS AND LEGS

Normally, with a standard cuff, the systolic blood pressure in the legs is about 20 to 40 mm Hg higher than that in the arms. With a large cuff (18 cm), the systolic blood pressure in the lower extremities is about the same (± 10 mm Hg) as that in the upper extremities. A large cuff is more accurate than a standard cuff for measuring the blood pressure in the legs. The femoral pulse should occur slightly earlier than the radial pulse and should be of equal or greater intensity. A diminished and delayed femoral pulse is a classic finding in coarctation of the aorta. Decreased femoral pulses may also occur because of occlusive disease in the terminal aorta or iliac arteries, aortic dissection, or aneurysm of the abdominal aorta. Decreased or absent popliteal and pedal pulsations with good preservation of the femoral pulses are indicative of occlusive peripheral vascular disease.

PULSE AND PRESSURE DIFFERENCES BETWEEN THE ARMS

Normally there is a difference of less than 15 mm Hg of systolic blood pressure between the two arms. An aberrant radial artery is the most common cause of unequal radial pulses. Pulse and pressure differences between the arms may also be due to other causes:

1. Acquired disease.
   a. Subclavian steal syndrome.

? **b.** Aortic arch syndrome (pulseless disease, Takayasu's syndrome).

   c. Thoracic outlet syndrome.

   d. Arterial thrombosis and embolism.

   e. Aneurysm of the thoracic aorta.

   f. Dissecting aneurysm.

   g. Incompressible brachial artery.

2. Congenital disease.

   a. Coarctation of the aorta.

   b. Supravalvular aortic stenosis (in more than 50 percent of cases, the pressure difference between the arms exceeds 20 mm Hg, with the right arm pressure greater except in dextrocardia).

✓ **c.** Patent ductus arteriosus.

   d. Anomalous subclavian artery.

Arterial Hypertension

H. Harold Friedman

NORMAL BLOOD PRESSURE

The maximum normal blood pressure is 140/90 mm Hg. In normal persons in the recumbent position, the popliteal blood pressure exceeds the branchial pressure by 20 to 40 mm Hg when determined by sphygmomanometry.

SYSTOLIC HYPERTENSION

Definition

Elevation of the systolic pressure without concomitant elevation of the diastolic pressure constitutes systolic hypertension.

Etiology

1. Decreased elasticity of the aorta due to aortic atherosclerosis (most common).

2. Increased cardiac output due to fever, anemia, thyrotoxicosis, hyperkinetic heart syndrome, arteriovenous fistula, Paget's disease, beriberi, or anxiety.

3. Increased stroke volume due to aortic insufficiency or complete heart block.

4. Coarctation of the aorta.

Symptoms

Symptoms, if any, are produced by the underlying disease and are not attributable to the hypertension per se.

Signs

Systolic hypertension is signified by a persistently elevated systolic pressure.

Diagnostic Approach

1. Rule out coarctation of the aorta by checking the blood pressure and pulses in both the upper and lower extremities. If the blood pressure in the legs is 20 to 30 mm Hg less than that in the arms or if the femoral pulse peak is delayed, or both, check further for evidence of aortic coarctation.

2. Rule out high-output states and conditions causing increased stroke volume.

3. If the foregoing conditions are excluded and the patient is middle-aged or elderly, aortic atherosclerosis is the most probable cause.

DIASTOLIC HYPERTENSION

Definition

Diastolic hypertension is defined as elevation of the diastolic pressure above normal values. It is almost always associated with concomitant elevation of the systolic pressure. The diagnosis of hypertension is not warranted unless blood pressure readings exceed normal values on at least three separate occasions after a 15- to 20-minute period of rest.

Etiology

1. Primary, or essential, hypertension (80 to 90 percent of cases).

2. Secondary hypertension.
   a. Endocrine disorders.
      (1) Adrenal.
         (a) Aldosteronism (1 to 2 percent of cases).
         (b) Pheochromocytoma (0.5 percent of cases).
         (c) Cushing's syndrome.
      (2) Thyroid: hypothyroidism.
      (3) Pituitary.
         (a) Acromegaly.
         (b) Cushing's disease.
      (4) Parathyroid: hyperparathyroidism.

b. Renal disease.

   (1) Renal artery lesions (at least 5 to 10 percent of cases).

   (a) *Intrinsic:* atherosclerotic plaque (most common); fibro-muscular hyperplasia; aneurysm, thrombosis or embolism; arteriovenous fistula; arteritis.

   (b) *Extrinsic* compression: tumor involving renal pedicle, congenital fibrous band, retroperitoneal fibrosis.

   (2) Parenchymal.

   (a) *Unilateral:* congenital hypoplastic kidney; pyelonephritis (pyogenic, tuberculous); irradiation, trauma, renal neoplasm, unilateral renal vein thrombosis; obstructive nephropathy.

   (b) *Bilateral:* glomerulonephritis; pyelonephritis; polycystic disease; connective tissue disease; amyloidosis; gouty nephropathy; nephrocalcinosis; obstructive nephropathy.

   (c) Coarctation of the aorta.

   (d) Toxemia of pregnancy.

c. Oral contraceptive agents.

d. Miscellaneous causes: polycythemia, burns, lead poisoning, CNS lesions (increased intracranial pressure, brain tumors, bulbar poliomyelitis).

Symptoms

1. The age and type of onset may provide clues to the etiology of hypertension.

a. A gradual onset between the ages of 35 and 55 years is typical of essential hypertension.

b. An acute onset in children or young adults suggests acute renal disease (e.g., acute glomerulonephritis).

c. Moderate to severe hypertension in the young is usually indicative of chronic renal disease (e.g., chronic glomerulonephritis).

d. A sudden onset in middle-aged or older persons suggests a renovascular cause.

e. A rapid onset of severe, progressive hypertension, or sudden acceleration of preexisting hypertension, may herald the onset of a malignant phase in either primary or secondary hypertension.

2. Elevated diastolic blood pressure per se is asymptomatic except possibly for morning occipital headache.

3. Symptoms in patients with essential hypertension are nonspecific or are related to the cardiovascular, cerebral, or renal complications of the disease.

4. Some types of secondary hypertension, such as primary aldosteronism, Cushing's syndrome, or pheochromocytoma, may be associated with symptoms or signs that are strongly suggestive of its cause.

5. Muscular weakness in association with hypertension suggests coexistent hypokalemia.

6. Symptoms of muscle weakness (sometimes with paralysis) in association with polyuria, nocturia, polydipsia, tetany, and hypertension are strongly suggestive of primary aldosteronism.

7. Attacks of headache, blurring of vision, sweating, palpitation, nausea, trembling, and pallor with either paroxysmal or persistent hypertension are suggestive of pheochromocytoma.

Signs

1. Delayed femoral pulses and blood pressures in the legs that are lower than those in the arms suggest coarctation of the aorta.

2. Decreased or absent femoral pulses may be indicative of occlusive disease in the abdominal aorta or iliac arteries or of coarctation of the aorta.

3. An abdominal bruit, audible anteriorly in the epigastrium or over the flank, is strongly suggestive of renal artery stenosis.

4. Bilaterally enlarged kidneys in patients with hypertension suggest polycystic disease.

5. An orthostatic drop in blood pressure suggests secondary rather than primary hypertension and is especially characteristic of pheochromocytoma.

6. The physical findings in some types of secondary hypertension (e.g., Cushing's syndrome) may be sufficiently characteristic to permit or at least suggest the correct diagnosis.

7. An assessment of the severity of the hypertension can be made from the degree of cardiac, cerebral, and renal involvement, and from the blood pressure readings:

Mild: diastolic pressure 100 mm Hg or less.
Moderate: diastolic pressure 100 to 120 mm Hg.
Severe: diastolic pressure above 120 mm Hg.
Malignant: diastolic pressure above 140 mm Hg.

8. The chronicity and severity of the hypertension may also be estimated by funduscopy:

Grade I: mild.
Grade II: moderately severe.
Grade III: severe.
Grade IV: malignant.

Initial Evaluation

The initial work-up in patients with hypertension has a threefold purpose: (1) to identify systemic complications of hypertension, (2) to establish an etiologic diagnosis, if possible, and (3) to screen for the fewer than 10 to 20 percent of hypertensives with potentially curable forms of the disease. Some work-up is indicated in every patient with hypertension. Under *ideal* conditions, every hypertensive patient should have the comprehensive rather than the limited basic work-up outlined in succeeding paragraphs. However, some selectivity is required because neither funds, personnel, nor facilities are available for a complete evaluation of every patient with hypertension. Furthermore, screening for the common causes of curable hypertension can usually be done on clinical grounds with simple procedures.

Limited Basic Work-up
In patients with stable, mild or moderate hypertension beginning above the age of 35 years, a satisfactory initial work-up can be limited to:

1. CBC.
2. Urinalysis.
3. Urine culture and sensitivity studies.
4. BUN or serum creatinine.
5. Serum electrolytes.
6. Blood sugar.
7. Blood uric acid.
8. Chest films.
9. Electrocardiogram.
10. Rapid-sequence intravenous pyelogram (IVP).

Comprehensive Basic Work-up
1. Urinalysis to screen for intrinsic renal disease. The urine usually shows no abnormalities in essential or renovascular hypertension and in primary aldosteronism unless the hypertension is severe, in which case there may be mild proteinuria or microscopic hematuria. On the other hand, it is rare to have primary renal disease without proteinuria and some abnormality of the urine sediment.

2. Urine culture and sensitivity studies to detect bacteriuria associated with pyelonephritis.

3. Serum electrolytes (Na, K, Cl, and CO_2) to detect hypokalemia and alkalosis caused by primary aldosteronism, Cushing's syndrome, or other diseases.

4. BUN or serum creatinine to screen for gross impairment of renal function.

5. Serum uric acid to detect hyperuricemia, gout, or related gouty nephropathy.

6. A 2-hour postprandial blood sugar or standard glucose tolerance test to detect diabetes or carbohydrate intolerance due to such other causes as pheochromocytoma, primary aldosteronism, or Cushing's syndrome.

7. Urinary vanillyl mandelic acid (VMA) determination to screen for pheochromocytoma.

8. Urinary 17-hydroxycorticosteroid determination to screen for Cushing's syndrome.

9. An electrocardiogram for evidence of left ventricular and left atrial enlargement. Other abnormalities due to myocardial damage from associated coronary artery disease may also be discovered.

10. Chest films to estimate heart size, detect pulmonary complications, or diagnose aortic coarctation.

11. A rapid-sequence IVP to help identify unilateral disease of the renal parenchyma, renovascular lesions, polycystic disease, pyelonephritis, etc. A normal result lends support to a diagnosis of essential hypertension.

Subsequent Evaluation

Negative Initial Work-up

Patients with mild to moderate hypertension that is familial and begins above the age of 35 years, with no abnormalities revealed by clinical history, examination, or initial limited or comprehensive work-up, are assumed to have *essential hypertension* and should be treated accordingly. No further work-up is necessary. When the initial work-up suggests a potentially curable form of hypertension, additional studies are justified only if the results to be obtained will materially alter the treatment program. The situation must be tailored to each patient. Thus, a complete work-up for pheochromocytoma is indicated if the clinical history and urinary VMA excretion suggest this diagnosis, because surgical removal of the tumor is necessary to effect a cure. On the other hand, a 65-year-old woman with a blood pressure of 160/100 mm Hg and no evidence of systemic complications does not need renal arteriography; even if renovascular disease were detected, surgical therapy probably is not warranted.

Abnormal Urinary Findings

1. If the urinalysis suggests *primary renal parenchymal disease* or if the BUN or the serum creatinine is elevated, a creatinine clearance test should be performed to estimate the degree of renal function impairment and to provide a baseline for future studies. More comprehensive studies for the diagnosis of primary renal parenchymal disease are discussed in the section Proteinuria, Chapter 7.

2. The presence of abnormal urinary findings such as proteinuria, white cells, and white cell clumps or casts, together with bacteriuria, sug-

gests the diagnosis of *chronic pyelonephritis*, although urinalysis may yield negative findings in this disease. Bacteriuria with over 100,000 colonies per milliliter of urine (from a clean-voided specimen) is considered significant. In chronic pyelonephritis, the IVP usually shows bilaterally shrunken kidneys with scarred and clubbed calyces.

HYPOKALEMIA AND HYPERTENSION

If the serum potassium level is low (3 mEq per liter or less) or borderline, further investigation for possible causes of hypokalemia and hypertension (listed below) is warranted. For practical purposes, if cases of essential hypertension on diuretics or other potassium-depleting drugs are excluded, the most common cause is primary aldosteronism. Adrenocortical hyperplasia and other rare syndromes of adrenocortical dysfunction are uncommon causes of hypokalemia in patients with hypertension.

Etiology

1. Essential hypertension with:
   a. Vomiting and diarrhea.
   b. Diuretic therapy.
   c. Oral contraceptive or estrogen therapy.
   d. Steroid therapy.

2. Renal disease.
   a. Accelerated or malignant hypertension.
   b. Renovascular hypertension.
   c. Potassium-losing nephropathies (e.g., chronic pyelonephritis).
   d. Renin-secreting renal tumor.
   e. Liddle's syndrome.

3. Adrenocortical dysfunction.
   a. Primary aldosteronism.
      (1) Aldosterone-producing adenoma.
      (2) Cortical hyperplasia.
   b. Cushing's syndrome and the ectopic ACTH syndrome.
   c. Endogenous mineralocorticoid excess (some adrenocortical tumors).
   d. Exogenous administration of mineralocorticoids.

4. Pseudoaldosteronism (excessive licorice ingestion syndrome).

Diagnostic Approach

The *first* step is to determine whether the potassium loss is the result of renal or extrarenal mechanisms. Extrarenal potassium depletion is easily recognized by the clinical picture and is correctable by replacement therapy with potassium salts. On the other hand, if there is renal potassium-wasting, then diuretics, kidney disease (parenchymal or vascular), primary aldosteronism, or other rare forms of adrenocortical dysfunction may be responsible. Before proceeding with additional laboratory studies, it is well to recheck the history and physical examination for diagnostic clues.

1. History.
   a. Inquire specifically for possible causes of potassium depletion: Has the patient been taking diuretics, laxatives, steroids, estrogens, or oral contraceptive agents? Is there a history of vomiting or diarrhea? Has potassium intake been reduced?
   b. Be sure that the patient is not a licorice ingestor, because the glycyrrhizinic acid in licorice may mimic the action of aldosterone by producing hypertension, alkalosis, and suppressed renin activity (but with low aldosterone secretion). Measurement of urinary aldosterone excretion will differentiate between primary aldosteronism and the syndrome of chronic licorice ingestion.
   c. Ask whether the patient has been on a low-sodium diet, because salt restriction may mask the hypokalemia of primary aldosteronism.

2. Physical examination.
   a. In primary aldosteronism, retinopathy is usually mild (Grade I or II) and edema is absent.
   b. A positive Trousseau's or Chvostek's sign in an untreated hypertensive patient is presumptive evidence of hyperaldosteronism.
   c. Lack of an abdominal bruit is an important sign favoring aldosteronism over renovascular hypertension.
   d. The Valsalva maneuver in primary aldosteronism does not elicit the characteristic hypertensive overshoot and bradycardia found in other types of hypertension.

3. Determining the mechanism of potassium loss.
   a. If the patient has been taking diuretics or other drugs that induce hypokalemia, these should be discontinued. Give 50 mEq of potassium (as the chloride) daily for 1 week. Stop the potassium chloride and recheck the serum potassium and sodium in 1 to 2 weeks. If the serum potassium is then normal, for practical purposes renal potassium-wasting and the diagnosis of primary aldosteronism can be ruled out. On the other hand, if the serum potassium is borderline or low, proceed as in paragraph **b** below.
   b. If the serum potassium is borderline or low and there is no obvious cause for the hypokalemia, check for potassium-wasting. Measure the 24-hour urinary excretion of potassium while the patient is on a regular salt intake (as reflected in a urinary sodium level of approximately 100 mEq/24 hours). Urinary potassium excretion of less than 20 mEq/24 hours is strong evidence against renal potassium-wasting and the diagnosis of primary aldosteronism, while a level of 60 mEq/24 hours or greater is strongly suggestive of renal potassium-wasting.
   c. If the serum potassium is initially low and the studies outlined in paragraphs **a** and **b** above show negative findings, it can be assumed that the patient does not have renal potassium-wasting or

primary aldosteronism, and further investigation for this diagnosis is not warranted.

d. If the preliminary results, as outlined in paragraphs **a** and **b** above, are suggestive of nondiuretic renal potassium-wasting, the two most likely possibilities are primary aldosteronism and renovascular hypertension. At this point the determination of plasma renin activity and aldosterone excretion are the next steps indicated.

(1) Plasma renin activity (PRA). The PRA test is done by comparing the plasma renin level under basal conditions with the level obtained after 4 hours of ambulation. The patient should be on a 20 mEq sodium diet for at least 4 days prior to the test. The normal response is a twofold or threefold rise in PRA after 4 hours of ambulation. Patients with primary aldosteronism show decreased plasma renin values, which typically fail to rise after activity. It must be remembered that about 25 percent of patients with essential hypertension have suppressed PRA, but aldosterone excretion is usually low or normal in these patients. Plasma renin activity is decreased in patients with excessive production of desoxycorticosterone or corticosterone, and is normal or elevated in patients with secondary aldosteronism.

(2) Aldosterone excretion. Measure the quantity of aldosterone in a 24-hour urine sample after the patient has been on a sodium intake of at least 200 mEq per day. Increased aldosterone secretion after salt-loading is found in primary and secondary aldosteronism (it may also occur, rarely, in essential hypertension). When aldosterone excretion is increased, elevated PRA suggests renovascular hypertension, and low PRA, primary aldosteronism. Aldosterone secretion is reduced in the 17-alpha-hydroxylase and 11-beta-hydroxylase deficiency syndromes and in Liddle's syndrome.

(3) Adrenal arteriography and venography. If the diagnosis of primary aldosteronism is established, adrenal arteriography or venography may be advisable in the preoperative evaluation of the patient for tumor localization. In some medical centers, tumor localization is attempted by catheterization of the adrenal veins bilaterally. Usually there is at least a twofold increase in the adrenal venous aldosterone levels on the side with the tumor.

Summary of the Results of Various Tests for Hypertension with Hypokalemia

1. If aldosterone excretion is increased and PRA is suppressed, the diagnosis is primary aldosteronism due to an aldosterone-producing adenoma, nodular hyperplasia, or adrenocortical hyperplasia (glucocorticoid remediable hypertension).

2. If aldosterone excretion is increased and PRA is normal or elevated, the diagnosis is secondary aldosteronism due to accelerated or malignant hypertension, renovascular hypertension, essential hypertension with diuretic therapy, or essential hypertension with oral contraceptive medications.

3. If aldosterone excretion is reduced and PRA is suppressed, mineralo-corticoids other than aldosterone, such as desoxycorticosterone and corticosterone, may be responsible for the hypertension.

   a. The 17-alpha-hydroxylase deficiency syndrome is characterized by hypertension, hypokalemic alkalosis, hypogonadism, primary amen-orrhea, little if any 17-hydroxycorticosteroids or aldosterone in the urine, and responsiveness to glucocorticosteroids.

   b. The 11-beta-hydroxylase deficiency syndrome is characterized by hypertension, hypokalemic alkalosis, sodium retention and edema, virilization in the female, precocious puberty in the male, reduced excretion of 17-hydroxycorticosteroids and aldosterone, and respon-siveness to glucocorticosteroids.

ABNORMAL INTRAVENOUS PYELOGRAM

The rapid-sequence IVP is the best screening procedure for determining the role played by the kidney in hypertension.

1. If the kidneys are reduced in size and scarred, and the calyces are clubbed, *chronic pyelonephritis* is probable.

2. If the kidneys are shrunken with normal calyces and pelves, *chronic glomerulonephritis* or *nephrosclerosis* is likely.

3. Grossly enlarged kidneys with spidery calyces are virtually pathog-nomonic of *polycystic disease*.

4. *Unilateral primary parenchymal disease*, not due to vascular impair-ment, is characterized by clubbed calyces and a thinned cortex on the affected side. In addition to the urographic findings, the evidence for unilateral parenchymal disease, rather than renovascular disease, as the cause of hypertension includes a history of urinary tract infections, decreased urine osmolality, and increased sodium concentration by split-function studies, normal renal vasculature by arteriography (ex-cept that the vasculature size will reflect the diminished function), and normal peripheral and renal plasma renin activity.

5. *Renovascular hypertension* is suggested by one or more of the follow-ing findings: (a) unilateral reduction in kidney size, exceeding 1.5 cm on the left or 1.0 cm on the right, (b) delayed appearance of the contrast medium on the affected side, (c) greater concentration of the radiopaque medium on the affected side when the contrast material finally does appear, and (d) notching of the pelvis or upper ureter on the affected side by collateral vessels. Even if renovascular hypertension is suggested by the urographic findings, it is unnecessary to do ad-

ditional studies unless surgery is contemplated. Ancillary studies available for the diagnosis of renovascular hypertension in addition to the IVP are the radioactive renogram, determination of plasma renin activity, aortography, catheterization of the renal veins for PRA, and differential renal function tests.

a. The radioactive renogram is a safe, easy test to perform. It is not a specific diagnostic study but provides a comparison of the blood flow to each kidney. Although positive renogram and IVP findings do not always coincide in the same patient, a combination of the two may identify renovascular disease in a larger number of cases than will either test alone.

b. Aortography should be performed by the femoral route with selective injection of the renal arteries. The mere presence of anatomic renal arterial lesions does not establish their functional significance. Proof of the functional significance of these lesions in the form of increased PRA should be obtained.

c. Plasma renin activity is usually increased in patients with renovascular hypertension both in the basal state and after 4 hours of ambulation.

d. Some authorities believe that the best technique for confirming the diagnosis of curable renovascular hypertension is the determination of PRA in blood samples from the renal veins of both kidneys. A level of PRA on the involved side that is at least one and a half times greater than that on the uninvolved side is considered significant.

e. Split kidney function tests, employing bilateral ureteral catheterization, are usually performed prior to surgery, primarily to be certain that if nephrectomy is required, the remaining kidney will function adequately. The diagnosis of renal ischemia may also receive additional support. Split kidney function tests generally show impairment of renal function on the affected side unless there are segmental lesions that are too small to produce measurable renal function impairment. In the interpretation of the tests, a 50 percent or greater decrease in urine volume, a 15 percent or greater decrease in sodium concentration, a lowered glomerular filtration rate, and an increased creatinine concentration on the affected side are considered diagnostic of renal ischemia. Bilateral lesions may not be detected with this technique, and both false-positive and false-negative responses may occur.

INCREASED EXCRETION OF VMA

1. Urinary excretion of VMA that is twice the normal rate is virtually pathognomonic of *pheochromocytoma*. False-positive and false-negative results may be produced by interfering drugs.

2. Clinically, pheochromocytoma is characterized by one or more of the following features: paroxysmal or persistent hypertension; attacks of headache, blurred vision, sweating, palpitation, trembling, and pallor; hyperglycemia and glycosuria; orthostatic hypotension; a tendency to cholelithiasis; a familial incidence in some cases; and an association with such diseases as carcinoma of the thyroid gland, parathyroid adenoma, neurofibromatosis, and neuroectodermal diseases (e.g., Lindau-von Hippel disease and tuberous sclerosis). Ninety percent of pheochromocytomas occur in the adrenal gland, and of these about 10 percent are bilateral. Two percent of extramedullary tumors are multiple. Malignancy is present in fewer than 10 percent of cases.

3. If VMA excretion is increased, the diagnosis should be confirmed by assay of catecholamines or metanephrines, or both, in a 24-hour urine specimen.

4. If excretion of VMA, catecholamines, or metanephrines is normal in a case with a high index of clinical suspicion, urine should be collected for a short, carefully timed period during and immediately after an attack and examined for catecholamines.

5. Pharmacologic tests such as the phentolamine, histamine, tyramine, and glucagon tests are unnecessary and inadvisable because they are hazardous and less accurate than urine assays.

6. Extraabdominal location of the tumor can be ruled out by physical examination of the neck and by chest films. Some adrenal pheochromocytomas are revealed by intravenous pyelography. Attempts at more detailed localization of the tumor do not appear to be necessary. If extraabdominal lesions are excluded, final localization of the tumor is by surgical exploration.

7. All patients with suspected pheochromocytoma should be evaluated preoperatively by an expert.

Precordial Pulsations and Movements

H. Harold Friedman

A great deal of useful clinical information is obtained by inspection and palpation of the precordium and chest wall. The apical impulse can be located and its characteristics defined. In addition, palpable sounds, murmurs, thrills and abnormal pulsations, and ventricular enlargement can be detected. For a complete examination, the patient should be examined while sitting, lying supine, and lying in the left lateral recumbent position. The heart sounds are the most useful reference points for timing cardiac pulsations.

APICAL IMPULSE

Normal

1. The location of the apex beat is determined most accurately in the sitting position. The normal apical impulse lies in or about the fifth intercostal space inside the midclavicular line at a distance no greater than 10 cm from the left sternal border. The impulse is confined to a single area no greater than 2 or 3 cm in diameter.

2. The normal apex beat is a systolic outward movement of brief duration (from S_1 to before S_2) that has a light, tapping quality. A somewhat more forceful beat is not abnormal in tense or thin-chested individuals.

3. The outward thrust of the apex beat is accompanied by slight inward movement of the chest wall overlying the right ventricle.

4. The apical impulse may not be palpable in many normal individuals.

Abnormal

1. Aside from its absence as a normal variant, the apical impulse may be impalpable because of disease (e.g., mitral stenosis, constrictive pericarditis). Thus, absence of the apex beat by itself has little diagnostic significance.

2. An apex beat that is not substantially displaced from its normal location but that is heaving, sustained (lasting from S_1 to S_2), forceful, and strong enough to lift the fingers against firm pressure, is indicative of left ventricular hypertrophy due to pressure loading (e.g., systemic hypertension, aortic stenosis). It is associated with increased systolic precordial retraction, producing the so-called left ventricular rock.

3. A sustained and abnormally bulging apical impulse, indistinguishable from the heave of left ventricular hypertrophy, may be encountered in myocardial infarction in the absence of hypertrophy.

4. An apex beat that is displaced laterally and downward is indicative of left ventricular dilatation, with or without hypertrophy.
   a. A sustained but weak apical impulse is indicative of dilatation.
   b. A hyperdynamic impulse, meaning one that is forceful, exaggerated, and abrupt (although prolonged beyond normal), is indicative of combined dilatation and hypertrophy due to volume overloading (e.g., aortic or mitral regurgitation, left-to-right shunt). A hyperdynamic impulse is also associated with a left ventricular rock.

5. Double apical impulses may be associated with an S_3 or S_4 gallop. In such cases, the ventricular impulse is systolic, and the additional impulse is diastolic.

6. Double apical thrusts, with both impulses occurring in systole, are strongly suggestive of idiopathic hypertrophic subaortic stenosis, but

they may also occur in some cases of myocardial infarction, angina pectoris, left ventricular aneurysm, or the systolic click syndrome associated with prolapse of the mitral valve into the left atrium.

7. The presence of asynchronous cardiac impulses palpable at both the xiphoid and apex suggests combined ventricular hypertrophy.

LEFT PARASTERNAL PULSATIONS

1. A slight precordial lift may occur normally in children and young adults.

2. Bulging of the precordium in a child generally denotes long-standing right ventricular enlargement.

3. A localized, sustained, heaving lift in the lower left parasternal region is indicative of right ventricular hypertrophy due to pressure loading (e.g., pulmonary hypertension from any cause, pulmonary stenosis). The lift is associated with conspicuous systolic retraction of the chest further to the left, producing the so-called right ventricular rock.

4. A hyperdynamic impulse over a relatively large area parasternally is indicative of right ventricular enlargement due to volume loading (e.g., atrial septal defect). This impulse is also associated with a right ventricular rock.

5. A left parasternal lift may be palpable in the absence of right ventricular hypertrophy or pulmonary hypertension when the right ventricle is pushed anteriorly by a giant left atrium.

6. Marked right ventricular dilatation may displace the right ventricular beat leftward to the site of the normal cardiac impulse. In such cases, identification of the impulse as right rather than left ventricular in origin is supported by the presence of a right ventricular lift, an accentuated P_2, and the demonstration of a left ventricular impulse, or the thrill and murmur of mitral valvular disease, in the left axilla.

OTHER SYSTOLIC PRECORDIAL PULSATIONS AND MOVEMENTS

1. A diffuse systolic depression of the precordium followed by a brisk diastolic rebound and a palpable or audible "knock" is characteristic of chronic constrictive pericarditis.

2. A diffuse systolic depression at the left side of the chest accompanied by an opposite pulsation at the right side is characteristic of tricuspid regurgitation.

3. Systolic depression of the midportion and right side of the chest may be found in marked aortic regurgitation.

4. Paradoxical sustained outward systolic movements, or bulges, are commonly palpable in patients with myocardial infarction or angina pectoris at some point medial to the apex beat. When present at the apex, however, they are indistinguishable from the apical thrust of a hypertrophied left ventricle. A bulge signifies the presence of ventricular asynergy or aneurysm.

PULSATIONS IN THE LEFT SECOND AND THIRD INTERCOSTAL SPACES

1. A faint, nonlifting, systolic pulsation may be normal in young people and patients with pes excavatum, and during tachycardia.
2. A systolic lifting pulsation in this area is indicative of pulmonary artery dilatation or increased pulmonary blood flow.

PULSATIONS IN THE SECOND RIGHT INTERCOSTAL SPACE

Pulsation in the second right intercostal space suggests dilatation of the aorta.

PULSATIONS OF THE STERNOCLAVICULAR JOINTS AND STERNUM

1. Pulsation of the right sternoclavicular joint may indicate a right-sided aortic arch.

2. Pulsation of either sternoclavicular joint occurs in aortic dissection or aneurysm.

3. Systolic outward pulsation of the upper half of the sternum is generally due to aneurysm of the ascending aorta. Aneurysm of the transverse aorta is usually not associated with visible pulsations but may cause displacement of the trachea or a tracheal tug.

EPIGASTRIC PULSATIONS

1. Epigastric pulsations may be helpful in the diagnosis of ventricular hypertrophy in patients with emphysema.

2. Pulsations in the epigastric region may originate in the aorta or result from an overactive or hypertrophied heart.

3. The pulsations of a hypertrophied right ventricle are palpable high in the epigastric area beneath the rib cage; those of a hypertrophied left ventricle, under the left costal margin. To be indicative of hypertrophy rather than simple overactivity or displacement, such pulsations should have a significant downward thrust.

THORACIC ARTERIAL PULSATIONS

1. Visible arterial pulsations over the back of the chest occur frequently in coarctation of the aorta from an increased collateral circulation. They are seen best with the patient leaning forward and the back illuminated by a light from above shining obliquely downward.

2. Pulsations in the right lower neck beneath the sternomastoid muscle are usually due to kinking of the common carotid artery rather than to aneurysm.

3. Other abnormalities of the arterial pulse are described in the section Arterial Pulse, earlier in the chapter.

HEART SOUNDS

The first sound and both components of the second sound, ejection sounds, the opening snap of mitral stenosis, pericardial friction rubs, and gallop sounds may all be palpable when present. They are identified by their characteristics and timing. Gallop sounds on occasion may be felt even when they are not heard. Left-sided gallops and the mitral opening snap may sometimes be felt more easily with the patient in the left lateral recumbent position.

THRILLS

Thrills are palpable vibrations associated with murmurs. The presence of a thrill indicates only that the accompanying murmur is loud. It has no other significance.

Heart Sounds
H. Harold Friedman

NORMAL HEART SOUNDS

Usually only two heart sounds, called the first sound and the second sound, are audible in normal persons (see Fig. 3-1, p. 47). The first sound (S_1)

is ordinarily louder at the apex than at the base. The converse is true of the second sound (S_2). At the apex, S_1 is usually louder than S_2 but may be of the same or even lesser intensity than S_2. At the base, S_2 is louder than S_1. Decreased intensity of the heart sounds may be due to poor conduction of the sounds because of such conditions as a thick chest wall, emphysema, or pericardial effusion. Increased intensity of the heart sounds may occur normally in children or thin-chested individuals. In the discussion that follows, only cardiac factors influencing the intensity of the heart sounds are considered.

THE FIRST HEART SOUND (S_1)

1. *Increased intensity* of S_1 may be found in the following conditions:
   a. Sinus rhythm with a short P-R interval (0.08 to 0.12 second).
   b. Hyperkinetic circulatory states.
   c. Mitral stenosis.

2. *Decreased intensity* of S_1 may occur when myocardial contractility is impaired or when hemodynamics are altered, as in shock, myocardial infarction, congestive failure, or terminal states. S_1 may be decreased in intensity in mitral or aortic regurgitation.

3. *Variation in the intensity* of S_1 is a common occurrence in arrhythmias such as atrial fibrillation, AV dissociation, ventricular tachycardia with AV dissociation, and complete AV block. The term *cannon sounds* refers to the very loud first sounds that occur intermittently in the last three conditions.

4. *Wide splitting* of S_1 may result from mechanical delays in mitral or tricuspid valve closure (e.g., mitral stenosis, Ebstein's anomaly, atrial septal defect).

5. S_1 may be *masked* by a loud systolic murmur (e.g., mitral regurgitation).

THE SECOND HEART SOUND (S_2)

The second heart sound (S_2) consists of aortic (A_2) and pulmonary (P_2) components. A_2 normally precedes P_2 and is the louder sound in adults. P_2 is usually audible in the pulmonary area; less commonly, it can be heard in the aortic area or left sternal border. It cannot normally be heard at the apex.

Intensity

1. P_2 is usually louder than A_2 up to the age of about 20 or 30 years; in persons above this age, A_2 is louder than P_2.

2. *Increased intensity of A_2* occurs when the systemic arterial pressure is elevated, as in essential hypertension. It may also be accentuated in

aortic dilatation or aneurysm and in some cases of aortic regurgitation. A tambour-like A_2 is characteristic of syphilitic aortitis.

3. *Decreased intensity of A_2* is commonly observed in hypotension, shock, and congestive failure. In valvular aortic stenosis, A_2 is usually diminished or absent.

4. *Increased intensity of P_2*, with P_2 louder than A_2, is found in pulmonary hypertension due to such conditions as mitral stenosis, left-sided heart failure, primary pulmonary hypertension, pulmonary emboli, and left-to-right shunts. In these conditions, P_2 is sometimes audible at the apex.

5. *Decreased intensity of P_2* or absence of P_2 is noted in pulmonary stenosis.

6. A_2 or P_2 may be masked by loud systolic murmurs (e.g., pulmonary stenosis and aortic stenosis, respectively).

Splitting

Normal Splitting
1. Normal or physiologic splitting of S_2 into earlier A_2 and later P_2 components is heard best in the pulmonary area or along the left sternal border.

2. The maximum normal split between A_2 and P_2 is about 0.03 second in expiration and 0.06 second in inspiration.

3. In normal young adults, in the recumbent position, S_2 is either single or narrowly split during expiration, and is audibly and more widely split during inspiration. However, in the upright position, expiratory splitting of S_2 should not be audible.

4. In adults, audible expiratory splitting of S_2 in the upright position is, with rare exceptions, suggestive of organic heart disease.

5. S_2 is often single in both expiration and inspiration. This pattern is observed more frequently with advancing age and is quite common in normal adults above the age of 50 years.

Wide Splitting
Splitting of S_2 that exceeds normal values may be caused by a delayed P_2, an early A_2, or a combination of the two.

1. A *delayed P_2* may be found in the following conditions:
   a. Right bundle branch block.
   b. Increased right ventricular stroke volume, as in left-to-right shunts (e.g., anomalous pulmonary venous drainage, atrial septal defect, ventricular septal defect) and pulmonary insufficiency.

   c. Increased resistance to right ventricular ejection (e.g., pulmonary stenosis, pulmonary hypertension, and pulmonary embolism).

   d. Structural abnormalities such as pes excavatum and the straight back syndrome.

2. An *early* A_2 may result from decreased resistance to left ventricular ejection or decreased left ventricular stroke volume, as in ventricular septal defect or mitral regurgitation.

Wide and Fixed Splitting

1. The term *fixed* splitting of S_2 refers to an already widely split S_2 that splits no further or splits by not more than 0.02 second during inspiration in either the recumbent or the sitting position.

2. Wide and fixed splitting of S_2 may be observed in atrial septal defects and some other left-to-right shunts, severe right-sided heart failure, acute massive pulmonary embolism, and cardiomyopathy.

3. The widely split S_2 of right bundle branch block is not fixed.

Reversed or Paradoxical Splitting

1. Reversed splitting of S_2 is rarely a normal finding. It results from delayed aortic closure so that A_2 follows rather than precedes P_2 during the entire respiratory cycle.

2. Usually the splitting narrows during inspiration and widens during expiration.

3. The most common cause of paradoxical splitting is left bundle branch block. Other conditions that sometimes produce reversed splitting are the following: right ventricular arrhythmias or pacing, aortic stenosis, the Wolff-Parkinson-White (WPW) syndrome, systemic hypertension, patent ductus arteriosus, cardiomyopathy, angina pectoris, myocardial infarction, and severe left ventricular failure from any cause.

SINGLE SECOND HEART SOUND

1. A single S_2 is a common normal variant in persons above the age of 50 years.

2. S_2 may be single because of changes in P_2:

   a. P_2 is faint or not detected (e.g., tetralogy of Fallot, tricuspid atresia, pulmonary atresia, pulmonary stenosis).

   b. P_2 is synchronous with A_2 (e.g., ventricular septal defect with Eisenmenger's syndrome, some cases of aortic stenosis, occasional instances of left bundle branch block).

   c. P_2 is masked by a systolic murmur (e.g., aortic stenosis).

3. S_2 may be single because of changes in A_2:
   a. A_2 is faint or not detected (e.g., aortic stenosis).
   b. A_2 is synchronous with P_2 (see paragraph **2b** above).
   c. A_2 is masked by a systolic murmur (e.g., pulmonary stenosis).

4. S_2 is single when there is only one semilunar valve (e.g., truncus arteriosus).

ABNORMAL AND EXTRA SOUNDS

The various abnormal and extra sounds that may be encountered are discussed below; their differential diagnosis is summarized in Tables 3-3 and 3-4.

The Third Heart Sound (Ventricular Gallop, S_3)

Normal
   1. The third sound (S_3) is commonly audible in normal children and young adults below the age of 30 years.

   2. The normal S_3 is a soft, low-pitched sound that is usually localized to the apex. It is heard best with the bell of the stethoscope with the subject in the left lateral recumbent position. The sound is louder in expiration than in inspiration.

Abnormal
   1. S_3 is abnormal above the age of 30 years and probably at any age in the presence of heart disease.

   2. S_3 occurs 0.12 to 0.18 second after A_2 and coincides with the descending limb of the V wave of the jugular venous pulse.

   3. S_3 may be accompanied by a palpable or visible apical shock or bulge.

   4. A left-sided S_3 (LS_3) is caused by left ventricular disease or failure; a right-sided S_3 (RS_3) by right ventricular disease or failure. LS_3 is heard best at the apex; RS_3, along the left sternal border, the tricuspid area, and occasionally in the right supraclavicular fossa. LS_3 is louder in expiration; RS_3, in inspiration.

   5. An S_3 sound may be the earliest sign of myocardial failure.

   6. The intensity of S_3 is decreased by sitting or standing and increased by brief exercise.

   7. An LS_3 is absent in pure or predominant mitral stenosis, but RS_3 may occur when there is pulmonary hypertension. If an LS_3 is heard in a patient with both mitral stenosis and regurgitation, it can be assumed that regurgitation is the predominant lesion.

TABLE 3-3. Differential Diagnosis: S_4 Preceding M_1 vs. Split S_1 (M_1 Preceding T_1)

Parameter	LS_4 Preceding M_1	RS_4 Preceding M_1	Split S_1 (M_1 and T_1)
Characteristics of sound	Faint, low-pitched sound (S_4) followed by higher-pitched sound (M_1)	Faint, low-pitched sound (S_4) followed by higher-pitched sound (M_1)	M_1 and T_1 about same in intensity and pitch
Effect of pressure with stethoscope diaphragm	LS_4 more faint or inaudible	RS_4 more faint or inaudible	M_1 and T_1 may be more faint but sharper and clicky
Area of maximum audibility	Apex, especially in left lateral recumbent position, with bell chest piece	Lower left sternal border, with bell chest piece	Lower left sternal border and medial to apex but not lateral to it, with bell or diaphragm
Interval between sounds	Usually 0.05 to 0.10 sec	Usually 0.05 to 0.10 sec	Usually about 0.03 sec
Precordial pulsations	Presystolic and systolic apical impulses	Right ventricular lift or heave	Single systolic apical impulse
Effect of respiration	LS_4 louder in expiration	RS_4 louder in inspiration	Splitting somewhat more evident in expiration
Effect of change in venous return			
Increase (e.g., leg raising)	LS_4 louder	RS_4 louder	Little or no effect
Decrease (e.g., sitting)	LS_4 more faint or inaudible	LS_4 more faint or inaudible	Little or no effect

LS_4 = left-sided S_4 M_1 = first audible component of S_1
RS_4 = right-sided S_4 T_1 = second audible component of S_1
S_1 = first sound

TABLE 3-4. Differential Diagnosis of Various Heart Sounds

Parameter	Split S_2, A_2 Preceding P_2	Opening Snap	S_3	S_4	Ejection Sound
Characteristics of sound	P_2 soft unless accentuated	Relatively loud, high-pitched	Faint, low-pitched	Faint, low-pitched	Sharp, clicking
Interval between sounds	A_2-P_2, 0.03 to 0.05 sec during inspiration	A_2-OS, 0.04 to 0.12 sec	A_2-S_3, 0.12 to 0.18 sec; S_3-S_1, 0.18 sec	S_4-M_1, 0.05 to 0.10 sec; S_2-S_4, >0.20 sec	M_1-ES, 0.04 to 0.09 sec; M_1-T_1, 0.03 sec
Area of maximum audibility	Localized to pulmonary area and LSB	Widespread: OSMV: 4-LICS, apex, and LSB; OSTV: lower LSB; OSMV: loud, snapping S_1 at apex and A_2, P_2, and OS audible in pulmonary area	Localized; LS_3: apex in LLRP; RS_3: LSB, tricuspid area, and supraclavicular fossa	Localized; LS_4: apex in LLRP, not transmitted; RS_4: lower LSB, sometimes lower RSB	Usually localized; PES: 2- and 3-LICS; AES: apex, LSB, aortic area
Precordial pulsations	P_2 sometimes palpable if accentuated; other pulsations depend on underlying conditions	OS may be palpable; apical impulse often impalpable in pure mitral stenosis	LS_3 palpable or visible, or both; RS_3 may have right ventricular heave or lift	LS_4: presystolic and systolic apical impulses; RS_4: right ventricular heave or lift	ES not palpable; other pulsations depend on underlying conditions

	Splitting increased unless fixed; P₂ louder on inspiration	OSMV louder on expiration; OSTV louder on inspiration	LS₃ decreased with inspiration; RS₃ increased with inspiration	LS₄ louder in expiration; RS₄ louder in inspiration	PES decreased and moves closer to S₁ with inspiration; AES not affected by respiration
Effect of respiration					
Effect of change in venous return					
Increase (e.g., leg raising)	P₂ louder, split increased	Little or no effect	Louder	Louder	Little or no effect
Decrease (e.g., sitting)	A₂ louder, split decreased	Little or no effect	Fainter	Fainter	Little or no effect

A_2 = aortic component of S_2
AES = aortic ES
ES = ejection sound
LICS = left intercostal space
LLRP = left lateral recumbent position
LS_3 = left-sided S_3
LS_4 = left-sided S_4
LSB = left sternal border
M_1 = mitral component of S_1
OS = opening snap
OSMV = OS mitral valve
OSTV = OS tricuspid valve
P_2 = pulmonary component of S_2
PES = pulmonary ES
RS_3 = right-sided S_3
RS_4 = right-sided S_4
RSB = right sternal border
S_2 = second heart sound
S_3 = third heart sound
S_4 = fourth heart sound
T_1 = tricuspid component of S_1

8. S_3 must be differentiated from the second component of a split S_2, an opening snap, and an S_4 (see Table 3-4).

9. The pericardial knock, a diastolic filling sound occurring somewhat earlier than the usual S_3 (0.06 to 0.12 second after A_2), is found in most cases of chronic constrictive pericarditis; it coincides with the end of the Y descent in the jugular venous pulse.

10. S_3 may coexist with S_4, producing a quadruple rhythm, whereas either sound alone, when combined with S_1 and S_2, produces a triple rhythm. When S_3 and S_4 coincide, the condition is called a summation sound, or gallop. Transient slowing of the heart rate by carotid massage may separate a suspected summation sound into its S_3 and S_4 components.

The Opening Snap

1. The opening of the mitral or tricuspid valves is normally inaudible. Audible opening of an AV valve occurs when it is stenosed. The sound produced is called an opening snap (OS).

2. The OS of the mitral valve (OSMV) is virtually pathognomonic of mitral stenosis and indicates that the valve is pliable. The OS disappears when the valve becomes rigid, fixed, or calcified. It may also disappear in the presence of aortic insufficiency or when mitral regurgitation is the predominant lesion. Surprisingly, the OS persists after commissurotomy. It is audible both in sinus rhythms and in atrial fibrillation.

3. The OSMV is a high-pitched, snapping sound that occurs between 0.04 and 0.12 second after A_2. The severity of mitral stenosis may be roughly estimated from the A_2-OS interval. As a rule of thumb, the stenosis is severe when the interval is short, and mild when it is long.

4. The OSMV is heard best at the lower left sternal border and at the apex, but it is also frequently audible at the base. The sound may be palpable as well as audible. Its timing coincides with the V wave of the jugular venous pulse. The intensity of the sound is not affected by respiration.

5. The mitral OS is associated almost always with a loud S_1 and frequently with a split S_2 and accentuated P_2.

6. An OS of the tricuspid valve (OSTV) may be heard in some patients with tricuspid stenosis. The auscultatory characteristics of this sound are similar to those of the mitral OS, but there are some differences. The OSTV is heard best over the lower end of the sternum or at the right lower sternal edge. The tricuspid A_2-OS interval is shorter than the mitral A_2-OS interval. The tricuspid OS is not appreciably affected by respiration. An OSTV is occasionally heard in atrial septal defects in the absence of tricuspid stenosis.

7. In severe MS, the A_2-OS interval may so short that the OS cannot be clearly differentiated from the components of S_2. Under such circumstances, the administration of phenylephrine may, by increasing the A_2-OS interval, separate the OS from S_2 enough to make it identifiable as a separate sound.

The Fourth Sound (Atrial Sound or Gallop, S_4)

1. The fourth sound (S_4) occurs about 0.12 second after the P wave, preceding S_1 by about 0.05 to 0.10 second when the P-R interval is normal. S_4 sounds, also called atrial or presystolic gallops, are usually indicative of myocardial abnormality. Atrial sounds are not audible in atrial fibrillation.

2. S_4 is usually a soft, low-pitched sound, hence it is heard best with the stethoscope bell applied lightly to the chest wall. It may be inaudible with the diaphragm.

3. S_4 may be left-sided or right-sided in origin.

Left-sided S_4

1. Left-sided S_4 (LS_4) is usually heard best at the cardiac apex with the patient in the left lateral recumbent position.

2. It is usually associated with a presystolic apical impulse.

3. LS_4 may wax and wane with respiration, becoming louder during expiration or becoming audible only during this phase of respiration.

4. Maneuvers that increase venous return (e.g., leg raising, exercise) tend to increase the intensity of the sound; those that decrease venous return (e.g., sitting) have the opposite effect.

5. LS_4 has been reported to occur in some normal individuals over 50 years of age, but it is more commonly associated with one of the following conditions:
  a. Disorders characterized by decreased compliance of the left ventricle (e.g., systemic hypertension, aortic stenosis or insufficiency, cardiomyopathy).
  b. Acute myocardial infarction (LS_4 is heard in an overwhelming majority of cases).
  c. Attacks of angina pectoris.
  d. AV block, of varying degree.
  e. Hyperkinetic circulatory states (e.g., hyperthyroidism, anemia).

6. LS_4 is ordinarily not audible in mitral valve disease, but it may occur in acute mitral regurgitation due to ruptured chordae tendineae.

Right-sided S_4

1. Right-sided S_4 (RS_4) is usually heard along the lower left sternal border and sometimes over the right internal jugular vein.

2. RS$_4$ is usually associated with a sustained left parasternal heave and a giant jugular A wave.

3. RS$_4$ may wax and wane during respiration, becoming loudest during inspiration.

4. Maneuvers that increase the venous return to the heart increase the intensity of S$_4$; those that decrease the venous return have the opposite effect.

5. RS$_4$ is heard in conditions in which there is either decreased compliance of the right ventricle or increased resistance to right ventricular filling:
   a. Pulmonary hypertension (e.g., atrial septal defect, ventricular septal defect, patent ductus arteriosus, pulmonary embolism, primary pulmonary hypertension).
   b. Pulmonary stenosis.
   c. Cardiomyopathy.

Systolic Sounds

Pulmonary Ejection Sounds

1. Pulmonary ejection sounds (PES) occur at the time blood is ejected from the right ventricle into the pulmonary artery. They follow M$_1$ by 0.04 to 0.09 second (range 0.02 to 0.14 second).

2. PES are heard best over the second or third left intercostal spaces. They are poorly heard or inaudible at the apex. They tend to decrease in intensity and move closer to S$_1$ during inspiration.

3. PES have a sharp clicking quality.

4. PES occur in most cases of pulmonary stenosis and in many cases of primary and secondary pulmonary hypertension.

Aortic Ejection Sounds

1. Aortic ejection sounds (AES) occur at the time of ejection of blood from the left ventricle into aorta. Their timing is similar to that of PES.

2. AES, in contrast to PES, are usually heard best at the apex and have no respiratory variation. They may also be heard along the left sternal border and in the aortic area.

3. AES are present in almost all cases of congenital valvular aortic stenosis, but not in infundibular, supravalvular, or idiopathic hypertrophic subaortic stenosis. AES may be heard in some cases of rheumatic aortic stenosis and in occasional instances of aortic insufficiency, coarctation of the aorta, aneurysm of the ascending aorta, and the tetralogy of Fallot.

Systolic Clicks

1. Clicks are systolic sounds. Although systolic clicks (SC) occur at any time during systole, they are more common in mid or late systole. They are usually single, but sometimes two or more sounds may be heard.

2. Systolic clicks are heard best in the midprecordium or at the apex, and may show respiratory or positional variation in intensity or even in timing from beat to beat.

3. Many clicks are benign. However, systolic clicks associated with mid or late systolic murmurs are indicative of nonrheumatic mitral regurgitation.

Pericardial Friction Rub

1. The pericardial friction rub is a rough, scratchy sound, often quite changeable in character from day to day or even minute to minute, audible over the precordium in most cases of acute pericarditis but rarely in chronic constrictive pericarditis. The rub is usually louder on inspiration. The sound may have systolic, diastolic, and presystolic components. When two or three components are present, the diagnosis is made easily. When the rub is heard only during systole, it may be mistaken for a murmur or an extracardiac sound. With continued observation the friction rub either assumes a to-and-fro character or disappears.

2. A pericardial friction rub should be differentiated from a *pleuropericardial friction rub* and from the to-and-fro *crunching sound of mediastinal emphysema*, which is coarser in quality and is often associated with crepitus of the soft tissues of the neck.

Heart Murmurs

H. Harold Friedman

Murmurs are related to several factors: (1) increased flow through normal or abnormal valves, (2) forward flow through narrowed or deformed valves, (3) backward or regurgitant flow through incompetent valves or septal defects, (4) more or less continuous flow through extracardiac and intracardiac shunts and narrowed or collateral vessels, and in vascular structures, and, less often, (5) vibration of loose structures within the heart. The following abbreviations are used in this section:

A_2 = aortic component of second heart sound
AES = aortic ejection sound(s) or click(s)
AR = aortic regurgitation
AS = aortic stenosis
ASD = atrial septal defect
CM = continuous murmur(s)

DM = diastolic murmur(s)
EM = ejection murmur(s)
ES = ejection sound(s) or click(s)
ICS = intercostal space
IE = infective endocarditis
IHSS = idiopathic hypertrophic subaortic stenosis
IPS = infundibular pulmonary stenosis
JVP = jugular venous pulse
LA = left atrium
LAE = left atrial enlargement
LICS = left intercostal space
LLRP = left lateral recumbent position
LLSB = lower left sternal border
LRSB = lower right sternal border
LSB = left sternal border
LV = left ventricle (-ular)
LVE = left ventricular enlargement
MR = mitral regurgitation
MS = mitral stenosis
OS = opening snap
OSMV = OS mitral valve
OSTV = OS tricuspid valve
P_2 = pulmonary component of second heart sound
PA = pulmonary artery
PDA = patent ductus arteriosus
PES = pulmonary ejection sound(s) or click(s)
PH = pulmonary hypertension
PPH = primary pulmonary hypertension
PR = pulmonary regurgitation
PS = pulmonary stenosis
RA = right atrium
RAE = right atrial enlargement
RICS = right intercostal space
RM = regurgitant murmur(s)
RSB = right sternal border
RV = right ventricle (-ular)
RVE = right ventricular enlargement
S_1 = first heart sound
S_2 = second heart sound
S_3 = third heart sound
S_4 = fourth heart sound
SC = systolic click(s)
SEM = systolic ejection murmur(s)
SM = systolic murmur(s)
SPH = secondary pulmonary hypertension
SRM = systolic regurgitant murmur(s)
T/F = tetralogy of Fallot
TR = tricuspid regurgitation
TS = tricuspid stenosis
ULSB = upper left sternal border
URSB = upper right sternal border
VAS = valvular aortic stenosis
VPS = valvular pulmonary stenosis
VSD = ventricular septal defect(s)

TYPES OF MURMURS

There are three basic types of murmurs: systolic, diastolic, and continuous. An SM begins with or after S_1 and ends before, at, or slightly beyond S_2. A DM begins with or after S_2 and ends before S_1. A CM begins in systole, continues through S_2 without interruption, and ends at some time in diastole.

Systolic Murmurs

Systolic Ejection Murmurs

1. *Mid systolic EM* are caused by normal or increased forward flow through either normal or abnormal right or left ventricular outflow tracts. They may be found in AS or PS, increased flow through a normal valve, ejection across a nonstenosed but deformed valve, dilatation of the aorta or pulmonary artery, or combinations of these. The murmur of AS is the prototype of left-sided mid systolic EM, and the murmur of PS, of right-sided EM. Such murmurs begin after S_1 and end before A_2 if left-sided, and before P_2 if right-sided. The murmurs are of variable intensity, high- to medium-pitched, noisy, rough or harsh in quality, and generally crescendo-decrescendo (diamond-shaped) in character.

2. *Early systolic EM* are primarily flow murmurs, beginning after S_1 and ending midway through systole. They tend to be decrescendo (kite-shaped) in character.

Systolic Regurgitant Murmurs

SRM are due to flow from high- to low-pressure chambers or vessels. Thus they occur in MR, TR, VSD, and some aortopulmonary communications. RM may be classified according to their timing as pansystolic (holosystolic), early systolic, mid systolic, or late systolic. *Pansystolic* RM start with S_1 and end with or beyond A_2. They are typical of the aforementioned conditions. *Early systolic* RM start with S_1 but end in mid systole. They occur in some VSD, in tight MS with slight MR, and in TR from IE. *Mid systolic* RM begin after S_1 and end before or at A_2. They are usually found in MR due to papillary muscle dysfunction, although any type of SRM may occur in this condition. *Late systolic* RM start about mid systole, often with an SC, and end at or beyond A_2. They occur most often in nonrheumatic MR associated with prolapse of one or both mitral leaflets into the LA, but they may sometimes be found in rheumatic MR and in calcification of the mitral annulus.

Diastolic Murmurs

DM may be classified as early diastolic, mid diastolic, or late diastolic (presystolic). *Early DM* are due to semilunar valve incompetence. *Mid and late DM* are due either to stenosis of the atrioventricular valves or to increased flow across these valves.

TABLE 3-5. The Effects of Physiologic and Pharmacologic Maneuvers on Murmurs

Murmur	Inspiration	Sudden Standing	Sudden Squatting	Amyl Nitrite	Vasopressors (Phenylephrine or Methoxamine)	Valsalva and Post-Valsalva Effect	Effect of Miscellaneous Maneuvers on Murmur
Aortic stenosis	NSC	D	I	I	D or NSC	D, with delayed return of intensity of murmur	I after extrasystole or pause, and leg raising
Idiopathic hypertrophic subaortic stenosis	NSC	I	D	I	D	I	I after extrasystole or pause, standing; D after leg raising
Pulmonary stenosis	I	NSC	I	PS: I (most cases); Tetralogy of Fallot: D	PS: NSC; Tetralogy of Fallot: I	D, with immediate return of intensity of murmur	. . .
Aortic regurgitation	D	NSC compared with sitting	I	D Austin Flint murmur: D	Austin Flint murmur: I	. . .	I when sitting, when leaning forward, and in expiration
Mitral regurgitation Pansystolic	NSC or D	D or NSC	I	D	I	D, with later I	Beat after extrasystole or pause: NSC

	Murmur starts earlier; is longer	Murmur starts earlier; is longer	Murmur starts later; is shorter	Murmur starts earlier; is longer	I	I, with later D	Murmur starts later; is shorter
Mid to late systolic (click syndrome)							
Papillary muscle dysfunction	NSC	NSC	Variable	Variable	Variable	...	D or NSC
Tricuspid regurgitation	I	D or NSC	I	I or NSC	NSC	D, with later I	...
Ventricular septal defect without pulmonary hypertension	NSC	NSC	I	D	I	NSC	...
Mitral stenosis	NSC or slight D; may reveal A_2-P_2-OS sequence	D	I	I	D; A_2-OS interval is widened	NSC	I after exercise and in left lateral recumbent position
Tricuspid stenosis	I	D	I	I	NSC	NSC	...
Pulmonary regurgitation	I or NSC	...	...	NSC	NSC	...	...

D = decreased intensity, I = increased intensity, NSC = no significant change in intensity.
SOURCE: Adapted from M. C. Dohan and M. G. Drisitiello, Physiologic and pharmacologic manipulations of heart sounds and murmurs, *Mod. Concepts Cardiovasc. Dis.*, 39:121, 1970.

83

Continuous Murmurs

CM begin after S_1, continue through S_2 without interruption, enveloping it, and end at some time in diastole before S_1. The murmur need not persist through all of diastole to be considered continuous. CM occur in extracardiac and intracardiac shunts but may be caused by flow through narrowed or collateral vessels or by increased flow in vascular structures.

DESCRIPTION OF MURMURS

Descriptions of murmurs should include their timing, intensity, pitch, quality, duration, location, and radiation. The most widely used system (Levine and Harvey) for grading the intensity of heart murmurs uses a six-point scale.

Grade 1: very faint.
Grade 2: faint.
Grade 3: moderately loud.
Grade 4: loud.
Grade 5: very loud.
Grade 6: loudest possible.

PHYSIOLOGIC AND PHARMACOLOGIC MANEUVERS

Physiologic and pharmacologic maneuvers may have effects on the intensity of murmurs that may have some diagnostic significance. The maneuvers and their effects on various murmurs are summarized in Table 3-5. Use of these maneuvers is often helpful in the differential diagnosis of specific auscultatory problems (see Table 3-6).

DIAGNOSTIC APPROACH TO MURMURS

The diagnostic evaluation of any heart murmur involves first, a decision as to whether the murmur is innocent or organic, and second, if organic, a determination of the anatomic lesion and its cause. The work-up of a patient with an organic murmur should include examination of the arterial and jugular venous pulses, inspection and palpation of the precordium and chest wall, and systematic auscultation of the heart, thorax, and related vascular structures. Also indicated in all cases are an electrocardiogram and chest films (preferably PA, lateral, and oblique views taken with a barium-filled esophagus). Cardiac fluoroscopy with image amplification is invaluable in studying motion and dynamic changes as well as in the detection of valvular or other calcifications.

Based on the aforementioned procedures, it is possible to make the correct cardiac diagnosis in the vast majority of cases. When this is not possible or for other legitimate reasons (e.g., confirmation of a diagnosis, preoperative evaluation), apexcardiography, external recordings of the jugular and carotid pulses, phonocardiography, echocardiography, cardiac cath-

TABLE 3-6.   Maneuvers Helpful in the Differential Diagnosis
of Similar Murmurs

Diagnostic Problem	Useful Maneuvers*
Mitral regurgitation vs. tricuspid regurgitation	Respiration, amyl nitrite, vasopressors
Aortic stenosis vs. idiopathic hypertrophic subaortic stenosis	Squatting, standing, Valsalva, amyl nitrite
Mitral regurgitation vs. idiopathic hypertrophic subaortic stenosis	Squatting, standing, amyl nitrite, vasopressors
Aortic stenosis vs. mitral regurgitation	Amyl nitrite, vasopressors, postextrasystolic beat
Aortic stenosis vs. mid to late systolic murmur of mitral regurgitation	Standing, amyl nitrite
Mitral stenosis vs. Austin Flint murmur	Amyl nitrite, vasopressors
Mitral stenosis vs. tricuspid stenosis	Respiration, amyl nitrite, vasopressors
Pulmonary stenosis vs. tetralogy of Fallot	Amyl nitrite
Pulmonary stenosis vs. small ventricular septal defect	Amyl nitrite, vasopressors

* The responses to these maneuvers are shown in Table 3-5.
Source: Adapted from M. C. Dohan and M. G. Drisitiello, Physiologic and pharmacologic manipulations of heart sounds and murmurs, *Mod. Concepts Cardiovasc. Dis.*, 39:121, 1970.

eterization and angiocardiography may be indispensable tools for diagnosis, differential diagnosis, or the study of cardiovascular hemodynamics. As a general rule, preference should be given to noninvasive techniques when the information yielded is comparable to that obtainable by catheter intervention. Since all of these supplementary techniques are highly technical and require special equipment, they usually are not performed by the nonspecialist in cardiology, hence are not discussed here.

In the presentation that follows, primary consideration is given to the more frequent, uncomplicated murmurs encountered in adults, omitting discussions of many complex congenital or acquired lesions. The murmurs are described according to their timing and site of maximum intensity.

INNOCENT MURMURS

Innocent murmurs are those not due to recognizable lesions of the heart. Although they may occur at any age, they are most common in children and adolescents. The characteristics of innocent murmurs in young people and their differential diagnosis are summarized in Tables 3-7 and 3-9. The aortic ejection murmur of middle and old age, although not innocent, is nevertheless benign. It is, so to speak, the innocent murmur of the elderly. It is discussed in paragraph **2d** below.

TABLE 3-7. Innocent Murmurs in Young People and Their Differential Diagnosis

Innocent Murmur	Maximum Site and Transmission	Features of Innocent Murmur	Organic Murmur To Be Differentiated	Features of Organic Lesion
Pulmonary ejection murmur	2LICS with radiation to LLSB and apex	Early to mid systolic, rough or blowing, low- to medium-pitched; increased in recumbency, held expiration, and after exercise; common in the straight back syndrome or pes excavatum; S_2 normally split; precordium quiet	Atrial septal defect	Murmur louder, longer, with wide fixed splitting of S_2; right ventricular impulse hyperdynamic
			Mild valvular pulmonary stenosis	Murmur louder, longer, harsher with thrill; S_2 widely split; sustained right ventricular lift
Vibratory murmur	Apicosternal region; may be widely transmitted	Early to mid systolic, medium-pitched, crescendo-decrescendo, vibratory, twangy, or groaning; louder with amyl nitrite; no significant change with vasopressors	Small ventricular septal defect	Murmur high pitched, blowing, holosystolic, with thrill in 3LICS or 4LICS; when early systolic, often no thrill, but murmur is high-pitched, blowing; softer with amyl nitrite; louder with vasopressors
			Mitral regurgitation	Murmur holosystolic, apical, transmitted to left axilla and scapula; softer with amyl nitrite; louder with vasopressors

Supraclavicular arterial bruit	Maximum on the right side of neck, and louder above the clavicle than below it	Short, low-pitched early systolic; louder with slight compression of the subclavian artery, decreased or obliterated by marked compression of the subclavian artery or hyperextension of shoulders; sounds and precordium normal	Aortic stenosis	Murmur maximum in 2RICS or apex, often with thrill; A_2 decreased or absent; sustained left ventricular lift
Venous hum	Neck, especially on the right side with head turned away from side being examined	Continuous, low- to medium-pitched, peaking after S_2; decreases or disappears with recumbency; obliterated by compression of jugular veins; louder with amyl nitrite; softer or no change with vasocompressors	Patent ductus arteriosus	Maximum over pulmonary area; not affected by position change or compression of jugular veins; peaks at S_2; softer with amyl nitrite; louder with vasopressors
Mammary souffle	RSB or LSB from 2ICS to 4ICS	Medium- to high-pitched, continuous, with systolic accentuation; occurs in late pregnancy and lactation, then disappears; obliterated by firm stethoscope pressure	Patent ductus arteriosus	See above
			Arteriovenous fistula of chest wall	Murmur louder, with thrill; usually not obliterated with stethoscope pressure; persists after pregnancy or lactation

SOURCE: Adapted from R. F. Castle, The innocent heart murmurs, *Rocky Mt. Med. J., 69*:45, 1972.

SYSTOLIC MURMURS ACCORDING TO SITE OF MAXIMUM INTENSITY

Second Right Intercostal Space (Aortic Area): Mid Systolic Ejection Murmurs

1. Etiology.
   a. Left ventricular outflow obstruction.
      (1) Congenital aortic stenosis.
         (a) Valvular.
         (b) Subvalvular (discrete).
         (c) Supravalvular.
      (2) Acquired aortic stenosis.
         (a) Rheumatic.
         (b) Nonrheumatic.
      (3) Idiopathic hypertrophic subaortic stenosis.
   b. Aortic ejection murmur of middle and old age (probably due to aortic valve sclerosis).
   c. Transmitted murmur of mitral regurgitation.
   d. Aortic flow murmur in free aortic regurgitation.
   e. Supraclavicular arterial bruit.
   f. Coarctation of the aorta (some cases).

2. Diagnostic features.
   a. The murmur of AS is the prototype of left-sided SEM. When a crescendo-decrescendo, loud, noisy, harsh aortic EM, which is transmitted upward to the right and into the carotids, occurs in association with a thrill, a faint or absent A$_2$, and an anacrotic or a small pulse with a delayed systolic peak, the diagnosis of AS is established. The presence of valvular calcification on fluoroscopy or x-ray is confirmatory.
   b. Isolated AS in persons under the age of 30 years is usually congenital, particularly if the valve is calcified. The younger the individual, the more likely it is that the lesion is congenital. In adolescence and adult life up to the age of about 50, AS is most commonly rheumatic. In the presence of concomitant mitral and tricuspid valvular disease, a rheumatic origin is almost certain. Isolated calcific AS in persons above the age of 50 may be rheumatic, idiopathic, or the result of calcification of a congenitally bicuspid valve. It is usually impossible to distinguish between these possibilities pathologically, let alone clinically. Aortic EM in persons above the age of 50 or 60 years are most commonly benign and are usually easy to identify (see paragraph **2d** below).
   c. The differential diagnosis of the various causes of AS is summarized in Table 3-8. It is especially important to differentiate between valvular AS and IHSS. Some important differences are as follows: The murmur of IHSS is medium-pitched and less rough than that of valvular obstruction. It is usually maximum at the LLSB or at the apex rather than in the 2RICS. The murmur, like that of AS,

is ejection in type except at the apex, where it is likely to be holo-systolic because of associated MR. Sudden squatting, the Valsalva maneuver, changes in position, amyl nitrite, and vasopressors may help differentiate between AS and IHSS when the auscultatory findings are similar. In IHSS, the thrill when present is maximum at the LLSB or at the apex, the ventricular impulse is sustained or double-peaked, the carotid pulse is brisk or bisferiens, S_3 and S_4 sounds are frequently audible, S_2 is single or paradoxically split, the murmur of AR is absent, and diagnostic abnormalities may be found in the ECG or echocardiogram, or on cardiac catheterization. IHSS must also be distinguished from MR due to other causes; for this purpose, compare the features of each in Tables 3-9 and 3-11.

d. The murmur of AS must also be differentiated from the benign nonobstructive aortic EM of middle and old age. The latter tends to be both less harsh and less intense than the murmur of AS. It shows little upward radiation but is commonly transmitted to the apex, where it may be louder than at the base. It retains the configuration of a mid systolic EM at all locations. The arterial pulse is normal unless the pulse pressure is increased by concomitant hypertension. The JVP, the apical impulse, and the heart sounds are normal. No extra sounds are audible. A thrill is rarely present. The diagnosis of this benign murmur is supported by the age of the patient, the presence of aortic dilatation or systemic hyper-tension, and the absence of murmurs of other valvular lesions. When the murmur is loudest at the apex, it may be mistaken for the murmur of MR, which differs in being higher-pitched, blowing, and pansystolic rather than mid systolic.

e. The differential diagnosis of the murmurs of AS and MR is dis-cussed in Table 3-12.

f. In free AR, it may be difficult to determine whether a mid systolic aortic EM is due to flow or to coexisting AS. Favoring stenosis over flow are the absence of peripheral signs of AR, a normal diastolic blood pressure, and the harshness and late peaking of the murmur. Either murmur may be loud and may be associated with a thrill.

g. The differential diagnosis between aortic EM and innocent supra-clavicular arterial bruits is given in Table 3-7.

h. The differential diagnosis of the murmurs of PS and AS is sum-marized in Table 3-10.

i. Coarctation of the aorta usually produces a basal SEM that may be heard in the 2RICS but that is more commonly heard better in the 2LICS or, rarely, at the apex. The murmur is heard as well or even better posteriorly in an area medial to the left scapula.

Left Sternal Border: Mid Systolic Ejection Murmurs

1. Etiology.
   a. Right ventricular outflow obstruction.
      (1) Congenital pulmonary stenosis.

TABLE 3-8. The Differential Diagnosis of Systolic Ejection Murmurs in the Second Right Intercostal Space

Parameter	Congenital Aortic Stenosis			Acquired Aortic Stenosis	Idiopathic Hypertrophic Subaortic Stenosis	Aortic Valve Sclerosis (Nonobstructive)	Supraclavicular Arterial Bruit
	Valvular (75% of Cases)	Subvalvular (Discrete)	Supravalvular				
Age	Youth	Youth	Youth	Adolescence to old age; rare below age of 10 years	Mostly young adults, but occurs at any age	Middle and old age	10 to 20 years
Sex		M:f = 4 or 5:1		M:F = 2:1	Familial: M = F; Nonfamilial: M:F = 4:1	M > F	M = F
Physical appearance	Normal	Normal	Typical facies	Normal	Normal	Normal	Normal
Arterial pulse	Small; slow rise to late systolic peak	Small; slow rise to late systolic peak	Right brachial and carotid greater than left; blood pressure in right arm greater than in left arm	Small; slow rise to late systolic peak	Brisk and unsustained, or bisferiens	Normal	Normal
Jugular venous A wave	Normal or increased	Normal or increased	Normal or increased	Normal or increased	Normal or increased	Normal	Normal
Apical impulse	Sustained heave	Sustained heave	Sustained heave	Sustained heave	Sustained heave or bifid impulse	Normal	Normal

Maximum thrill	1st or 2nd RICS	1st or 2nd RICS	Just beneath right clavicle and right neck	1st or 2nd RICS	Lower left sternal border of apex	Uncommon; 1st or 2nd RICS	Supraclavicular
Aortic ejection sound	Common	Rare	Rare	Rare	Rare	Absent	Absent
Splitting of S_2	Single or narrowly split; sometimes paradoxical	Single or narrowly split; sometimes paradoxical	Single or narrowly split; sometimes paradoxical	Single or narrowly split; sometimes paradoxical	Usually single, but paradoxical splitting common	Single or narrowly split	Normal
Intensity of A_2	Normal or increased	Normal or increased	Normal or increased	Usually decreased or absent, sometimes normal	Normal or decreased	Normal	Normal
Audible or palpable S_4	Uncommon in mild to moderate stenosis; common in severe	Uncommon in mild to moderate stenosis; common in severe	Uncommon in mild to moderate stenosis; common in severe	Uncommon in mild to moderate stenosis; common in severe and over age of 40 years	Common	Absent	Absent

TABLE 3-8. (*Continued*)

Parameter	Congenital Aortic Stenosis			Acquired Aortic Stenosis	Idiopathic Hypertrophic Subaortic Stenosis	Aortic Valve Sclerosis (Nonobstructive)	Supraclavicular Arterial Bruit
	Valvular (75% of Cases)	Subvalvular (Discrete)	Supravalvular				
Systolic murmur	Maximum 1st or 2nd RICS; harsh; ejection	Maximum 1st or 2nd RICS; harsh; ejection	Often maximum 1st RICS; harsh; ejection	Maximum 1st or 2nd RICS; harsh; ejection	Maximum lower left sternal border or apex; less harsh, medium-pitched; ejection; but may be pansystolic at apex	Maximum 1st and 2nd RICS, but sometimes at apex; rough ejection; early peak, short duration	Maximum above rather than below clavicle; usually right-sided; rough ejection; early peak, short duration
Murmur of aortic regurgitation	10 to 20% of cases	55 to 100% of cases	25% of cases	Common	Absent	Absent	Absent
Effect of maneuvers on systolic murmur:							
Sudden squatting	Increased	Increased	Increased	Increased	Decreased	Maneuvers usually not performed	Maneuvers usually not performed

Valsalva	Decreased	Decreased	Decreased	Decreased	Increased
Amyl nitrite	Increased	Increased	Increased	Increased	Increased
Vasopressors (phenylephrine or methoxamine)	Increased	Increased	Increased	Increased	Decreased or absent
Electrocardiogram	Left ventricular enlargement (LVE) with ST-T changes			LVE, later with ST-T changes; left atrial abnormality; may mimic anteroseptal myocardial infarction (MI)	LVE: ST-T changes, left or biatrial abnormality; abnormal Q waves simulating MI common; Wolff-Parkinson-White common	Normal
						Normal
X-ray findings	Concentric left ventricular hypertrophy (LVH); poststenotic dilatation of the aorta; valvular calcification common	Concentric LVH; poststenotic dilatation usually absent	Concentric LVH; poststenotic dilatation absent	Concentric LVH; poststenotic dilatation of aorta may be present; valvular calcification common, increasing with advancing age	LVH; poststenotic dilatation of aorta absent	Normal

TABLE 3-9. Differential Diagnosis of Systolic Ejection Murmurs at Left Sternal Border
Part I

Parameter	Congenital Pulmonary Stenosis (Uncomplicated)	Tetralogy of Fallot (Uncomplicated)	Idiopathic Dilatation of Pulmonary Artery	Atrial Septal Defect	Innocent Murmurs
Clinical features	Murmur present from birth; growth and development normal; chubby, round facies typical	Cyanosis present at rest or after exercise; most common type of cyanotic congenital heart disease above the age of 4 years; dyspnea and squatting common	Asymptomatic in healthy young people	Asymptomatic; F >M; mostly young people	Normal in young people; also in straight back syndrome (SBS) and pes excavatum (PE)
Arterial pulse	Normal, or decreased if severe	Normal	Normal	Normal or small	Normal
Jugular venous pulse	Mild: normal A waves Moderate to severe: large A waves	Normal; large A waves occur if PS is severe and the VSD is small; large A and V waves in CHF	Normal	Usually normal; large A waves in PH or LV failure	Normal
Precordial pulsations	Valvular: sustained RV lift reaching to 3LICS; no impulse over 2LICS Infundibular: sustained RV lift, not reaching 3LICS	Slight RV lift below 3LICS	PA impulse palpable 2LICS; RV impulse not palpable	Hyperdynamic RV impulse: systolic pulsation of enlarged pulmonary trunk	Normal
Maximum thrill	Valvular: 2LICS or occasionally 3LICS Infundibular: 3LICS or more commonly 4LICS	Usually 3LICS	None	Usually absent, but may be felt over PA	None

Ejection sounds	Valvular: Mild: PES present or absent Moderate to severe: PES 2LICS, which decreases and moves toward S_1 with inspiration Severe: may be absent Infundibular: absent	PES rare because PS is usually infundibular; AES present in 2RICS only in severe PS or atresia	PES 2LICS	Absent unless PH is present	None PES in SBS
Heart sounds	S_1: normal S_2: narrowly split in mild PS; widely split in more severe PS; widely split in infundibular PS P_2: valvular Mild: normal or increased Moderate to severe: decreased or absent Infundibular: usually absent RS_4: in moderate to severe PS	S_1: normal Mild: widely split S_2; P_2 decreased or absent Moderate: P_2 absent A_2 loud Severe: P_2 absent A_2 loud RS_4: absent	S_1: normal S_2: narrowly or widely split	S_1: normal, or loud and split with $T_1 > M_1$ S_2: wide, fixed splitting P_2: normal or increased and audible at apex RS_4: sometimes present RS_3: sometimes present	S_1: normal; may be loud in SBS or PE S_2: normally split; may be widely split with increased P_2 in SBS or PE RS_4: may be present in SBS or PE
Systolic murmur	Harsh, long crescendo-decrescendo; Valvular: Mild: ends before A_2 Moderate: ends with A_2 Severe: ends after A_2 Maximum: 2LICS or 3LICS, radiating upward and to the left Infundibular: maximum 3LICS or 4LICS Intensity increases with amyl nitrite; unchanged with vasopressor	Harsh, shorter than in VPS Mild: loud, late peak, ends at A_2 Moderate: loud, mid systolic peak, ends before A_2 Severe: short, early, faint If IPS, maximum in 3LICS or 4LICS If VPS (uncommon), PES with long systolic murmur Intensity decreases with amyl nitrite and increases with vasopressor	Short, maximum in 2LICS	Medium-pitched; short; or extends to S_2; usually maximum in 2LICS	EM: rough blowing; early to mid systolic, short, 2LICS Vibratory (Still's murmur): medium-pitched, groaning, in apicosternal region Cardiorespiratory: LSB or apex louder in inspiration; disappears with breath holding Murmurs widely transmitted

TABLE 3-9. (*Continued*)
Part I

Parameter	Congenital Pulmonary Stenosis (Uncomplicated)	Tetralogy of Fallot (Uncomplicated)	Idiopathic Dilatation of Pulmonary Artery	Atrial Septal Defect	Innocent Murmurs
Other murmurs	Presystolic or PR murmurs occur, but are rare	Continuous murmur in pulmonary atresia	PR in some cases	Tricuspid diastolic flow murmur common in large shunts; murmur of PR in pulmonary hypertension	None
Electro-cardiogram	RAD; RAE; RVE	RAD; RVE with dominant R wave in V_1	Normal	P waves: normal or peaked; P_{II} may be inverted in sinus venosum defect QRS: rSr´ in V_1 Secundum: RAD, CW loop in FP; Primum: LAD, CCW loop in FP	Normal
X-ray findings	Valvular: normal or decreased pulmonary blood flow; post-stenotic dilatation of main PA and LPA; Infundibular: PA not dilated	Pulmonary vascularity normal or increased; *coeur en sabot*	Dilated pulmonary trunk	Pulmonary plethora, small aorta; marked dilatation of main PA and RPA; dilatation of RA and RV	Normal

TABLE 3-9.
Part II

Parameter	Flow Murmurs (High Output States)	Primary Pulmonary Hypertension	Secondary Pulmonary Hypertension	Small Ventricular Septal Defect (Uncomplicated)	Coarctation of the Aorta in Adults (Uncomplicated)	Idiopathic Hypertrophic Subaortic Stenosis
Clinical features	Hyperkinetic state; occurs at any age	Healthy, acyanotic young women; effort syncope, angina-like pain, dyspnea, fatigue common	Associated with left-to-right shunts (ASD, VSD, PDA) or mitral stenosis; cyanosis and clubbing common in congenital cases	Normal; usually recognized in childhood	Generally normal; M >F; arterial hypertension common	Mostly young adults, but occurs at any age
Arterial pulse	Bounding	Small; pulse pressure narrow	Normal	Normal	Small and delayed femoral pulse; blood pressure in arms greater than in legs; carotid pulses often prominent	Brisk and unsustained, or bisferiens
Jugular venous pulse	Normal	Large A waves	Large A waves	Normal	Normal	Normal or increased A waves
Precordial pulsations	Brisk LV impulse	Presystolic distention of RV; RV lift; 2LICS: systolic impulse of dilated main PA, palpable P₂ and sometimes palpable PES	Depends on underlying lesion	Normal except for systolic thrill	Collaterals common around scapula; LV impulse normal or sustained heave; Pulsations of dilated ascending aorta often palpable in 2RICS or 3RICS	Sustained LV heave or double systolic apical impulse
Maximum thrill	None	None	Whether thrill is present depends on nature of primary lesion	Usually present at 3LICS or 4LICS near sternum; may be absent	Suprasternal common	LLSB or apex

TABLE 3-9. (*Continued*)
Part II

Parameter	Flow Murmurs (High Output States)	Primary Pulmonary Hypertension	Secondary Pulmonary Hypertension	Small Ventricular Septal Defect (Uncomplicated)	Coarctation of the Aorta in Adults (Uncomplicated)	Idiopathic Hypertrophic Subaortic Stenosis
Ejection sounds	None	PES in 2LICS and 3LICS, decreasing with inspiration	PES sometimes audible	Absent	AES commonly present and may be palpable; suggests bicuspid aortic valve	AES rare
Heart sounds	S_1: normal S_2: normally split as a rule	S_1: normal S_2: normally split; may be widely split in RV failure P_2: markedly accentuated RS_3: may be present RS_4: present in RV failure	S_1: normal S_2: narrow, or widely split P_2: markedly accentuated OS and increased S_1 when MS is present RS_4: common	S_1: normal S_2: normally split as a rule	S_1: normal S_2: single or normally split A_2: accentuated LS_4: common LS_3: occasionally present	S_1: normal S_2: usually single, but paradoxical splitting common A_2: normal or decreased LS_4: common
Systolic murmur	Short, early, maximum in 2LICS	Mid systolic EM in 2LICS	Mid systolic EM in 2LICS	Soft, early, SEM; high-frequency; decrescendo or crescendo-decrescendo; ends in mid systole, maximum at 3LICS or 4LICS Decreased by amyl nitrite and increased with vasopressors	Murmur most prominent at LSB and often transmitted to apex and along subclavian arteries; may be audible below clavicles on both sides Murmur often louder posteriorly than anteriorly Presence of AES and SEM in 2RICS and murmur of AR-bicuspid aortic valve	SEM maximum lower LSB or apex; may be pansystolic at apex Murmur decreased or disappears with squatting or vasopressors; increased with Valsalva or amyl nitrite

Other murmurs	None	May have PR and TR	Diastolic flow murmurs (mitral or tricuspid) common; PR and TR may occur; In MS: mid diastolic, with presystolic crescendo accentuation	None	AR (see above)	None
Electro-cardiogram	Normal	Normal axis or RAD; RAE; RVE	Biatrial and bi-ventricular enlargement common in shunts	Normal	Normal or LVE	LVE, ST-T changes; left or biatrial enlargement, abnormal Q waves and WPW common
X-ray findings	Normal	Dilatation of main PA and its branches; RVE, RAE clear peripheral lung fields	Depends on primary disease, but pulmonary plethora, biatrial and bi-ventricular enlargement common in shunts	Normal or slight LVE: little or no increase in pulmonary vasculature	Notching of ribs, especially in 3rd to 8th posterior ribs; retrosternal notching due to dilated internal mammaries	LVE; no post-stenotic dilatation of aorta

CCW = counterclockwise, CW = clockwise, FP = frontal plane, LAD = left axis deviation, RAD = right axis deviation.

99

TABLE 3-10. Differential Diagnosis of Murmurs of Pulmonary and Aortic Stenosis

Parameter	Pulmonary Stenosis	Aortic Stenosis
Effect of inspiration on murmur with patient standing	Louder	Fainter
Maximum site	Left sternal border	2RICS or apex
Post-Valsalva effect	Immediate return of intensity of murmur	Delayed return of intensity of murmur
Effect of inspiration on ejection sound	Pulmonary ejection sound may decrease and move toward S_1 or disappear	Aortic ejection sound unchanged
S_2	Usually widely split except in very mild stenosis, when splitting is narrow	Usually single or narrowly split; reversed splitting may be present in severe stenosis
S_4	Right-sided S_4 often present	Left-sided S_4 often present

      (2) Tetralogy of Fallot.
      (3) Acquired pulmonary stenosis.
         (a) Rheumatic fever.
         (b) Carcinoid syndrome.
   b. Idiopathic dilatation of the pulmonary artery.
   c. Atrial septal defect.
   d. Ventricular septal defect (some cases with small left-to-right shunts).
   e. Pulmonary hypertension.
      (1) Primary.
      (2) Secondary.
         (a) Left-to-right shunts.
         (b) Mitral stenosis.
   f. Coarctation of the aorta.
   g. Idiopathic hypertrophic subaortic stenosis.
   h. Pulmonary flow murmurs in hyperkinetic circulatory states (e.g., fever, anemia, thyrotoxicosis).
   i. Innocent murmurs.
      (1) Pulmonary ejection murmur.
      (2) Vibratory or Still's murmur.
      (3) Cardiorespiratory murmur.
 2. Diagnostic features.
   a. As may be seen from paragraph **1** above, a large number of murmurs may have their sites of maximum intensity along the LSB. The murmur of VPS with an intact ventricular septum is the prototype

of the SEM of pulmonary outflow obstruction, but similar murmurs may occur in other conditions. By attention to the various parameters listed in Table 3-5, including physiologic and pharmacologic maneuvers, it is often possible to distinguish between them. There will remain nevertheless a fair number of cases in which the diagnosis can be established only by cardiac catheterization.

b. The differential diagnosis of innocent murmurs is considered in Tables 3-7 and 3-9.

c. At times it may be difficult to distinguish between the murmurs of PS and AS. The differentiating features are listed in Table 3-10.

Apex and Lower Left Sternal Border: Pansystolic Regurgitant Murmurs and Their Variants

1. Etiology.

  a. Mitral regurgitation.

    (1) Congenital: as an isolated lesion, part of an endocardial cushion defect, Marfan's syndrome, Ehlers-Danlos syndrome, IHSS, or anomalous left coronary artery arising from the pulmonary artery.

    (2) Acquired.

      (a) Rheumatic.

      (b) Nonrheumatic.

        i) Papillary muscle dysfunction or rupture.

        ii) Infective endocarditis.

        iii) Ruptured chordae (rheumatic, infective endocarditis, trauma, unknown etiology).

        iv) "Click" syndrome with prolapse of mitral leaflets into left atrium.

        v) Calcification of the mitral annulus.

        vi) Left ventricular dilatation (e.g., cardiomyopathy, aortic valve disease).

  b. Tricuspid regurgitation.

    (1) Rheumatic (organic or relative, or both).

    (2) Nonrheumatic.

      (a) Right ventricular dilatation (e.g., cardiomyopathy, severe left-sided heart failure).

      (b) Pulmonary hypertension.

      (c) Trauma.

      (d) Carcinoid syndrome.

  c. Ventricular septal defect.

    (1) Congenital.

    (2) Acquired (e.g., septal rupture in acute myocardial infarction).

2. Diagnostic features.

  a. The murmur of rheumatic MR is the prototype of the pansystolic RM. The murmur starts with S_1, which is typically decreased or

masked by the murmur, and ends with or beyond A$_2$. It is high-
to medium-pitched, blowing, and usually plateau-shaped, although
it may be crescendo, decrescendo, or crescendo-decrescendo. S$_2$ is
split narrowly when MR is mild, and widely when it is moderate
or severe. An accentuated P$_2$ is common and a loud S$_3$ is often
present. For practical purposes, a holosystolic murmur that is maximal at the apex, regardless of its characteristics, is virtually diagnostic of MR.

b. The murmur of MR must be differentiated from the murmurs of
TR and VSD (see Table 3-11). MR due to IHSS should be distinguished from MR due to other causes (compare Tables 3-9 and
3-11).

c. The murmur of rheumatic TR should be distinguished from the
usually coexisting murmur of MR. This may be difficult, but attention to the intensity of the murmur during inspiration and
expiration usually provides the answer. The murmur of TR is louder
in inspiration, whereas that of MR is unchanged or slightly diminished. Also, the former is louder at the LLSB, and the latter, at
the apex.

d. Sometimes the murmurs of AS and MR masquerade one for the
other, as occurs when the former is louder at the apex or the latter
is louder at the base. Table 3-12 should help in differential diagnosis between the two.

e. Once the diagnosis of MR is established, its cause should be determined.

   (1) The congenital varieties, with the exception of IHSS, are
   usually found at an early age and are rarely problems in adult
   medicine.

   (2) Rheumatic valvulitis is by far the most common cause of MR,
   and a history of rheumatic fever or chorea can almost always
   be obtained.

   (3) IE appears in other systemic manifestations or a history of
   same.

   (4) MR caused by ruptured chordae tendineae is usually acute if
   the etiology is nonrheumatic, as in IE, trauma, or idiopathic
   cases. Rheumatic fever and IE account for about half the
   cases, but in about one-third, the cause is unknown. In addition to the loud holosystolic murmur, distinctive features of
   ruptured chordae (in contrast to conventional rheumatic
   MR), include the sudden onset of dyspnea and pulmonary
   edema, sinus rhythm, minimal left atrial enlargement, mild
   cardiomegaly, and a fourth heart sound. Radiation of the
   murmur to the base and carotid arteries is produced by rupture
   of the posterior leaflet. When the anterior leaflet ruptures, the
   murmur radiates to the axilla, posterior thorax, and vertebral
   column.

   (5) MR due to rupture of a papillary muscle is most commonly
   caused by myocardial infarction. If the patient survives, congestive heart failure dominates the clinical picture. Survival

depends not only on the severity of the MR but also on the state of the myocardium. Coronary and left ventricular angiography are indicated whenever MR is acute to assess the severity and possible causes of the lesion with a view to surgical intervention. The differential diagnosis between a ruptured papillary muscle and perforation of the interventricular septum in myocardial infarction is discussed in paragraph **(12)** below.

(6) MR due to papillary muscle dysfunction is common in coronary artery disease both in angina pectoris and in myocardial infarction. The murmur is variable. It may be pansystolic or midsystolic (simulating an SEM), and it may change from time to time in the same patient. Atrial sounds are commonly audible. When the murmur is mid systolic, S_1 is often normal and SC may be heard.

(7) The mid systolic click–late systolic murmur syndrome comprises patients who have one or both of these findings. The condition is nonrheumatic and is the consequence of mitral valve dysfunction with regurgitation resulting from the prolapse of one or both mitral leaflets into the left atrium. The MR is demonstrable by left ventricular cineangiography. It is important to identify the syndrome because it is usually relatively benign and associated with a good prognosis.

(8) Nonrheumatic calcification of the mitral annulus is a not unusual cause of MR in elderly females. The hallmark of this condition is a J-, U-, or oval-shaped calcification at the site of the mitral annulus, demonstrated best by fluoroscopy under image amplification.

(9) MR or TR, or both, may occur in cardiomyopathy. In this condition, there are usually "unexplained" cardiomegaly and S_3 and S_4 gallops, accompanied by congestive failure. The RM of cardiomyopathy, whether mitral or tricuspid, tends to become fainter or vanish when failure ceases, whereas the murmurs of MR and TR due to other causes remain the same or become louder with restoration of compensation.

(10) MR may result from LV dilatation. The mechanism is not clear, but it may involve such factors as dilatation of the mitral annulus and papillary muscle dysfunction. The presence of a quiet precordium, marked lateral displacement of the cardiac apex, a nondynamic LV impulse, little left atrial enlargement, and a soft pansystolic murmur suggest LV dilatation rather than valvular disease as the cause of MR.

(11) TR is most often rheumatic and is more a functional than an anatomic lesion. Rheumatic TR is always associated with mitral and often with aortic valvular disease. Thus its cause is established by the company it keeps. In pulmonary hypertensive TR, there is usually good evidence of obliterative pulmonary vascular disease, persistent wide splitting of S_2 on expiration, and prominent A as well as V waves in the JVP (versus prominent V waves only in rheumatic TR). Traumatic

TABLE 3-11. Differential Diagnosis of Pansystolic Regurgitant Murmurs

Parameter	Mitral Regurgitation	Tricuspid Regurgitation	Ventricular Septal Defect
Arterial pulse	Abrupt and collapsing	Reflects associated left-sided lesions	Brisk, bounding, or bisferiens
Jugular venous pulse	Normal	Large V waves with a rapid Y descent, often with systolic expansion of liver	Normal; large A waves in PH
Precordial pulsations	Hyperdynamic LV impulse; apical systolic thrill	Hyperdynamic RV impulse; diffuse systolic depression on left side of chest with opposite pulsation on right; systolic thrill LLSB	Hyperdynamic LV impulse; systolic thrill at 3LICS or 4LICS
Heart sounds	S_1: normal or decreased S_2: wide expiratory splitting that is not fixed P_2: often accentuated LS_3: common LS_4: rare OS: rare	S_1: normal, increased or decreased in tricuspid area S_2: normal or wide splitting; paradoxical in early pulmonary closure OS: rare RS_3: common RS_4: rare	S_1: normal S_2: normal, or widely split with large shunts; with PH, P_2 increased and splitting normal or narrow LS_3: often present LS_4: absent
Systolic murmurs	Typical pansystolic, maximum at apex; high- to medium-pitched, blowing, and usually plateau-shaped. May be crescendo, decrescendo, or crescendo-decrescendo, radiation to left axilla and scapula. Mid or late nonpansystolic murmurs common in nonrheumatic types; may start with SC	Murmur is similar to that of MR but maximum at 4LICS or 5LICS; radiation to xiphoid, LRSB, and pulmonary area, but when RVE is marked, may be heard at apex	Harsh, plateau-shaped, maximum at 3LICS or 4LICS; with high VSD, may be maximum at 2LICS; the murmur may be early systolic rather than holosystolic when the VSD is small

	MR	TR	AR
Diastolic murmurs	Rumbling mid diastolic flow murmur may be heard at apex in pure, severe MR	Rumbling mid diastolic flow murmur may be heard at LLSB in pure, severe TR	A rumbling mid diastolic flow murmur may be heard at apex in large shunts. Murmur of AR indicates incompetence of medial aortic cusp
Effect of maneuvers on systolic murmur:			
Inspiration	Unchanged or decreases slightly	Increased	Unchanged
Amyl nitrite	Rheumatic: softer Mid to late (click syndrome): softer, starts earlier, lasts longer Papillary muscle dysfunction: variable effect	Increased	Small with PH: decreases Large with hyperkinetic PH: louder Large with pulmonary vascular disease: little change
Vasopressor (phenylephrine or methoxamine)	Rheumatic: louder Mid to late (click syndrome): increased Papillary muscle dysfunction: variable effect	NSC	Small: louder Large: unchanged or paradoxical increase
Electrocardiogram	Atrial fibrillation common; LVE and LAE, and sometimes RVE	Atrial fibrillation usual; RVE and sometimes LVE	Small: normal Large: LVE, RVE, LAE, RAE
X-ray findings	LVE and LAE	RVE, RAE, often with prominent great veins	Small: normal Large: pulmonary plethora, large PA, LVE, RVE, LAE, RAE

TABLE 3-12.   Differential Diagnosis of Aortic Stenosis and Mitral
Regurgitation Masquerading One for the Other

Parameter	Aortic Stenosis	Mitral Regurgitation
Arterial pulse	Small, delayed upstroke and peak	Brisk, collapsing
Precordial pulsations	Sustained LV heave; thrill over carotid arteries or 2RICS	Hyperdynamic LV impulse; apical thrill
Heart sounds	S_1: normal S_2: normally decreased or absent; may be single, narrowly split, or para-doxically split AES: may be present LS_3: may be present in LV failure LS_4: may be present	S_1: decreased or masked by murmur S_2: normal or widely split AES: absent LS_3: commonly present without LV failure LS_4: absent; present only in MR due to ruptured chordae
Systolic murmur	Ejection type regardless of location; trans-mitted to carotid arteries even with apical radiation Murmur usually louder after long pauses (as in ventricular premature contractions or atrial fibrillation)	Holosystolic in pure rheumatic mitral regurgi-tation; usually trans-mitted to left axilla; radiates to base when posterior mitral leaflet is incompetent Mid to late systolic murmur almost always maximal at apex Murmur unchanged after long pauses
Phonocardiogram	Murmur ends before A_2	Murmur ends at or after A_2
Amyl nitrite	Murmur louder	Murmur softer
Phenylephrine	Murmur softer	Murmur louder

TR is rare. TR is sometimes caused by the carcinoid syndrome (see p. 111).

(12) VSD is congenital but may sometimes result from rupture of the interventricular septum in myocardial infarction. A post-infarctional VSD must be distinguished from a papillary mus-cle rupture with a similar cause. With septal rupture, the murmur and thrill are usually maximum at the LLSB, with the clinical picture dominated by right-sided heart failure. In papillary muscle rupture, the murmur is usually not as intense and is loudest at the apex. A thrill is uncommon, and left-sided heart failure is the dominant clinical manifestation. Often the correct diagnosis can be made only by cardiac cath-eterization.

(13) Systolic whoops and honks are short, loud, somewhat incon-stant, systolic murmurs, often preceded by systolic clicks, having auscultatory characteristics corresponding to the de-scriptive terms. Most whoops and honks are caused by MR.

DIASTOLIC MURMURS

Early Diastolic Murmurs at the Base and Sternal Borders

1. Etiology.
   a. Aortic regurgitation.
      (1) Rheumatic fever.
      (2) Infective endocarditis.
      (3) Calcific aortic stenosis.
      (4) Senile aortic dilatation.
      (5) Disease of the aorta.
         (a) Dissecting aneurysm.
         (b) Arterial hypertension.
         (c) Marfan's syndrome.
         (d) Miscellaneous diseases.
      (6) Syphilis.
      (7) Congenital lesions.
         (a) Bicuspid aortic valve.
         (b) Coarctation of the aorta.
         (c) Ventricular septal defect.
         (d) Other congenital defects.
      (8) Postsurgical and posttraumatic.
      (9) Miscellaneous causes (e.g., ankylosing spondylitis, other rheu-
          matoid variants).
   b. Pulmonary regurgitation.
      (1) Congenital.
         (a) Congenital pulmonary valve incompetence.
         (b) Absence of the pulmonary valve.
         (c) Idiopathic dilatation of the pulmonary artery.
      (2) Acquired.
         (a) Disease of the pulmonary valve.
            i) Rheumatic.
            ii) Postsurgical.
            iii) Infective endocarditis.
         (b) Pulmonary hypertension.
            i) Primary.
            ii) Secondary: mitral stenosis (most common cause of
                PR); cor pulmonale; or Eisenmenger's syndrome.

2. Diagnostic features.
   a. The murmur of AR is the prototype of the murmur of semilunar
      valve incompetence. The diagnosis is based on the presence of a
      high-pitched, blowing, but sometimes harsh or musical DM, be-
      ginning immediately after A_2 and lasting through most or all of
      diastole. The murmur is heard best at the 3LICS with the patient

seated, leaning forward, and holding his breath in expiration. Transmission of the murmur is to the LSB, the apex, and sometimes to an area above the apex in the anterior axillary line. The murmur may also be audible in the 2RICS. Radiation of the murmur along the RSB rather than the LSB should suggest an uncommon cause of AR, such as disease of the proximal aorta or of the aortic valve, in association with dilatation and displacement of the aortic root. In the former category are such conditions as aneurysm, dissection, Marfan's syndrome, cystic medial necrosis of the aorta, and aneurysm of the sinus of Valsalva. The latter group comprises cases of aortic valve disease due to IE, trauma, VSD with AR, and syphilis. A musical murmur of AR is usually caused by eversion of an aortic cusp, most commonly of syphilitic or rheumatic origin. AR causes widening of the pulse pressure, except in mild cases, giving rise to peripheral signs such as a bounding or collapsing arterial pulse, pistol-shot sounds or double sounds (Traube's sign) over large superficial arteries, Duroziez's to-and-fro murmur, and capillary pulsation; none of these findings is specific for AR. Pulsation in the 2RICS is usually due to dilatation of the aorta. Pulsation of the sternoclavicular joints suggests aortic aneurysm or dissection. The apical impulse is hyperdynamic, and in some severe cases may show a double outward movement in diastole. In marked AR, systolic depression of the midportion and right side of the chest may be seen. S_1 may be diminished or absent. A_2 is commonly accentuated but may be decreased when AS is present. An AES may be audible. Other murmurs that may occur in AR include an aortic SEM due to flow or concomitant AS (see p. 89), an apical holosystolic murmur due to anatomic or relative MR, and the rumbling Austin Flint mid diastolic murmur probably due to relative MS.

b. The murmur of PR, originally described by Graham Steell, must be distinguished from the murmur of AR, which has similar characteristics. Acquired PR is almost always due to dilatation of the pulmonary valve ring secondary to PH. In the presence of MS, the differentiation of AR from PR may be difficult or impossible. Aortic valvulography may be useful in establishing the diagnosis of AR but not in ruling PR in or out. Amyl nitrite may be of some help because it decreases the intensity of the murmur of AR but has no effect on the murmur of PR. In general, a basal DM should be attributed to AR if there are peripheral signs of AR, if AS is present, if the murmur is decreased with amyl nitrite, if LVE is noted, or if the aorta is large and pulsatile; and to PR if there is an accentuated P_2, if RVE but not LVE is present, if the murmur is unaffected by amyl nitrite, or if the lesion is secondary to PPH. PR may occur in the absence of PH following surgical treatment of VPS or IE, or from congenital incompetence of the pulmonary valve.

c. The Austin Flint murmur of AR must be distinguished from the murmur of MS, which is often associated with rheumatic AR. The patient with both AR and MS is more likely to be female, fibrillating, and having marked exertional dyspnea, hemoptysis, or both. Usually S_1 is accentuated, P_2 is loud, an OS is present unless the valve is calcified or inflexible, S_3 is absent, and the murmur is longer. An apical DM associated with calcification of the mitral valve should be attributed to MS whether an OS is present or not. In the absence of mitral valvular calcification or an OS, an apical DM should also be considered of stenotic origin if the SM of MR is audible. In contrast to the foregoing, the patient with the Austin Flint murmur is typically male, usually in sinus rhythm, with only moderate exertional dyspnea and no history of hemoptysis. The murmur is early to mid diastolic, relatively short, S_1 is decreased, P_2 is commonly normal or only slightly accentuated, and S_3 is often present. No OS is audible. If a rheumatic origin can be excluded, an apical DM in AR should be considered an Austin Flint murmur. The Austin Flint murmur is decreased, and the murmur of MS increased, with amyl nitrite. In MS, the ECG is more likely to show RAD and RVE; in AR, LVE.

d. For practical purposes, AR is most commonly due to rheumatic fever, IE, calcific AS, or senile ectasia of the aorta, with rheumatic cases constituting about 75 percent of the total. Clues to the cause of AR may be found in the history, especially with respect to the time of discovery of the murmur. Murmurs beginning in childhood suggest a congenital origin; those discovered in the second or third decade are most often rheumatic; those found in the fourth or fifth decade or somewhat later are usually due to calcific disease of the aortic valve; and those discovered late in life are usually caused by aortic dilatation. A history of rheumatic fever is helpful when positive, but it is often absent in rheumatic cases. When mitral valvular disease coexists with AR, the cause is almost certainly rheumatic. A history of syphilis or of its treatment, a positive serology, calcification of the ascending aorta, and a tambour-like A_2 suggest a syphilitic origin. IE is diagnosed by the usual criteria for the disease. In the presence of familial disease, particularly if supported by appropriate clinical data, Marfan's syndrome, the mucopolysaccharidoses, and the Ehlers-Danlos syndrome should be considered as causes of AR. Ankylosing spondylitis and other rheumatoid variants may sometimes cause AR. AR due to aortic dilatation is not associated with other valvular lesions, but systemic hypertension is a common accompaniment. It is probably the most common cause of AR in the elderly.

Mid and Late Diastolic Murmurs at the Apex and Lower Left Sternal Border

1. Etiology.
   a. AV valve obstruction.
      (1) Mitral stenosis.
      (2) Tricuspid stenosis.
      (3) Atrial myxomas.
      (4) Left atrial ball-valve thrombus.

    b. Increased flow across the AV valves without obstruction (relative stenosis).

       (1) Mitral valve.

          (a) Active rheumatic valvulitis (Carey-Coombs murmur).

          (b) Mitral regurgitation (some cases).

          (c) AR with the Austin Flint murmur.

          (d) Patent ductus arteriosus.

          (e) Ventricular septal defect.

       (2) Tricuspid valve.

          (a) Tricuspid regurgitation.

          (b) Atrial septal defect.

    c. Miscellaneous causes.

       (1) Hyperthyroidism.

       (2) Anemia.

       (3) Complete heart block.

       (4) Left ventricular dilatation secondary to hypertensive or arteriosclerotic heart disease, or both.

       (5) Atypical verrucous endocarditis.

       (6) Chronic or adhesive pericarditis.

       (7) Eisenmenger's syndrome.

       (8) Primary pulmonary hypertension.

       (9) Coarctation of the aorta with aortic stenosis.

2. Diagnostic features.

    a. The murmur of MS is typically a low-pitched, rumbling, mid diastolic murmur with presystolic crescendo accentuation. The earliest murmur is usually a mid diastolic murmur, although sometimes it is only presystolic. In atrial fibrillation, the presystolic component disappears. S_1 is loud and sharp. P_2 is normal or accentuated, and an OS is present unless the valve is rigid, fibrosed, or calcified. S_3 and S_4 sounds are not present. The murmur is maximum at the apex and often confined to its vicinity. It is heard best with the bell chest piece at the site of the apical impulse with the patient lying in the left lateral recumbent position. When not clearly audible, it may become more discernible after exercise. The murmur is generally unaffected by respiration but may decrease slightly with inspiration. In pure MS, the apical impulse is often normal. An RV lift means PH or TR.

    b. When MS and MR are combined, SM and DM are usually audible, but S_3 and S_4 sounds or an OS are not heard. S_1 is usually decreased. If an S_3 sound is present, it can be assumed that MR is the predominant lesion. (See also paragraph **g** below.)

    c. The differential diagnosis between the Austin Flint murmur and that of MS is discussed on pages 108 and 109.

    d. The murmur of MS must be distinguished from that of left atrial myxoma, a condition in which, contrary to the situation in MS, the DM tends to vary with body position and an OS is not present. There is often a variable and at times musical SM. Irregular clicks may be heard throughout systole and diastole. Fever and embolic phenomena are common. Left atrial myxoma can be diagnosed by echocardiography or angiocardiography.

e. An atrial ball-valve thrombus may simulate MS but should be suspected if severe pulmonary congestion and embolic phenomena are associated with syncope, relief of symptoms in the upright position, murmurs changing with body position, tachycardia, and at times episodes of coldness, cyanosis, and numbness of the hands and feet.

f. The differential diagnosis of true MS and relative MS is summarized in Table 3-13. Also helpful in the diagnosis of relative rather than true MS is evidence of a primary condition capable of causing the relative stenosis (p. 110).

g. The presence of a DM in patients with MR may raise the question of whether the DM is due to the MR itself or is the result of associated MS. Favoring pure MR as the cause of the DM is clinical evidence of severe regurgitation manifested by a large LV, a hyperdynamic apical impulse, wide splitting of S_2 on expiration, a soft S_1, and a DM that is loud and blowing and that starts with the S_3 sound. Favoring coexisting MS as the cause of the DM are the following: an earlier, longer, rumbling DM that begins after the OS, absence of S_3, normal splitting of S_2, a normal or increased P_2, calcification of the valve, and a normal-size or minimally enlarged heart.

h. The murmur of TS is similar in its characteristics to that of MS. It differs in that it is maximal at the LLSB rather than at the apex and is louder on inspiration. The murmur of MS is unaffected or decreases slightly with inspiration.

i. The carcinoid syndrome is commonly associated with stenotic or regurgitant lesions of the tricuspid and pulmonary valves. Systemic manifestations, such as cutaneous flushing and telangiectasia, intestinal hypermotility, bronchoconstriction, and hypotensive crises, in association with RV failure, are clues to the diagnosis. Con-

TABLE 3-13.   Differential Diagnosis of True and Relative Mitral Stenosis

Parameter	Mitral Stenosis	Relative Mitral Stenosis
Right ventricular lift	Often present	Absent
Left ventricular lift	Absent	Present
Apical thrill	Sometimes present	Absent
Loud, sharp S_1	Present	Absent
P_2	Usually increased	Variable
OS	Present	Absent
S_3	Absent	Present
Diastolic murmur	Rumbling; starts after opening snap; longer	Blowing; starts with S_3; shorter

firmation may be obtained by finding increased urinary excretion of 5-hydroxyindoleacetic acid.

CONTINUOUS MURMURS OVER THE THORAX

1. Etiology and site of maximum intensity.
   a. Extracardiac shunts.
      (1) Patent ductus arteriosus (2LICS or immediately below left clavicle).
      (2) Pulmonary AV fistula: congenital or acquired (lower lobes or right middle lobe).
      (3) Systemic AV fistula (directly over the fistula).
      (4) Some cases of aortopulmonary septal defect (2LICS or 3LICS).
      (5) Postsurgical shunts in the tetralogy of Fallot (to the right or left of the upper sternum).
   b. Intracardiac shunts.
      (1) Sinus of Valsalva aneurysm with rupture into right atrium or ventricle (4LICS).
      (2) Coronary arteriovenous fistula with connection to the right atrium or ventricle (apicosternal region).
      (3) Small atrial septal defect with tight mitral stenosis: Lutembacher's syndrome (LLSB).
      (4) Total anomalous pulmonary venous drainage (ULSB).
   c. Arterial stenosis.
      (1) Coarctation of the aorta (posterior chest).
      (2) Pulmonary artery branch stenosis (SM or CM over site of stenosis).
      (3) Aortic arch syndrome (over affected vessel).
   d. Increased flow through normal or dilated vessels.
      (1) Jugular venous hum (neck, above the clavicle).
      (2) Mammary souffle (2LICS to 4LICS, or 2RICS to 4RICS).
      (3) Increased bronchial collateral circulation (posterior chest).
         (a) Truncus arteriosus.
         (b) Severe tetralogy of Fallot.
         (c) Other congenital malformations.

2. Diagnostic features.
   a. The murmur of PDA is the prototype of CM associated with extracardiac shunts. It starts with S_1, continues through S_2 without interruption, and fades steadily during diastole. Systolic accentuation of the murmur is quite characteristic. The murmur usually has a machinery-like quality. It is loudest in the 2LICS or immediately below the left clavicle. A thrill may be present. When PDA is associated with moderate to large left-to-right shunts, a DM due to flow may be heard at the apex. S_1 is usually normal. An S_3 sound

is common. If PH develops, the diastolic component of the CM decreases or disappears, so that only an SM remains. P_2 becomes accentuated, a PES may be heard, and the murmurs of PR and TR may appear.

b. When a patient presents with the clinical picture of a left-to-right shunt with PH and only an SM at the 2LICS or the 3LICS, the diagnostic possibilities include PDA, VSD, ASD, and an aorto-pulmonary window.

c. With CM, the location of the maximum site of the murmur may be of some diagnostic significance (see paragraph **1** above).

d. Rupture of an aortic sinus with a right-sided communication is suggested by the sudden appearance of a CM in a young adult following trauma or exertion. The murmur is maximal at the LLSB.

e. Coronary arteriovenous fistula with connection to the RA or RV is manifested by a superficial CM with diastolic accentuation, loudest in the apicosternal region, and is commonly associated with a thrill. The murmur is decreased by the Valsalva maneuver. In contrast, the CM of extracardiac shunts (e.g., PDA) shows systolic accentuation and is unaffected by the Valsalva maneuver.

f. The to-and-fro murmurs of AS and AR, or of PS and PR, may be mistaken for CM. The chief differentiating point is that CM envelop S_2 but to-and-fro murmurs do not. By careful auscultation in to-and-fro murmurs, it will be found that the SEM ends before S_2 and the DM begins after S_2. There is thus a hiatus between the two murmurs, a condition that does not exist in CM.

g. The characteristics and differential diagnosis of the jugular venous hum and the mammary souffle, both of which are innocent CM, may be found in Table 3-7.

Cardiomyopathy

Lane D. Craddock

Cardiac enlargement, with few exceptions, is a sign of organic heart disease. Its etiology can usually be ascertained from the history, physical examination, and laboratory data (including the electrocardiogram, chest films, echocardiogram, radioisotope scanning, angiocardiogram, and cardiac catheterization). Assuming that artifactual enlargement is excluded (e.g., cardiac displacement, transverse position of the heart, thoracic deformity, pericardial fat pads or cysts, faulty roentgenographic techniques), cardiomegaly, in actual clinical practice, is most often due to the conventional etiologic forms of heart disease (e.g., coronary artery disease, hypertension, rheumatic fever). However, there remain a significant number of cases of cardiomegaly that are not due to the usual causes. Many of these appear to be the result of some type of cardiomyopathy (disease of the heart muscle). This presentation will consider the etiology, classification, clinical features, and differential diagnosis of the cardiomyopathies.

DEFINITION

The terms *cardiomyopathy, myocardosis,* and *myocardiopathy* refer to disease of the heart muscle. It is characterized anatomically by cardiomegaly due to hypertrophy or dilatation, or both, and functionally by a clinical picture consistent with congestive failure (congestive cardiomyopathy), cardiac hypertrophy with or without ventricular outflow obstruction (hypertrophic cardiomyopathy), or simulating constrictive pericarditis (restrictive or obliterative cardiomyopathy).

ETIOLOGY

Cardiomyopathy may be primary (idiopathic) or secondary. The primary cardiomyopathies are myocardial diseases of unknown cause, probably due to multiple causes and not related to any known systemic disorder. Secondary cardiomyopathies are those in which the myocardial involvement is secondary to a systemic illness even when the cause of this disease is not understood (e.g., amyloidosis). It should be noted that some authorities use the term *primary myocardial disease* to indicate any myocardial disorder, idiopathic or secondary, in which cardiac involvement is the major clinical manifestation. A combined etiologic and clinical classification of the cardiomyopathies is shown in Table 3-14.

CLINICAL FEATURES

Congestive Cardiomyopathy

The clinical presentation is most commonly that of biventricular failure, although sometimes the picture of left or right ventricular failure predominates. Dyspnea, orthopnea, paroxysmal nocturnal dyspnea, and dependent edema are thus common symptoms. Other presentations include syncope (due to arrhythmia or heart block), arrhythmia, embolic phenomena, and occasionally angina. Sudden death is distressingly frequent. On physical examination, the usual signs of congestive failure may be noted. Cardiomegaly—predominantly left ventricular in most cases—reduced intensity of the heart sounds, regurgitant systolic murmurs, and gallop rhythm (S_3, S_4, or summation gallop) are characteristic. A decreased arterial pulse with a narrow pulse pressure is common. Cyanosis is rare.

Hypertrophic Cardiomyopathy

Obstructive (Idiopathic Hypertrophic Subaortic Stenosis)

1. Patients in this group have left ventricular hypertrophy in association with muscular ventricular outflow obstruction. The disease is often familial and is common in young and middle-aged adults.

2. Many cases are discovered before the onset of symptoms because of the detection, on routine examination, of left ventricular enlargement or a heart murmur, or both. Individuals with symptoms generally complain of exertional dyspnea, syncope, or angina.

TABLE 3-14.   Etiologic and Clinical Classification of the Cardiomyopathies

A. Primary cardiomyopathy
  1. Congestive
    a. Idiopathic
    b. Familial
    c. Peripartal
  2. Hypertrophic (familial and nonfamilial)
    a. Obstructive
    b. Nonobstructive
  3. Restrictive
    a. Endomyocardial fibrosis
    b. Endocardial fibroelastosis
B. Secondary cardiomyopathy*
  1. Connective tissue disease (e.g., systemic lupus erythematosus, scleroderma, dermatomyositis, rheumatoid arthritis)
  2. Neuromuscular diseases (e.g., Friedreich's ataxia, myotonia atrophica, progressive muscular dystrophy)
  3. Vascular disease (e.g., ischemic cardiomyopathy)
  4. Metabolic disease (e.g., hyperthyroidism, hypothyroidism, hemochromatosis, glycogen storage disease, mucopolysaccharidoses, amyloidosis)
  5. Neoplastic diseases (e.g., lymphomas, leukemia, metastatic carcinoma)
  6. Nutritional diseases (e.g., beriberi, kwashiorkor)
  7. Myocarditis
    a. Viral
    b. Parasitic
    c. Protozoal
    d. Other
  8. Sarcoidosis
  9. Drugs, chemicals, and toxins (e.g., emetine, arsenic, carbon monoxide poisoning)
  10. Posttraumatic disorders

* Secondary cardiomyopathies usually present with a clinical picture of congestive failure; less often, with restrictive features. Ischemic heart disease may present clinically as a congestive cardiomyopathy, hence its inclusion in the classification.

3. On physical examination it is observed that the apical impulse is typically forceful and often bifid, the arterial pulse is brisk and bisferiens, an S_4 sound is present, a systolic ejection murmur is audible at the mid or lower left sternal border, and a mitral regurgitant murmur is often heard at the apex (see the preceding section, Heart Murmurs).

Nonobstructive

1. In addition to the aforementioned clinical patterns, there are patients with myocardial disease who present primarily with evidence of hypertrophy (usually concentric) of the left ventricle. A history of syncope, palpitation, angina, or dyspnea may be obtained. Most such cases are familial, although isolated nonfamilial cases do occur. There are no characteristic murmurs. An atrial gallop is commonly heard.

2. Some of these patients eventually develop evidence of left ventricular outflow obstruction. It would thus appear that hypertrophic cardiomyopathy can exist with or without obstruction. Recent echocardio-graphic observations suggest that asymmetric septal hypertrophy is the pathognomonic anatomic abnormality and the common denominator of both the nonobstructive and obstructive forms.

Restrictive Cardiomyopathy

1. A very small number of patients with myocardiopathy, notably those due to diseases such as amyloidosis, leukemia, and polyarteritis nodosa may present with a picture resembling that of constrictive pericarditis.

2. The major features are an elevated venous pressure, deep X and Y descents in the jugular venous pulse, severe right-sided heart failure, clear lung fields, and only moderate cardiomegaly.

3. Endomyocardial fibrosis and endocardial fibroelastosis are also primary cardiomyopathies. The former condition is seen almost exclusively in Africans; the latter, in children.

LABORATORY STUDIES

Electrocardiogram

1. The electrocardiogram is almost invariably abnormal in the cardio-myopathies.

2. Nonspecific ST segment and T wave abnormalities are common.

3. Almost any type of arrhythmia may occur, but ventricular premature systoles and atrial fibrillation are seen most frequently. Abnormalities of AV conduction are not uncommon.

4. P wave abnormalities, especially left atrial and biatrial enlargement, are often present.

5. Left ventricular hypertrophy is quite common, but right ventricular hypertrophy is infrequent. All types of ventricular conduction defects, especially left bundle branch block and left anterior fascicular block, are often present. Ventricular preexcitation is a common accompaniment of familial forms of cardiomegaly.

6. Pseudoinfarction patterns occur frequently in idiopathic hypertrophic subaortic stenosis and amyloidosis.

Chest Films

1. The chest x-rays usually reveal only cardiomegaly.

2. When congestive heart failure supervenes, evidence of pulmonary vascular congestion and pleural effusion may appear.

Cardiac Catheterization

1. Cardiac catheterization is of greater value in ruling out valvular, congenital, and other types of heart disease than in establishing the diagnosis of a cardiomyopathy.

2. Hemodynamic studies may be helpful in differentiating between obstructive and nonobstructive forms of cardiomyopathy.

3. The finding of restricted filling (secondary to a noncompliant ventricle or a partially obliterated ventricular cavity, or both) supports the diagnosis of a restrictive cardiomyopathy, but it is also seen in constrictive pericarditis.

4. Coronary arteriography may be helpful in differentiating ischemic heart disease from other types of myocardial disease. A normal arteriogram excludes coronary artery disease as a cause of cardiomyopathy.

CRITERIA FOR THE DIAGNOSIS OF CARDIOMYOPATHY

1. Cardiomegaly due to left ventricular or biventricular enlargement without evidence of valvular calcification.

2. An abnormal electrocardiogram.

3. The presence of an S_3 or S_4 gallop rhythm, or both.

4. Absence of sustained arterial hypertension and, almost always, absence of diastolic murmurs.

5. Exclusion of other causes of heart disease: rheumatic or other valvular disease, congenital heart disease, constrictive pericarditis, pericardial effusion, cor pulmonale, hypertensive heart disease, and coronary artery disease.

DIFFERENTIAL DIAGNOSIS OF CARDIOMYOPATHY

Coronary Heart Disease

Ischemia of the myocardium may produce a clinical picture indistinguishable from that found in other types of cardiomyopathy. An unequivocal, documented history of myocardial infarction or angina pectoris, or both, establishes the diagnosis of coronary artery disease. However, it should be recognized that typical or atypical angina may occur in cardiomyopathy. Ischemic cardiomyopathy is usually found in older patients. When it occurs in younger patients, the premature coronary heart disease is most often familial and is generally associated with abnormal serum lipid concentrations and abnormal lipoprotein electrophoretic patterns. Many such patients are diabetic or at least show abnormal findings on glucose tolerance tests. Physical findings are rarely helpful, although the presence of systolic precordial bulges due to ventricular asynergy or aneurysm are indicative of ischemic heart disease. The electrocardiogram may be helpful if diagnostic infarction patterns are present, but pseudoinfarction patterns are occasionally seen in cardiomyopathy. When it is not possible to distinguish between coronary heart disease and cardiomyopathy on clinical grounds, selective coronary arteriography, ventriculography, and hemodynamic studies may be of assistance.

Congenital Heart Disease

Congenital heart disease is rarely a problem in differential diagnosis. Patients with hypertrophic cardiomyopathy and either left or right ventricular outflow obstruction may have murmurs mimicking aortic or pulmonary stenosis, respectively. (See the preceding section, Heart Murmurs, for further details.) The correct diagnosis can be established by cardiac catheterization and angiographic studies. In rare instances, an Eisenmenger complex of long duration (e.g., with atrial septal defect) may show marked cardiomegaly without the identifying features of the congenital lesion and thus may be mistaken for a cardiomyopathy. However, cardiac catheterization will reveal the bidirectional shunting. Moreover, the associated arterial oxygen unsaturation will not be corrected by the administration of 100 percent oxygen. Sometimes the mitral regurgitant murmur of a cardiomyopathy may be mistaken for the murmur of a ventricular septal defect. Here again, cardiac catheterization and angiocardiography will establish the correct diagnosis.

Rheumatic Heart Disease

The diagnosis of rheumatic heart disease is based on a history of rheumatic fever accompanied by a characteristic structural lesion of the heart (e.g., mitral stenosis) or on evidence of a characteristic structural lesion even in the absence of a history of rheumatic fever. Rheumatic heart disease is often suspected as the cause of murmurs of mitral or tricuspid regurgitation in patients with congestive heart failure. When compensation is restored in such patients, murmurs due to cardiomyopathy tend to diminish or disappear, whereas rheumatic murmurs tend to become louder. The murmur of mitral stenosis is virtually diagnostic of rheumatic heart disease, although diastolic rumbles have been reported in a few patients with cardiomyopathy. Other diastolic murmurs (e.g., due to aortic insufficiency) virtually exclude cardiomyopathy. The presence of valvular calcification also eliminates cardiomyopathy. In doubtful cases, cardiac catheterization may be indicated.

Hypertensive Heart Disease

Occasionally confusion occurs between cardiomyopathy and hypertensive heart disease when the blood pressure is elevated. However, the arterial hypertension is much milder (diastolic pressure 90 to 110 mm Hg) in cardiomyopathy and is not sustained. It tends to disappear when congestive heart failure improves. In patients with systemic hypertension, it is usually possible to document a long history of elevated blood pressure with corroborative changes in the ocular fundi. In hypertensive heart disease, there is a rough correlation between the heart size and the severity and duration of the hypertension, whereas in cardiomyopathy the cardiomegaly is out of proportion to the mildness of the hypertension.

Pericardial Disease

Patients with cardiomyopathy often present with a clinical picture that may be confused with constrictive pericarditis or pericardial effusion. Some clinical features may be of assistance in the differential diagnosis. An apical impulse that is displaced downward and to the left favors myocardial rather than pericardial disease. The presence of the pansystolic murmurs of mitral or tricuspid regurgitation also support the diagnosis of cardiomyopathy rather than pericarditis. Gallop rhythms are common in cardiomyopathy, although they must be differentiated from the early diastolic knock of pericarditis. In pericardial disease, there is a tendency to low voltage in the electrocardiogram; in cardiomyopathy, the findings are as described previously (p. 116). Echocardiography, radioisotope scanning, cardiac catheterization, and angiocardiography may be of assistance in making the diagnosis. Sometimes the problem can be resolved only by exploratory thoracotomy. The differences in hemodynamics between restrictive cardiomyopathy and constrictive pericarditis are listed in Table 3-15.

Primary Pulmonary Hypertension

Primary pulmonary hypertension may present with cardiac enlargement and right-sided heart failure, simulating a cardiomyopathy. Clues to the diagnosis

TABLE 3-15. Hemodynamics of Myocardial and Pericardial Disease

Parameter	Constrictive Pericarditis	Cardiomyopathy
Left atrial pressure	Tends to equal RAP	10 to 20 mm Hg >RAP
Right atrial pressure	Usually >15 mm Hg with prominent Y trough	Usually <15 mm Hg: normal if wedge pressure normal
Cardiac output	Tends to normal with normal AV difference	Usually low with increased AV difference
Right ventricular pressure	Consistent early diastolic dip	Early diastolic dip may disappear with therapy
Diastolic right ventricular pressure	Tends to equal or exceed ⅓ of systolic pressure	Usually does not equal ⅓ of systolic pressure
Pulmonary artery pressure	Systolic pressure usually <40 mm Hg	Systolic pressure often 45 to 65 mm Hg
Respiratory variation in pressures	Tends to be absent	Usually present
Diastolic pressure plateau	RAP = RVDP = PADP = PWP	PWP >RAP

RAP, right atrial pressure; AV, arteriovenous; RVDP, right ventricular diastolic pressure; PADP, pulmonary arterial diastolic pressure; PWP, pulmonary wedge pressure.
Source: N. O. Fowler, Pericardial Disease. In J. W. Hurst and R. B. Logue (Eds.), *The Heart*, 2d ed. New York: McGraw-Hill, 1970. P. 1267.

are an accentuated P_2, dilated pulmonary arteries and clear lung fields in the chest films, and electrocardiographic evidence of right ventricular enlargement.

Hyperkinetic Heart Syndrome

This is an uncommon entity. It is uncertain at present whether it should be regarded as a cardiomyopathy. The distinguishing features are a high cardiac output, an increased rate of ventricular ejection, slight cardiac enlargement, and a wide pulse pressure with brisk pulses.

DIFFERENTIAL DIAGNOSIS OF PRIMARY AND SECONDARY CARDIOMYOPATHY

Since the clinical features of primary and secondary cardiomyopathy are similar, the differentiation is made only by excluding those systemic ailments known to produce myocardial disease. Some of the more important secondary cardiomyopathies and their distinguishing features are discussed below.

Connective Tissue Diseases

The diagnostic features of these diseases are described in the sections Peripheral Joint Arthritis and Myalgia, Chapter 8.

Neuromuscular Diseases

1. *Friedreich's ataxia* is characterized by ataxia, progressive skeletal deformities, and speech disturbances, beginning in adolescence and terminating in congestive failure or infection within 20 years after its onset. Heart disease occurs in 30 to 50 percent of cases and may be the initial manifestation of the disease.

2. *Myotonia atrophica* is characterized by atrophy involving primarily the muscles of the face, neck, forearms, and thighs, increased muscle tone, cataracts, premature baldness, and gonadal atrophy. Although the neuromuscular defects are usually apparent before evidence of heart disease appears, the latter may be the presenting feature.

3. *Progressive muscular dystrophy* is characterized by weakness of the proximal musculature of the extremities, a waddling gait, a "climbing up the legs" phenomenon when arising from a sitting position, muscles that are hypertrophied or atrophied, and skeletal deformities.

Hyperthyroidism

Thyrotoxic heart disease is characterized by goiter, tachycardia, exophthalmos, warm moist skin, tremor, and arrhythmia, notably atrial fibrillation. The diagnosis can be confirmed by thyroid function tests.

Myxedema

Myxedema commonly causes pericardial effusion and is often associated with coronary artery disease. Whether it can cause myocardial disease is disputed. Clinically, myxedema is suggested by cold intolerance; hoarseness; a low-pitched voice; sluggishness, weakness, and fatigue; a dry, yellow, puffy skin; hair loss; a thick tongue; slow pulse; and decreased tendon reflexes. It is easily confirmed by determination of the serum T_4 level, the radioactive iodine uptake, or other thyroid function tests.

Hemochromatosis

This disease is characterized by a combination of liver disease, diabetes mellitus, hyperpigmentation of the skin, and heart disease.

Amyloidosis

Amyloidosis is one of the less common causes of cardiomyopathy. It should be considered in any elderly patient with unexplained cardiac enlargement and congestive failure. Purpura, waxy skin deposits, peripheral neuropathy, macroglossia, and nephrosis are other features of the disease. The presence of a disease known to cause secondary amyloidosis (e.g., rheumatoid arthritis, ulcerative colitis, chronic suppuration, tuberculosis) should alert the physician to this type of cardiomyopathy. The diagnosis can often be established by gingival or rectal biopsy.

Neoplasms

The presence of lymphoma, leukemia, or neoplasm should raise the question of secondary cardiomyopathy if the heart is enlarged or if it shows pericarditis. Arrhythmias are common.

Myocarditis and Pericarditis

Myocarditis may occur in association with many vital, bacterial, rickettsial, and parasitic diseases. The clinical evidence of myocarditis generally appears as the initial manifestations of the systemic infection begin to subside. Fever is characteristic. Fatigue, dyspnea, palpitation, and precordial discomfort may occur. Cardiac enlargement, murmurs, tachycardia, arrhythmias, and conduction defects are commonly observed. Embolic phenomena may be evident. Cardiomyopathy with congestive failure may occasionally occur in the wake of the benign idiopathic pericarditis syndrome.

Sarcoidosis

Cardiomyopathy due to sarcoidosis should be considered in heart disease of obscure origin in young Negroes. Tachycardia, cardiac enlargement, pericarditis, heart block, arrhythmias, and congestive heart failure may be noted. Cutaneous lesions, hilar and cervical adenopathy, and pulmonary infiltrates are common. Hyperglobulinemia and hypercalcemia may occur.

Alcoholic Cardiomyopathy

The consumption of large quantities of alcohol over a period of many years may cause myocardial disease in some individuals. The clinical spectrum is wide. Cardiac beriberi occasionally occurs in the alcoholic. It is manifested by moderate cardiomegaly, congestive failure, nutritional deficiencies, and responsiveness to thiamine. Beer-drinkers' cardiomyopathy, characterized by right-sided heart failure, massive cardiac dilatation, and other symptoms, is no longer seen since the addition of cobalt to beer was discontinued. The most common manifestations of alcoholic cardiomyopathy are cardiac dilatation and congestive failure, neither of which is responsive to thiamine. This type of cardiomyopathy may be observed in malnourished or obese heavy drinkers.

DIAGNOSTIC APPROACH TO CARDIOMYOPATHY

1. The diagnosis of cardiomyopathy should be considered in all cases of heart disease of obscure cause.

2. The diagnosis of cardiomyopathy is made by excluding other causes of heart disease and is based on the criteria listed earlier in this section (p. 117).

3. Once the diagnosis of cardiomyopathy is established, one must make every effort to distinguish between primary and secondary forms. In the examination of the patient, search carefully for systemic illness that may produce myocardial involvement. Each of the causes of secondary cardiomyopathy should be excluded. This can usually be accomplished by the history and physical examination, supplemented by selected laboratory tests.

4. The following work-up is suggested for cardiomyopathy:
   a. CBC.
   b. ESR.
   c. Urinalysis.
   d. Chest films.
   e. Electrocardiogram.
   f. Biochemical screening.
   g. Protein electrophoresis.
   h. Immunoglobulins.
   i. Serologic test for syphilis.
   j. LE preparation or ANA, or both.
   k. Rheumatoid factor.
   l. Muscle enzymes (CPK, aldolase).
   m. T_4 or other thyroid function tests.

5. Other procedures sometimes needed to establish an etiologic diagnosis are as follows:

   a. Tissue biopsy (lymph nodes, bone marrow, skin, muscle, rectal mucosa, gingiva).

   b. Cardiac catheterization.

   c. Angiocardiography.

   d. Echocardiography.

   e. Radioisotope scans.

   f. Pulmonary function studies.

Palpitation and Disorders of the Heartbeat

David Shander

DEFINITION

The term *palpitation* refers to any conscious sensation of cardiac activity. It is generally an unpleasant feeling. Palpitation is not directly related to the presence or absence of heart disease or to any specific arrhythmia. It may occur even when the heartbeat is normal.

ETIOLOGY

Normal

Palpitation may occur normally as a result of increased heart rate and vigor of myocardial contraction associated with physical activity or emotional stress. The cardiac rhythm is sinus tachycardia and needs no further discussion. Awareness of cardiac activity is common at night in most individuals who sleep on their sides. The heartbeat frequently is audible in the dependent ear and is probably the result of direct sound transmission to the ear.

Neurocirculatory Asthenia (Cardiac Neurosis)

An awareness of the heartbeat occurs in some individuals in the absence of physical exertion or consciousness of any emotional stress. Such persons are usually neurotic and frequently have other psychosomatic complaints. The episodes of palpitation are commonly associated with shortness of breath, lightheadedness, and precordial pain. The respiratory difficulty is frequently described as an inability to "get enough air in" or a feeling of suffocation. There may be an overwhelming sense of terror, which tends to perpetuate the symptoms. In some instances, deliberate hyperventilation may reproduce all of the symptoms. It is well to remember that cardiac neurosis is often associated with real cardiovascular disease. Such patients are understandably anxious, and sometimes perceive minor symptoms out of proportion to their significance, precipitating an acute anxiety reaction associated with palpitation and breathlessness.

TABLE 3-16.   Causes of Palpitation without Arrhythmia

1. Noncardiac disorders
   a. Anxiety
   b. Anemia
   c. Fever
   d. Thyrotoxicosis
   e. Hypoglycemia
   f. Pheochromocytoma
   g. Aortic aneurysm
   h. Migraine
   i. Arteriovenous fistula
   j. Drugs (epinephrine, amphetamines, digitalis, nitrates, ganglionic blocking agents)
2. Cardiac disorders
   a. Aortic regurgitation
   b. Aortic stenosis
   c. Patent ductus arteriosus
   d. Ventricular septal defect
   e. Atrial septal defect
   f. Marked cardiomegaly
   g. Acute left ventricular failure
   h. Hyperkinetic heart syndrome
   i. Tricuspid insufficiency

Palpitation Not Associated with Cardiac Arrhythmia

The conditions that may cause palpitation in the absence of arrhythmia are listed in Table 3-16.

Palpitation Associated with Cardiac Arrhythmia

Cardiac arrhythmias, including premature contractions, paroxysmal and non-paroxysmal tachycardias, marked bradycardias, and advanced AV block, are the most common causes of palpitation.

Premature Contractions

Many patients with premature contractions do not use the term *palpitation* to describe their complaint, but rather describe the premature systoles as "flip-flop" sensations in the chest, stoppage of the heart, or skipped beats.

Premature contractions may occur in the presence or absence of organic heart disease. They may be ventricular or supraventricular in origin. The clinical significance of such beats varies. Some are completely benign, whereas others may have serious or even grave prognostic importance. While physical examination and close scrutiny of the jugular venous pulse may assist in determining the origin of the beats, the final diagnosis of their etiology is based on the electrocardiographic findings. Criteria for the identification of the various types of premature beats are summarized in Table 3-17.

Supraventricular premature contractions (atrial and AV junctional) may occur in normal individuals. Other important causes include infectious disease and other febrile states, organic heart disease particularly with atrial involvement (e.g., mitral valvular disease, pericarditis), chronic obstructive

TABLE 3-17. Electrocardiographic Differential Diagnosis of Premature Contractions

Premature Contractions	Initial Deflection	P Wave	P-R Interval	QRS Complex	Compensatory Pause
Atrial (APC)	P wave	Premature; different from sinus P wave; usually upright but may be retrograde (inverted in leads II, III, and aVF, and upright in lead aVR)	Normal or prolonged	May be absent if APC is nonconducted; usually normal but may be wide and bizarre because of aberrant ventricular conduction or preexisting intraventricular block	Not fully compensatory unless sino-atrial (SA) node is suppressed by discharge of the APC
AV Junctional (JPC)	P wave or QRS complex	Retrograde	0.10 sec to negative; R-P interval variable; diagnostic if R-P interval $\leq$0.10 sec, even if QRS is abnormal	Usually normal but may be wide and bizarre because of aberrant ventricular conduction or preexisting intraventricular block	Not fully compensatory unless SA node is suppressed by discharge of the JPC or if sinus P is dissociated from a QRS that is not conducted back to the atria
Ventricular (VPC)	QRS complex	Sinus if dissociated from QRS; retrograde if ventricular impulse is conducted to atria	Absent if P and QRS are dissociated; if retrograde, R-P interval is >0.10 sec	Wide, bizarre	Fully compensatory unless retrograde conduction is present or beat is interpolated

NOTE: It is not possible by surface leads to distinguish absolutely between (1) VPCs and (2) JPCs showing aberrant ventricular conduction.

airway disease, and digitalis effect. Atrial premature beats are frequent precursors of atrial fibrillation, tachycardia, or flutter.

Ventricular premature beats are also frequently benign, but underlying myocardial disease or drug effects should be suspected if they occur frequently (more than one or two per minute), are paired or grouped, arise from more than one focus in the ventricles, or are very closely coupled to the preceding beat. Ventricular premature systoles in myocardial infarction may be harbingers of ventricular fibrillation, especially if they encroach upon the vulnerable period (the region at or about the peak of the T wave). In general, ventricular premature beats in nonischemic conditions are less ominous and the risk of sudden death is considerably less. An exception to this statement is ventricular premature contractions due to digitalis intoxication.

Paroxysmal Tachycardias

Most patients who experience bouts of paroxysmal tachycardia complain of palpitation, yet some, surprisingly, are completely unaware of their existence. Paroxysmal tachyarrhythmias may occur in normal individuals as well as in those with diseased hearts. Some are drug induced; digitalis is the most notable offender in this group. Attacks of paroxysmal tachycardia may last from less than a minute to hours or days, and may be recurrent. As in the case of extrasystoles, paroxysmal tachycardias may be supraventricular or ventricular in origin. Prolonged episodes of paroxysmal tachycardia may give rise to faintness, lightheadedness, syncope, dyspnea, angina, and congestive heart failure. The clinical evaluation of paroxysmal tachycardia is summarized in Table 3-18. The electrocardiographic differential diagnosis is considered in paragraph **8** below.

Bradycardias

Bradycardias may produce consciousness of the heartbeat when cardiac contraction is forceful as a result of increased stroke volume. Should the cardiac output decline, as a result of either very slow rates or weakened myocardial contractility, faintness or syncope may occur. The major causes of a slow pulse rate are sinus bradycardia, sino-atrial block, AV junctional rhythms, extrasystolic bigeminy, and AV block.

DIAGNOSTIC APPROACH

1. As a first step, physiologic causes of palpitation, disorders not associated with arrhythmia, and neurocirculatory asthenia should be ruled out as causes of palpitation. This can usually be accomplished by the history, physical examination, and selected laboratory tests.

2. All patients in whom arrhythmia is suspected as the cause of palpitation should be evaluated for the presence or absence of heart disease. Chest films and an electrocardiogram should be included in such an evaluation.

3. Although the correct diagnosis of an arrhythmia may sometimes be surmised from the history and physical examination, one should not

rely solely on these procedures. An electrocardiographic recording of
the arrhythmia in question is mandatory for correct diagnosis. In
those instances in which the conventional electrocardiogram or special
monitor leads are not decisive, right atrial or esophageal leads, or a
recording of the His bundle electrogram, may be of assistance.

4. In any patient complaining of palpitation, specific inquiry should
be made as to whether the symptom is continuous when present or
is related to isolated beats. The former situation suggests a paroxysmal
arrhythmia, and the latter, premature beats.

5. When rapid heart action is suggested by the history, additional features may help to distinguish between sinus and ectopic rhythms. A
tachycardia with a rate above 140 per minute, that starts and ends
abruptly and that can be terminated by vagal maneuvers performed
by the patient, suggests the diagnosis of paroxysmal rather than sinus
tachycardia. Also, tachyarrhythmias that awaken a patient from sleep
are more likely to be ectopic than sinus in origin.

6. Every patient with palpitation should be questioned concerning the
use of tea, coffee, tobacco, or drugs, since these may be precipitating
factors in any arrhythmia.

7. Associated symptoms or signs may provide clues to the presence of
coexisting disease (e.g., hyperthyroidism, pheochromocytoma) that
may be responsible for palpitation and dysrhythmia. Recurrent episodes of supraventricular tachycardia in otherwise healthy individuals
should lead to a search for the Wolff-Parkinson-White syndrome.

8. When a patient presents during an arrhythmic episode, an electrocardiogram should be recorded at once. The diagnosis may then be
obvious from the electrocardiogram. Not infrequently, however, particularly in paroxysmal tachycardias, the electrocardiogram may present diagnostic problems. Under such circumstances, attention to
the points listed below may be helpful in unraveling the correct diagnosis. It is useful to divide paroxysmal tachycardias into those characterized by normal QRS durations and those in which the QRS
duration is prolonged.

   a. Tachycardia with normal QRS duration.
      (1) The supraventricular origin of a tachycardia is established if
      the QRS complexes are of essentially normal configuration
      and duration. However, supraventricular tachycardia may be
      associated with abnormal QRS complexes. This variety is con-
      sidered separately in paragraph **b** below.
      (2) A tachycardia is atrial in origin if it is initiated by a premature,
      abnormal P wave and followed by a QRS complex at an ap-
      proximately normal P-R interval.
      (3) A tachycardia is AV junctional in origin if the P waves are
      inverted (retrograde) in leads II, III, and aVF, and up-

TABLE 3-18. Clinical Differential Diagnosis of the Tachycardias

Tachycardias	Rate Atrial	Rate Ventricular	Regularity	Onset and Termination
Sinus tachycardia	100 to 150 but may be faster	100 to 150 but may be faster	Regular	Gradual
Paroxysmal atrial tachycardia	140 to 250	140 to 250	Usually regular	Abrupt
Paroxysmal atrial tachycardia with block	120 to 250; usually 120 to 180 with 2:1 block	Variable	Regular or irregular	Gradual
Multifocal atrial tachycardia (chaotic atrial rhythm)	100 to 180	100 to 180	Irregular	Gradual
Atrial flutter	220 to 350; 2:1 block usually present if untreated	Variable	Regular or irregular	Abrupt
Atrial fibrillation	>350	Variable	Irregular; if regular, indicative of advanced or complete AV block	Abrupt
Paroxysmal AV junctional tachycardia	140 to 250 with AV dissociation, usually NSR	140 to 250	Regular	Abrupt
Nonparoxysmal AV junctional tachycardia	Depends on atrial mechanism; AV dissociation often present	65 to 130	Regular	Gradual
Paroxysmal ventricular tachycardia	With AV dissociation, usually NSR; may have retrograde atrial activation	140 to 200; May be slower with idioventricular or parasystolic ventricular tachycardia	Regular or slightly irregular	Abrupt

AV = atrioventricular, NSR = normal sinus rhythm, S_1 = first heart sound, S_2 = second heart sound.

Etiology	Physical Signs		Response to Carotid Sinus Massage
	Jugular Venous Pulsations	Heart Sounds	
Physical or emotional stress; increased sympathetic tone; decreased vagal tone; drugs; hypoxemia; shock; hyperkinetic circulatory states; congestive heart failure; myocardial disease	Normal	Normal	Gradual slowing, with return to previous rate
Most commonly noncardiac; may occur in normal subjects; hypoxemia; shock; pulmonary disease; any type of heart disease, especially mitral valvular disease	Normal or cannon A waves	S_1 constant in intensity	No effect, or abrupt termination
Most often due to combination of digitalis excess and potassium depletion; may also occur in coronary heart disease, rheumatic heart disease, and pulmonary disease	A waves at rapid, slightly irregular rate; may exceed ventricular rate	S_1 may vary in intensity	May increase degree of AV block and slow ventricular rate; contraindicated in most situations
Acute and chronic pulmonary disease, especially with respiratory failure and hypoxia; organic heart disease may be associated	May not be visible	S_1 may vary in intensity	No effect, or gradual slowing
Almost always associated with organic heart disease; hypoxemia; shock; acute or chronic pulmonary disease	Flutter waves may be visible at multiples of ventricular rate	S_1 may vary in intensity if rhythm is irregular	May increase degree of AV block, slow ventricular rate, and reveal flutter waves
Almost always associated with organic heart disease (especially rheumatic or coronary heart disease); hyperthyroidism	Irregular pulsations	S_1 varies in intensity	Gradual slowing, with return to previous rate
Same as for paroxysmal atrial tachycardia	Regular or irregular cannon A waves commonly occur	S_1 constant; varies in intensity if AV dissociation is present	No effect, or abrupt termination
Digitalis toxicity; coronary heart disease, especially inferior infarction; rheumatic carditis, postcardiac surgery	Regular or irregular cannon A waves commonly present	S_1 constant; varies in intensity if AV dissociation is present	No effect, or gradual slowing, with return to previous rate; contraindicated in most situations
Coronary heart disease, especially myocardial infarction; congestive heart failure; drug toxicity (digitalis, quinidine, epinephrine)	Irregular cannon A waves when AV dissociation is present	S_1 varies in intensity; S_2 widely split	No effect

right in lead aVR, if the P-R interval is 0.10 second or less, or if retrograde P waves follow the QRS complexes.

(4) During a continuous tachycardia with retrograde P waves and a P-R interval of 0.12 second or more, it is not possible to determine whether the tachycardia is atrial or AV junctional in origin. To distinguish between the two it is necessary to record the onset or termination of the tachycardia. If the paroxysm begins with a retrograde P wave and the P-R interval is 0.12 second or more, or if it ends with a QRS complex, then the tachycardia is considered to be atrial in origin. On the other hand, if the arrhythmia begins with a QRS complex that is followed by a retrograde P wave, or if it terminates with such a P wave, then the tachycardia is regarded as AV junctional in origin.

(5) Atrial flutter is recognized by the presence of a sawtooth appearance of the baseline.

(6) Atrial fibrillation is characterized by absence of P waves, rapid irregular oscillations of the baseline, and an irregularity of the ventricular response (unless advanced or complete AV block is present).

(7) Supraventricular tachycardia of undetermined origin is the correct designation for a regular tachyarrhythmia in which P waves are not identifiable.

(8) Carotid sinus massage, vagal maneuvers, and cholinergic drugs are often helpful in diagnosis. Vagal maneuvers other than carotid sinus pressure (e.g., eyeball pressure, induction of vomiting) are not recommended. Edrophonium chloride (Tensilon), in a dose of 10 mg intravenously, is the safest of the cholinergic drugs to administer. Any of these interventions may slow or terminate or have no effect on supraventricular arrhythmias. Carotid sinus massage is the most widely used procedure. In sinus tachycardia, it generally produces a gradual slowing of the heartbeat, which usually reverts to its original rate after the pressure is released; sometimes sinus tachycardia is unaffected by this maneuver. Carotid sinus massage either terminates or has no effect on most paroxysmal atrial or AV junctional tachycardias. In atrial flutter, carotid sinus pressure increases the degree of AV block so that fewer flutter impulses are conducted to the ventricles. With a lesser number of ventricular complexes, the F waves are more clearly revealed, making this a very useful maneuver when the diagnosis of atrial flutter is uncertain. Carotid sinus massage should always be performed with caution, particularly in the elderly, and under electrocardiographic control. The procedure is contraindicated in cerebral vascular disease, heart block, and digitalis intoxication.

b. Tachycardia with abnormal QRS duration.

(1) Tachycardia with abnormally wide QRS complexes may be supraventricular or ventricular in origin. All of the electrocardiographic manifestations of ventricular arrhythmia may be mimicked by supraventricular arrhythmia associated with QRS complexes that are abnormally wide as a result of aberrant ventricular conduction, bundle branch block, or ventricular preexcitation.

(2) Tachycardia with abnormal QRS complexes are supraventricular in origin if they are initiated by premature, ectopic P waves, regardless of the configuration of the QRS complexes.

(3) Tachycardias initiated by abnormal QRS complexes may be ventricular or AV junctional in origin. In the latter case, the QRS complexes may be bizarre because of the presence of the conditions listed in paragraph **(1)** above.

(4) A tachycardia that occurs after a premature beat interrupts the T wave of the preceding beat (R on T phenomenon) is regarded as ventricular in origin.

(5) The regularity of the tachycardia and its rate are of limited help in differential diagnosis.

(6) The configuration of the QRS complexes may provide a clue, but it rarely permits absolute differential diagnosis between aberrant ventricular conduction and ventricular ectopy. Favoring aberrant conduction are a triphasic RBBB pattern with an RSR' pattern in V_1 and a qRS pattern in V_6. Favoring ectopy are monophasic or diphasic complexes, a qR or RR' pattern with R greater than R' in V_1, a QS or rS pattern in V_6, an LBBB pattern with a wide r wave in V_1, or complexes that are positive in all of the precordial leads (preexcitation excluded) or negative in all of them. If the configuration of the QRS complexes during the tachycardia is the same as that during a known supraventricular rhythm, the tachycardia is considered supraventricular in origin.

(7) In the presence of AV dissociation, an atrial arrhythmia can be excluded, but an AV junctional mechanism with aberration or a ventricular rhythm remains as a diagnostic possibility.

(8) Retrograde conduction to the atria may occur in AV junctional or ventricular tachycardias.

(9) The most useful criteria for diagnosis of ventricular tachycardia in the conventional electrocardiogram are the presence of early ventricular capture or fusion beats, or both. Unfortunately, neither of these is absolutely pathognomonic of ventricular tachycardia because they sometimes occur in supraventricular tachycardias. Absence of fusion or capture beats does not rule out ventricular tachycardia.

(10) Since ventricular tachycardia is unaffected by carotid sinus massage, a response to this maneuver (such as termination of the tachycardia or slowing of the ventricular rate) is virtually diagnostic of supraventricular arrhythmia.

(11) The only method available at present for differentiating between supraventricular and ventricular arrhythmias is the

His bundle electrogram. With this recording, in supraventricular rhythms, an H deflection is seen to precede each QRS complex at a normal or prolonged H-V interval; and in ventricular rhythms, the QRS complexes are not preceded by H deflections.

9. The diagnosis of arrhythmia may pose a real problem if it is not present at the time of examination. One solution, if the condition is not serious, is to ask the patient to return when the rhythm disturbance returns. However, if the episodes occur infrequently or are of brief duration even when frequent, it may not be possible to catch the patient during an arrhythmic episode. Under such circumstances, the diagnosis must await a more propitious opportunity for examination, or the patient may be monitored.

10. Patients with serious arrhythmia problems, particularly when associated with other cardiovascular symptoms and organic heart disease, should be monitored if the rhythm disturbance cannot be diagnosed in any other way. Monitoring can be performed either on an inpatient or an outpatient basis. In the hospital, radiotelemetry (if available) is the most suitable method for monitoring patients since it permits them to be ambulatory. Direct connection to a nonportable unit is less desirable because the patient must be confined to bed. For outpatients, there is available portable apparatus that can tape-record continuously for 10 hours the patient's electrocardiogram while he goes about his normal activities. When the tape is later played back, the arrhythmias that occurred can be identified and reproduced on electrocardiographic paper to obtain permanent records.

Peripheral Vascular Disorders

Gilbert Hermann

ARTERIAL DISEASE

Acute Arterial Occlusion

Symptoms

The symptoms of acute arterial occlusion occur acutely or fairly rapidly (1 to 2 hours), often in a previously asymptomatic extremity. The pain may begin as numbness or tingling but, depending on the level of occlusion, will progress within hours to steady, severe pain. Coldness, numbness, pallor, and weakness are usually apparent.

Pertinent Past History

1. The patient may have heart disease associated with intracardiac clots as the source of peripheral arterial emboli.

   a. Rheumatic heart disease with subsequent atrial fibrillation.

b. Myocardial infarction, although a history of infarction may or may not be elicited.

2. Symptoms of chronic peripheral vascular insufficiency may be present. A sudden acute increase in symptoms may be secondary to thrombosis of a vessel previously compromised by atherosclerosis.

Signs

1. Determination of *temperature change* can be evaluated best by gently feeling the affected extremity with the back of the hand. The level of demarcation of temperature change can be decided by comparison with the opposite, uninvolved extremity. In general, the level of demarcation of temperature change is distal to the site of occlusion. For example, the level of temperature change from a warm to a cool extremity resulting from a sudden occlusion of the femoral artery in the upper thigh occurs at or below the knee; the level for popliteal artery occlusion is in the distal leg at or above the ankle. As side branches begin to occlude, the temperature demarcation level ascends more proximally in the extremity. Patients with a great deal of sympathetic activity may have a cool extremity on that basis alone.

2. Asymmetric *pulses* are extremely important signs, although they are not infallible evidence of vascular occlusion. The posterior tibial artery is more consistent anatomically than the dorsalis pedis artery (98 percent vs. 85 to 90 percent). Occasionally, pulsations just proximal to a recent occlusion may be much more pronounced than in the corresponding artery in the opposite, unobstructed side.

3. The affected limb is usually *paler* than the unaffected extremity, particularly in the dependent position.

4. *Sensation* to pain or touch diminishes progressively as the duration of occlusion is prolonged.

5. *Muscle strength* is decreased and is often manifested in inability to move the digits of the affected extremity.

6. The presence of *cardiac arrhythmias*, particularly atrial fibrillation, favors embolic rather than thrombotic occlusion.

Diagnostic Procedures

While the diagnosis of sudden occlusion is usually made easily by the history and physical examination, occasionally it is necessary to determine the extent of the occlusion and the status of the proximal and distal arterial tree by other methods.

1. The Doppler ultrasound is a valuable noninvasive technique for determining the point along the course of a major artery at which pulsatile flow either has ceased or is markedly diminished.

2. Although not indicated preoperatively in every patient, most vascular surgeons obtain postoperative arteriograms while the patient is still in the operating room to make certain that the distal arterial network is patent.

Chronic Arterial Occlusion

Etiology

1. Atherosclerosis.   Primary, or associated with such generalized conditions as diabetes, hypertension, or hyperlipidemia.

2. Arteritis.   Buerger's disease, a disorder primarily affecting younger adults, characterized by involvement of the medium-size arteries. Some believe that the disease is actually a form of early atherosclerosis.

3. Vasospastic disorders.
   a. Raynaud's phenomenon, usually part of a symptom complex associated with the connective tissue diseases and only rarely a primary disease.
   b. Drug-related disorders (e.g., ergot, propranolol).

Symptoms

The symptoms listed below are usually related to large vessel occlusion secondary to atherosclerosis, which is responsible for 90 to 95 percent of all chronic occlusive arterial disease.

1. Pain.
   a. Intermittent claudication.   The character of the pain associated with peripheral vascular insufficiency is unique and should not be confused with leg or buttock pain arising from skeletal or neurologic disease. Claudication is pain that typically begins after an increase in metabolic requirement (e.g., ambulation) and is relieved promptly with rest. It cannot be elicited by any other stimulus, such as palpation of the part or a change in its position.
   b. Rest pain occurs with far advanced vascular insufficiency and implies a pregangrenous state. Characteristically, the patient obtains some relief by dangling the affected extremity over the edge of the bed or by assuming a sitting position with both legs dependent.

2. Redness of the toes or foot on dependency implies moderate or severe arterial occlusive disease.

3. Coolness.   Do not place too much reliance on this symptom, because many perfectly healthy patients complain of "cold feet."

4. Nonhealing or slowly healing ulcers may occur spontaneously or may be secondary to minor trauma. They are generally painful.

Pertinent Past History
1. Diabetes mellitus.

2. Hypertension.

3. Family history of early atherosclerosis complications.

4. Drug use, particularly of substances known to predispose to vasospastic problems, such as ergot or propranolol.

Signs
1. The presence or absence and the quality of all *peripheral pulses* should be noted. The carotid, brachial, radial, aortic (if palpable), femoral, popliteal, dorsalis pedis, and posterior tibial pulses should be examined. The peripheral pulses may be normal in patients with predominantly small vessel disease. Arteriosclerotic vessels generally feel hard and non-compressible.

2. *Dependent rubor* is the most usual color change noted.

3. The *temperature* of the limb varies a great deal depending on the status of sympathetic activity. The ambient temperature obviously is a factor. A difference in temperature between the two limbs is significant.

4. Heavy *hair growth* on the digits is evidence against the diagnosis of chronic arterial insufficiency. Conversely, the absence of hair may reflect a genetic characteristic and is not necessarily indicative of chronic ischemia.

5. *Venous filling time* can be estimated by having the patient assume the supine position and having the examiner elevate the patient's legs to 45° for 1 to 2 minutes. The patient is then allowed to sit up with his feet dangling over the edge of the examining table. There should be definite venous filling in 15 to 20 seconds. A venous filling time greater than 1 minute is definitely abnormal.

6. Ischemic *ulcers* generally occur on the lateral aspect of the lower leg, although they may occur in other sites.

7. Abdominal *bruits* are compatible with but not diagnostic of aortic, iliac, or renal artery disease. Femoral or carotid bruits are abnormal and indicate arterial pathology.

Diagnostic Procedures
1. A Doppler ultrasound test should confirm the physical examination findings with respect to the level of arterial occlusion.

2. Arteriography is the most accurate diagnostic procedure for determining the anatomic status of the arterial tree. Since there are risks involved with the procedure, it should be done only when the need for recon-

structive surgery is apparent and a delineation of the anatomic situation before surgery is necessary.

VENOUS DISEASE

Superficial Phlebitis

Symptoms
A sudden onset of pain over some portion of the course of the greater saphenous vein is typical, although superficial phlebitis can occur in any superficially varicosed vein. No edema or systemic symptoms are observed.

Signs
A tender, red, swollen cord is palpable over the affected superficial vein. Occasionally, the swelling takes the form of ovoid nodules. There is no swelling except along the course of the vessel. The arterial pulses are usually present.

Deep Phlebitis: Acute

Symptoms
1. Sudden onset of thigh or lower leg edema, or both.

2. Pain that is aching in character, not related to exercise, and somewhat relieved by elevation of the affected extremity.

3. Bluish mottling of the skin, most marked in the dependent position.

4. Generalized malaise but no shaking chills.

Signs
1. *Edema.*   The legs should be measured at the ankles, calves, and thighs bilaterally and the comparative findings recorded.

2. *Tenderness,* especially over the affected deep veins. Gentle palpation rather than forceful squeezing usually elicits this sign in a meaningful manner.

3. *Dilated* superficial veins.

4. *Increased warmth* of the affected extremity.

5. *Mottling* of the leg, particularly prominent in the dependent position.

Differential Diagnosis
1. Phlegmasia alba dolens with obliteration of the arterial pulses can sometimes be mistaken for acute arterial occlusion.

2. Rupture of the plantaris tendon or partial tear of the gastrocnemius muscle. Characteristically, the pain occurs suddenly while the patient is engaged in strenuous physical exercise.

Diagnosis
1. Venography.
2. Doppler ultrasound.
3. Fibrinogen tagged with radioactive iodine.

Deep Phlebitis: Chronic

Symptoms
1. Swelling, most pronounced after prolonged upright position.
2. Enlarged superficial veins.
3. Ulceration of the lower leg.

Signs
1. Edema, usually confined to the lower leg.
2. Subcutaneous fibrosis: The skin is very thickened and brawny.
3. Stasis dermatitis.
4. Ulceration, usually on the lower one-third of the medial aspect of leg; not as painful as ischemic ulcers.

Diagnosis
1. A past history consistent with acute iliofemoral thrombosis, which is often postpartum or postsurgical.
2. Physical examination.
3. Venography.

4.

Respiratory Problems

Dyspnea

Marvin I. Schwarz
Paul M. Cox

DEFINITION

Dyspnea is shortness of breath accompanied by objective evidence of difficult, labored, or uncomfortable breathing. Other forms of breathlessness, such as hyperventilation, sighing respirations, and the subjective sensation of inability to take deep breaths, are thus excluded.

ACUTE DYSPNEA
Etiology

1. The more common pulmonary diseases that present with acute dyspnea include the pneumonias, thromboembolic disease, spontaneous pneumothorax, asthma, foreign body aspiration, noncardiac pulmonary edema (including noxious gas inhalation, high-altitude pulmonary edema, and neurogenic pulmonary edema), and the adult respiratory distress syndrome (fat embolization, shock lung).

2. The major nonpulmonary cause of acute dyspnea is cardiogenic pulmonary edema.

History

1. Pneumonia. Patients with pneumonia from any cause (tuberculous, viral, or bacterial) may present with purulent sputum, pleuritic chest pain, fever, chills, and a prodrome of upper respiratory tract symptoms.

8 – 965

2. Acute pulmonary embolism.   Patients with pulmonary embolism may have a characteristic clinical setting, such as prolonged immobilization, recent surgery, congestive heart failure, or recent trauma, particularly to the lower extremities. A predisposition to thromboembolism occurs in patients with a previous history of thrombophlebitis, women on oral contraceptives, and individuals with sickle cell anemia or polycythemic states.

3. Spontaneous pneumothorax.   Spontaneous pneumothorax is more apt to occur in young, tall, thin individuals. The patient usually gives a history of a sudden onset of chest pain and dyspnea brought on by strenuous exertion, coughing, or air travel. Predisposing factors include emphysema, recent chest trauma, and interstitial lung disease, particularly eosinophilic granuloma.

4. Acute bronchial asthma.   Acute asthma may begin at any age but is more frequent in patients with a past or family history of atopic disease. It may be seasonal in nature and may be associated with specific events or inciting agents.

5. Foreign body aspiration.   In the patient who has aspirated a foreign body, usually the history is obvious. However, the patient may not recall the event, especially if he was under the influence of alcohol at the time.

6. Noncardiogenic pulmonary edema.
   a. Noxious gas inhalation.   There is usually a history of accidental exposure to a poisonous gas (chlorine, phosgene, smoke).
   b. High-altitude pulmonary edema.   This condition usually occurs in young adults engaging in vigorous activity at high altitude prior to acclimatization.
   c. Neurogenic pulmonary edema.   This type of edema may be seen in epileptic patients during the postictal period and in patients with increased intracranial pressure.

7. Adult respiratory distress syndrome.   The adult respiratory distress syndrome includes many conditions that produce the same pathophysiologic disturbance in the lung. The diagnosis can be made if the clinical setting is recognized. The predisposing conditions include: fat embolization following severe trauma; shock secondary to gram-negative sepsis or blood loss; cardiopulmonary bypass during cardiac surgery; near-drowning; and severe infectious or aspiration pneumonia.

8. Cardiogenic pulmonary edema.   The patient usually presents with the characteristic symptoms of congestive heart failure. A previous history of heart disease should be sought. Not infrequently, previously undetected mitral stenosis may be discovered after an initial episode of pulmonary edema.

Physical Findings

Tachycardia, tachypnea, cyanosis, and fever may be noted in any patient who presents with acute dyspnea.

1. Pneumonia.   In the *bacterial* pneumonias, there are the signs of consolidation, including bronchial breath sounds, increased tactile and vocal fremitus, and egophony. There may be an associated decrease in breath sounds and fine rales heard over the involved area. If a pleural effusion accompanies the pneumonia, the physical findings may include a pleural friction rub, decreased to absent breath sounds, decreased fremitus, and flatness to percussion. In contrast, the *viral* pneumonias characteristically show a paucity of physical findings. Sometimes only rales are heard.

2. Acute pulmonary embolism.   Pulmonary emboli present with a variety of physical findings. The examination may reveal such signs as rales heard over the involved area, a pleural friction rub, and evidence of pleural effusion. Splinting of the involved side may be present and manifested by elevation of the diaphragm and a generalized decrease in breath sounds. Cardiac examination may reveal signs of right ventricular failure, including a right-sided third heart sound, the murmur of pulmonary regurgitation, or increased intensity of the pulmonary component of the second heart sound. Frequently, however, there are only the nonspecific findings of tachypnea and tachycardia.

3. Pneumothorax.   The physical findings of pneumothorax are decreased breath sounds, increased resonance, and decreased fremitus on the involved side. There may be shift of the trachea and heart to the opposite side. Distention of the neck veins may be visible if the pneumothorax is under tension. Hamman's sign (mediastinal crunch) may be heard in the presence of a left-sided pneumothorax.

4. Bronchial asthma.   Patients with asthma have hyperresonance to percussion and wheezing during their attacks. If bronchospasm is severe, the chest may be silent to auscultation.

5. Foreign body aspiration.   A patient who aspirates a foreign body may have localized wheezing and decreased breath sounds on the involved side. There may be air trapping during expiration (hyperresonance to percussion on the affected side following forced expiration).

6. Noncardiogenic pulmonary edema.
   a. Noxious gas inhalation.   Such patients usually have conjunctivitis, pharyngitis, acute bronchitis, and wheezing. Later on, diffuse, bilateral moist rales appear as the clinical picture of pulmonary edema evolves.
   b. High-altitude pulmonary edema.   Fine, moist bibasilar rales are commonly audible, although there is no evidence of heart failure.

    c. Neurogenic pulmonary edema. The findings are the same as in paragraph **b** above in association with evidence of neurologic injury. Systemic hypertension may develop acutely.

  7. Adult respiratory distress syndrome. Clinical evidence of shock may be present. Conjunctival and axillary petechiae are commonly seen in fat embolism. Rales may be heard.

  8. Cardiogenic pulmonary edema. There may be evidence of previous hypertension or heart disease. Cardiomegaly is suggested by lateral and downward displacement of the apical impulse: A third heart sound or summation gallop and murmurs may be heard. Examination of the lungs may reveal fine moist rales, particularly at the bases. Wheezes may also be heard.

Roentgenographic Findings

  1. Pneumonia.

    a. Lobar consolidation with air bronchograms is usually present in bacterial pneumonia. Pleural effusion, which may be infrapulmonary or interlobar, is sometimes seen.

    b. Viral and mycoplasma pneumonias may be lobar in distribution but are more likely to be diffuse and nonlobar in character. Pleural effusions occur less frequently than in bacterial pneumonias. Uncommonly, hilar adenopathy may occur.

  2. Acute pulmonary embolism. The chest roentgenogram may be normal or may show evidence of splinting (a raised diaphragm and basilar atelectasis). Pleural effusion or pulmonary infiltrates may be seen after infarction of the lung. A lobar consolidation similar to bacterial pneumonia may be present. Vascular changes occur frequently in acute pulmonary embolism but are difficult to interpret. Vascular cutoffs and decreased blood flow may sometimes be demonstrated, particularly if previous x-ray films are available for comparison. With large central pulmonary emboli, a sausage-shaped dilatation of the involved pulmonary artery may be seen.

  3. Spontaneous pneumothorax. The chest roentgenogram of pneumothorax is virtually diagnostic, if examined carefully. Occasionally, a small pneumothorax may not be seen unless inspiratory and expiratory films are evaluated. It is necessary to determine whether or not the pneumothorax is under tension. The classic findings of a tension pneumothorax are depression of the diaphragm on the affected side and a shift of the mediastinum to the opposite side.

  4. Bronchial asthma. In asthma, there may be radiologic signs of hyperinflation, such as flat diaphragms and an increase in the retrosternal and retrocardiac air spaces. When an infectious process precipitates an asthmatic attack, evidence of pneumonia may be seen on the chest roentgenogram.

5. Foreign body aspiration. Rarely, the foreign body is radiopaque and can be visualized. The chest roentgenogram usually shows nothing abnormal. There may be evidence of unilateral air trapping, which is demonstrated best by fluoroscopy and expiratory films. Consolidation collapse of the lung distal to the foreign body may occur after a period of time.

6. Noncardiogenic pulmonary edema. Early in the course of noxious gas inhalation, neurogenic and high-altitude pulmonary edema, and the adult respiratory distress syndrome, the chest x-ray may be normal. Eventually, the films may show evidence of pulmonary edema without cardiomegaly.

7. Adult respiratory distress syndrome. The findings are similar to those described for noncardiogenic pulmonary edema (see paragraph **6** above).

8. Cardiogenic pulmonary edema. The chest roentgenogram will show cardiomegaly except in some cases of acute myocardial infarction and mitral stenosis. Specific chamber enlargement is seen in valvular and congenital heart disease. An alveolar infiltrate showing a butterfly pattern is typical of this form of pulmonary edema. Distended veins to the upper lobes, Kerley lines, and a peripheral or hilar haze or both, may also be seen.

Laboratory Data

1. CBC. The hematocrit and hemoglobin values are normal in all of these conditions unless altered by coexisting disease. The white cell count is usually elevated, with a shift to the left, but it is rarely above 16,000 per cubic millimeter except in bacterial pneumonias. Asthma may be associated with a significant eosinophilia. Marked derangements in all formed blood elements may be seen in severely ill patients with the acute adult respiratory distress syndrome.

2. Urinalysis. Hematuria, proteinuria, formed elements, and casts may be seen in the pneumonias, congestive heart failure, and conditions associated with the adult respiratory distress syndrome. All of these findings are nonspecific.

3. Serum electrolytes. A low serum sodium may be seen in the infectious pneumonias. This may be associated with increased excretion of sodium in the urine. In patients with tuberculosis and Addison's disease, signs of adrenocortical insufficiency may develop.

4. Electrocardiogram. The electrocardiogram may be diagnostic if it demonstrates the classic pattern of acute myocardial infarction. Findings of right axis deviation, an $S_1 Q_3 T_3$ pattern, or right ventricular strain provide supportive evidence for the diagnosis of pulmonary embolism. However, atrial arrhythmias may be seen with pneumonias. Right axis deviation and the right ventricular strain pattern may also be seen in any case of acute dyspnea.

5. Examination of the sputum.

   a. Gross examination. Pink frothy sputum is often seen in cardiogenic or noncardiogenic pulmonary edema. Blood streaking is usually not helpful. The presence of mucus plugs may suggest asthma. Grossly purulent sputum suggests a bacterial pneumonic process, whereas a mucoid sputum is seen more frequently in viral and mycoplasma pneumonias.

   b. Gram stain. An adequate, freshly obtained sputum sample should be examined. The gram stain should demonstrate large numbers of polymorphonuclear leukocytes. Only if a predominant organism can be identified should it be tentatively considered the etiologic agent.

   c. Acid-fast stain. Acid-fast organisms should be sought carefully under oil immersion.

   d. Wright's stain. Eosinophilia may predominate in the sputum samples in asthmatic patients.

   e. Sputum cultures. Routine cultures for bacteria, tuberculosis, and fungi should be obtained. Facilities for culture of viruses and mycoplasma are not available except in specialized laboratories.

   f. Blood cultures. Blood cultures should be drawn from the febrile patient with acute dyspnea.

   g. Arterial blood gases. Arterial blood gases are of no value in differentiating between the various entities under consideration, but they are helpful in the management of patient care, since all of these conditions may present with varying degrees of hypoxemia.

   h. Cold agglutinins. Cold agglutinins may be elevated in mycoplasma pneumonia. Specific titer rises may be seen in viral pneumonias.

Further Studies

When the aforementioned studies are completed, the most likely diagnosis should be apparent, and treatment should be instituted. If pulmonary embolism is a prime consideration, perfusion and inhalation lung scans or pulmonary angiography, or both, should be performed. If foreign body aspiration is suspected, early bronchoscopy is probably indicated. If asthma is the apparent diagnosis, treatment should be instituted and the work-up completed when the patient's condition has stabilized.

CHRONIC DYSPNEA

Etiology

1. Pulmonary causes of chronic dyspnea.

   a. Chronic obstructive airway disease. (*Note:* Although there is usually considerable overlap between these three entities, the classic forms are described in the discussion that follows.)

   (1) Emphysema.

   (2) Chronic bronchitis.

   (3) Chronic bronchial asthma.

b. Restrictive lung diseases.

(1) Interstitial lung disease (the most common of which are sarcoidosis, rheumatoid lung, scleroderma lung, the pneumoconiosis, histiocytosis X, lymphangitic carcinomatosis, and idiopathic fibrosing alveolitis).

(2) Chest wall deformities (e.g., kyphoscoliosis and thoracoplasty).

(3) Pleural fibrosis.

(4) Alveolar-filling diseases (alveolar proteinosis, alveolar cell carcinoma, desquamative interstitial pneumonia, lipoid pneumonia, and alveolar microlithiasis).

2. Nonpulmonary causes of chronic dyspnea.

a. Congestive heart failure.

b. Anemia.

c. Hyperthyroidism.

d. Upper airway disease.

e. Obesity.

History

1. Pulmonary causes.

a. Chronic obstructive airway disease.

(1) Patients with emphysema usually give a long history of steadily worsening dyspnea. There may be a family history of emphysema or other obstructive lung disease.

(2) In chronic bronchitis, a productive cough is present for at least 3 months of every year for a consecutive 2-year period. Chronic bronchitis is usually associated with a long history of cigarette smoking, a "smoker's cough," wheezing, and repeated pulmonary infections.

(3) The history of patients with chronic asthma is similar to that noted in cases of acute asthma.

b. Restrictive lung disease.

(1) A complete discussion of the different causes of interstitial lung disease is beyond the scope of this text. In some conditions, diagnostic clues may be found in the history. In the connective tissue diseases, such as scleroderma, rheumatoid arthritis, and polymyositis, there may be a history or symptoms suggestive of the diagnosis. Sometimes, however, the disease presents with interstitial fibrosis and the systemic manifestations develop later. Patients with eosinophilic granuloma may have a history of recurrent pneumothorax or diabetes insipidus, or both. Patients with sarcoidosis, who are likely to be Negroes, may relate a history of arthralgias and painful erythematous nodules on the shins. In the pneumoconioses, the occupational history is of prime importance. In lymphangitic carcinomatosis, symptoms relating to a primary carcinoma of the stomach, breast, prostrate lung, or other organs may be disclosed.

(2) In patients with thoracic deformities, the history is obvious.

(3) Patients with pleural fibrosis may give a history of previous tuberculosis, a severe bacterial pneumonia, chest trauma, or surgery for tuberculosis.

(4) Among the alveolar-filling diseases, alveolar proteinosis and alveolar cell carcinoma may have significant sputum production. In lipoid pneumonia, there may be a history of inhalation of oily nose drops.

2. Nonpulmonary causes.
   a. Congestive heart failure. See Cardiogenic Pulmonary Edema (p. 140).
   b. Anemia. Progressive dyspnea is a common symptom of anemia and should be considered particularly if the patient complains of blood loss, pallor, and weakness.
   c. Hyperthyroidism. In thyrotoxic individuals, dyspnea may be the predominant presenting symptom. Usually these patients will have classic symptoms of thyrotoxicosis.
   d. Upper airway disease. Patients with upper airway disease usually have had an endotracheal tube or tracheostomy. They may complain of audible wheezing or upper airway rattling.
   e. Obesity. Corpulence is seldom the sole reason for a patient's complaint of dyspnea unless the obesity is severe or the weight gain has been rapid.

Physical Examination

1. Chronic obstructive airway disease.
   a. Emphysema. Usually the emphysematous patient is thin and asthenic, the AP diameter of the chest is increased, and hypertrophy of the accessory muscles of respiration is visible. There is hyperresonance to percussion with depressed immobile diaphragms. Auscultation reveals decreased breath sounds and a prolongation of the expiratory phase of respiration.
   b. Chronic bronchitis. The patient with chronic bronchitis tends to be short and stocky. He may appear plethoric or cyanotic, or both, because of erythrocytosis. Auscultation may reveal rhonchi, wheezing, and a prolonged expiratory phase of respiration. In more advanced stages, physical evidence of cor pulmonale may appear.
   c. Chronic bronchial asthma. Wheezing is a characteristic physical finding, and it may be associated with signs of hyperinflation of the lungs.
   d. Restrictive lung disease.
      (1) Interstitial lung disease. In interstitial fibrosis, clubbing may be noted. The chest examination may be normal except for dry inspiratory bibasilar rales. Signs of associated systemic diseases (e.g., arthritis, skin rash, lymphadenopathy, splenomegaly) may be seen. Evidence of a primary carcinoma may be found in lymphangitic carcinomatosis.

(2) Thoracic deformities. The diagnosis of kyphoscoliosis or a previous thoracoplasty is evident on inspection.

(3) Pleural fibrosis. There may be diminished expansion of the chest wall. Dullness of percussion, decreased fremitus, and decreased breath sounds may be noted on the involved side.

(4) Alveolar-filling diseases. There are no specific physical findings. Rales may be heard in occasional cases.

2. Nonpulmonary causes.

a. Congestive heart failure. Elevated venous pressure, bibasilar rales, and anasarca are the cardinal signs.

b. Anemia. Aside from pallor, there are no specific signs of anemia, although there are specific signs associated with different causes of anemia.

c. Hyperthyroidism. A goiter in association with tremor, moist skin, exophthalmos, and tachycardia are classic signs of Graves' disease.

d. Upper airway disease. Wheezing or stridor may be appreciated, and a tracheostomy scar may be present.

e. Obesity. Adiposity is usually obvious by inspection.

Roentgenographic Findings

1. Pulmonary causes.

a. Chronic obstructive airway disease.

(1) Emphysema usually shows bullous changes, evidence of hyperinflation of the lungs, and attenuation of the pulmonary vasculature on the chest roentgenogram.

(2) Chronic bronchitis may reveal roentgenographic evidence of cor pulmonale (right ventricular hypertrophy associated with pulmonary hypertension). There may be evidence of previous pneumonias manifested as localized areas of fibrosis. However, the chest roentgenogram may be within normal limits.

(3) In chronic bronchial asthma, the chest roentgenogram usually shows signs of hyperinflation, and sometimes diffuse fibrosis or chronic segmental fibrosis secondary to old infectious processes. Occasionally, evidence of mucoid impaction of the bronchi may be seen.

b. Restrictive lung disease.

(1) In the interstitial lung diseases, the chest roentgenogram demonstrates a linear, fibronodular, or fibroreticular infiltrate. Lytic lesions of the ribs or pneumothorax may be seen in histiocytosis. Kerley lines, pleural effusion, and mediastinal lymph node enlargement may be seen in lymphangitic carcinomatosis. A lung mass may also be demonstrable. In the interstitial lung disease due to connective tissue disease, pleural effusion or scarring may be seen. In scleroderma, a mediastinal air-fluid level may be demonstrated when the esophagus is involved. In sarcoidosis, hilar lymphadenopathy may be present. Silicosis may present with multiple interstitial nodules, which often coalesce in the upper lobes. Cavitary disease due to a superimposed mycobacterial infection may be present. In asbestosis, there can be seen a linear interstitial pattern, which may be associated with calcified plaques in the diaphragmatic pleura.

(2) In kyphoscoliosis, or after thoracoplasty, obvious skeletal deformity may be seen on the chest films.

(3) In pleural fibrosis, the pleural line is thickened and may be calcified.

(4) Alveolar-filling diseases demonstrate a characteristic acinar-filling pattern with air bronchograms, rosettes, and obliteration of the vascular markings. Early lipoid pneumonia and desquamative interstitial pneumonitis involve primarily the lower lobes.

2. Nonpulmonary causes.

a. Congestive heart failure. The radiographic picture of congestive heart failure is described on page 163.

b. Anemia. The chest roentgenogram is usually normal, although cardiomegaly may be present.

c. Hyperthyroidism. The chest films are usually normal, although the heart may be enlarged.

d. Upper airway disease. The chest roentgenogram may be normal, or there may be evidence of air trapping.

e. Obesity causes no significant pulmonary parenchymal infiltration, although cardiomegaly may be present. Because of the adiposity, the lung parenchyma may appear to be diffusely infiltrated if the chest films are underpenetrated.

Laboratory Data

1. CBC. Erythrocytosis may be seen in any pulmonary cause of chronic dyspnea. Low hemoglobin and hematocrit values are the diagnostic features of anemia. Leukocytosis may be seen in patients with chronic airway disease who have superimposed infection; it may also be seen in chronic congestive heart failure. Stress or spurious erythrocytosis may be seen in the obese hypertensive patient. Lymphocytosis is common in thyrotoxicosis, anemia, and connective tissue diseases. Abnormalities of the white blood cells may be seen in certain types of anemia. Eosinophilia may occur in chronic asthma.

2. Urinalysis. Changes in the urine sediment may be seen in the various connective tissue diseases, but these are nonspecific.

3. Blood chemistries. In chronic obstructive airway disease with alveolar hypoventilation, the serum bicarbonate may be increased. Dilutional hyponatremia may be seen in congestive heart failure. The serum calcium may be elevated in sarcoidosis. Serum creatinine and BUN may be elevated in renal failure due to the connective tissue diseases.

4. Sputum examination.   In chronic asthma, eosinophils are usually seen with the Wright's stain. The periodic acid Schiff stain is frequently positive in alveolar proteinosis. Sputum cytologic findings may be abnormal in alveolar cell carcinoma. In lipoid pneumonia, the Sudan III stain may be positive for fat-laden macrophages.

5. Electrocardiogram.   The electrocardiogram may show evidence of right axis deviation, right ventricular strain, atrial arrhythmia, and P pulmonale in all forms of chronic pulmonary disease. Evidence of left ventricular disease may be seen in chronic left-sided heart failure. Sinus tachycardia is frequently present in thyrotoxicosis and anemia.

6. Blood gases.   In all pulmonary causes of chronic dyspnea, hypoxemia may be present. Hypoventilation (defined as CO_2 retention) is seen more commonly in chronic bronchitis and thoracic cage deformities. Hyperventilation (low pCO_2) may be seen in interstitial lung disease. Hypoxemia, with or without CO_2 retention, may be seen in congestive heart failure. Arterial blood gases are usually normal in anemia, thyrotoxicosis, or upper airway disease. In obesity there may be mild hypoxemia.

7. Serum protein electrophoresis.   Electrophoresis may occasionally show a decrease or absence of alpha-1-globulin, particularly in younger patients with emphysema. If the alpha-1-globulin level is abnormal, specific assays for alpha-1-antitrypsin deficiency may be indicated.

Further Studies

From the foregoing data it should be possible to determine whether dyspnea is of pulmonary or nonpulmonary origin. Patients with pulmonary dyspnea should have ventilatory pulmonary function studies performed. In chronic obstructive airway disease, the ventilatory functions will show evidence of airway obstruction such as diminished FEV_1 and MMEF. Vital capacity may be normal or decreased, and there is usually an increase in the residual volume. In patients with a predominantly restrictive component (such as in interstitial fibrosis, chest wall deformities, and pleural diseases), ventilatory function usually shows a reduction in vital capacity and total lung capacity, but good flow rates (FEV_1, MMEF) are maintained. Lung biopsy may be indicated for medicolegal reasons in suspected pneumoconiosis, in the differential diagnosis of the alveolar-filling diseases, and in selected patients with interstitial fibrosis.

Wheezing
Marvin I. Schwarz
Paul M. Cox

Wheezing is a common complaint in patients with pulmonary disease. It may be caused by any of the following:

1. Large airway obstruction.
   a. Laryngeal stridor.
   b. Tracheal stenosis.
   c. Foreign body aspiration.

2. Endobronchial tumors and granulomas.

3. Bronchial asthma (including postexercise wheezing).

4. Acute bronchitis.

5. Chronic airway obstruction.

6. Acute left ventricular failure (cardiac asthma).

7. Pulmonary embolism.

Cough

Marvin I. Schwarz
Paul M. Cox

ACUTE COUGH

All the causes of acute dyspnea, with the possible exception of pneumothorax, may also present with cough of acute onset. The most frequent cause of this symptom in a previously healthy patient is acute bronchitis. The diagnosis of acute bronchitis is based on evidence of a preceding upper respiratory infection, followed by cough productive of mucoid or purulent sputum. Myalgias, headaches, malaise, fever, and an influenzal syndrome may be associated. The physical examination usually reveals nothing abnormal except evidence of upper respiratory tract inflammation, including the presence of rhonchi on auscultation. The chest roentgenogram is normal. Laboratory abnormalities, if any, are nonspecific.

CHRONIC COUGH

Etiology

Chronic cough is frequently found in the conditions causing chronic dyspnea. However, patients with pure emphysema, thoracic wall deformities, and pleural fibrosis, and patients with nonpulmonary causes of dyspnea may present without associated cough. Additional causes of chronic cough are bronchogenic carcinoma, benign endobronchial tumors, chronic granulomatous diseases including tuberculosis, sarcoidosis, fungal diseases, and lung abscess. Bronchiectasis, an important cause of chronic cough, is discussed in the following section, Hemoptysis.

History

1. Bronchogenic carcinoma.   Patients with bronchogenic carcinoma usually are heavy cigarette-smokers. In addition to cough, they may have hemoptysis and weight loss. Asbestosis and exposure to radioactive materials, as in uranium mining, frequently predispose individuals to development of bronchogenic carcinoma.

2. Bronchial adenoma.   Systemic symptoms are usually absent. Patients may complain of wheezing or give a history of recurrent pneumonia. Hemoptysis may be present.

3. Chronic granulomatous disease.   Persistent cough may be the only symptom. However, increased sputum production, hemoptysis, weight loss, fever, and night sweats are commonly associated. Patients with endobronchial sarcoidosis may have the same symptoms as those with fungal or tuberculous granulomatous disease. In addition, they may present with systemic symptoms such as arthralgias, arthritis, erythema nodosum, or a skin rash. Erythema nodosum may occur in histoplasmosis.

4. Lung abscess.   Patients with lung abscess are often alcoholics. Recent dental procedures, episodes of unconsciousness, and history of recent pneumonia due to staphylococci or gram-negative bacilli, in particular, are common antecedents. Halitosis, foul-smelling sputum, and fever are frequent complaints.

Physical Examination

1. Bronchogenic carcinoma.   In bronchogenic carcinoma, there may be evidence of malnutrition and weight loss. Lymphadenopathy may be present in the supraclavicular and infraclavicular areas. Bony metastases may be noted in the chest wall. Auscultation of the chest may reveal evidence of endobronchial obstruction manifested by localized wheezing, atelectasis, or pneumonia. Clubbing may be present. Evidence of metastatic disease may be noted in other organs, including the skin and the liver.

2. Bronchial adenoma.   In bronchial adenoma, abnormal physical findings are unusual. Occasionally there is evidence of unilateral or localized wheezing. Evidence of atelectasis is sometimes present on physical examination.

3. Granulomatous disease.   Granulomatous diseases may present without abnormal physical findings. Since the distribution of such diseases is usually apical and posterior, rales may be heard in these areas. When large cavities are present, characteristic cavernous breath sounds may be present. The symptoms in sarcoidosis are described in paragraph **3** above.

4. Lung abscess.   Clubbing, halitosis, rales, and cavernous breath sounds may be present.

Roentgenographic Findings

1. Bronchogenic carcinoma.   The chest roentgenograms of bronchogenic carcinoma may demonstrate a hilar mass associated with mediastinal lymphadenopathy or a single coin lesion. If the tumor partially or totally occludes a bronchus, evidence of volume loss in the form of elevation of the diaphragm or a shift of the lung fissures and hilar structures may appear. Another radiographic sign is a pneumonia distal to the obstruction. Lytic lesions may be seen in the ribs. Pleural effusion may also be present. If there is lymphangitic spread of the tumor, evidence of diffuse interstitial disease and Kerley lines may be seen.

2. Bronchial adenoma.   The most characteristic appearance of bronchial adenoma is that of a centrally placed, circumscribed mass with atelectasis distal to the lesion. A small number of cases may present as peripheral coin lesions.

3. Granulomatous diseases.   Evidence of a primary complex, i.e., a calcified mediastinal or hilar node on the same side as a calcified parenchymal lesion, may be noted in tuberculosis. Posterior and apical infiltrative disease or cavitary disease, or both, may be present. An apical pleural reaction and pleural effusion are commonly seen. In the more chronic cases, there may be evidence of upper lobe volume loss such as fibrotic streaking and retracted hilar structures. In sarcoidosis, the roentgenographic findings are variable. Bilateral and symmetric mediastinal and hilar lymphadenopathy is the most common radiographic presentation. This may be associated with alveolar or interstitial infiltrates, or both, early in the course of the disease. Pleural disease is rarely seen. In the more chronic stages of the disease, there is usually a diffuse interstitial infiltrate that may be linear or nodular, or a combination of the two. With further progression of the disease, bilateral upper lobe retraction with fibrotic streaking and cystic transformation may be seen.

4. Lung abscess.   Lung abscesses present radiographically as cavitary lesions, usually with air-fluid levels. An infiltrate may surround the cavity.

Laboratory Data

1. CBC.   Anemia may be seen in bronchogenic carcinoma, tuberculosis, fungus diseases, sarcoidosis, or lung abscess. The anemia may be hemolytic or may have the characteristics of anemia found in many chronic debilitating diseases. The white cell count may be elevated in all of these disorders, particularly if there is an associated infectious process. Leukemoid reactions have been reported in tuberculosis.

2. Urinalysis.   In patients with renal tuberculosis, white blood cells, with blood cell casts, proteinuria, and hematuria may be seen singly or in any combination. In patients who have bronchogenic carcinoma

associated with inappropriate antidiuretic hormone (ADH) secretion, dilute urine with low specific gravity and decreased osmolality may be excreted.

3. Electrolyte and serum enzyme abnormalities.

   a. Hyponatremia may occur in bronchogenic carcinoma with inappropriate ADH secretion or when adrenal insufficiency occurs as a result of adrenal metastasis. Hyponatremia is also not uncommon in tuberculosis. Although it may be secondary to inappropriate ADH secretion or adrenal insufficiency due to tuberculous involvement of the adrenal cortex, frequently no specific cause can be found. It usually disappears when treatment of the tuberculosis is instituted.

   b. Hypercalcemia may be seen in bronchogenic carcinoma, sarcoidosis, and certain bronchial carcinoid tumors.

   c. In bronchogenic carcinoma, sarcoidosis, and tuberculosis, abnormalities of liver function may occur as a result of liver involvement.

4. Sputum examination.   Sputum cytologic study may be diagnostic in carcinoma of the lung. Acid-fast stains are frequently positive in active tuberculosis, but they may be negative even when the culture is positive. Fungus organisms may be seen with special staining techniques. The sputum should be cultured for *Mycobacterium tuberculosis* and fungi. Gram stains may reveal the etiologic organism in lung abscess, but aerobic and anaerobic bacterial cultures should be obtained.

5. Electrocardiogram.   Electrocardiographic evidence of pericarditis may be seen in tuberculosis, sarcoidosis, and bronchogenic carcinoma with pericardial involvement. In sarcoidosis, the electrocardiogram may resemble that of myocardial infarction. Arrhythmias and atrioventricular conduction disturbances are seen commonly.

6. Skin testing and serologic study.

   a. PPD-S (Tween stabilized, TU or intermediate strength): Greater than 10 mm induration at 48 to 72 hours is strong evidence of infection with tuberculosis. However, a positive result does not necessarily indicate active tuberculosis or that tuberculosis is the cause of the patient's symptoms. False-negative findings may be due to anergy, improper technique, and other factors that are poorly understood. A negative skin test finding does not rule out tuberculosis. First- and second-strength PPD are not useful in the diagnosis of tuberculosis and should not be employed.

   b. Fungus skin tests probably should not be employed if active disease is suspected because they may affect the complement-fixation titers. Sera for fungus complement-fixation titers may be very helpful and are available anywhere in the United States through the Center for Disease Control in Atlanta, Georgia.

7. Other diagnostic procedures.

    a. With the new fiberoptic bronchoscopes, bronchoscopy has become a much safer, more comfortable procedure. It should be performed whenever the aforementioned tests do not lead to diagnosis and to determine the extent and resectability of tumors. A biopsy should be done at the time. Bronchial brushings may also be obtained. Postbronchoscopy sputa should be collected for cytologic study, acid-fast and fungus stains, and cultures, since they may be positive even when bronchoscopy or brush biopsy is negative. Bronchoscopy and brush biopsy may be necessary in lung abscess to restore drainage and obtain cultures.

    b. If bronchoscopy and bronchial brushing findings are normal, bronchography may be employed. This procedure is particularly helpful in outlining submucosal masses such as adenomas.

    c. Mediastinoscopy is useful for determining the resectability of bronchogenic carcinoma and for the diagnosis of sarcoidosis.

    d. In very rare instances, the procedures listed above may not lead to a diagnosis. Diagnostic thoracotomy may then be necessary.

Hemoptysis

Marvin I. Schwarz
Paul M. Cox

DEFINITION

Hemoptysis is the expectoration of blood or bloody sputum.

ETIOLOGY

Some of the important causes of hemoptysis have been described in earlier sections. These include infectious pneumonias, pulmonary embolism, bronchogenic carcinoma, mitral stenosis, chronic obstructive pulmonary disease, and tuberculosis and other granulomatous diseases. Other causes of hemoptysis include bronchiectasis, pulmonary arteriovenous malformations, pulmonary sequestration, idiopathic hemosiderosis, Goodpasture's syndrome, coagulation disorders, and intracavitary fungus balls (aspergillosis). Bronchitis is the most common cause.

HISTORY

    1. Bronchiectasis. Characteristically there is a history of repeated episodes of pneumonia or bronchitis. Chronic production of foul-smelling sputum is a classic finding, but it is not always present. Sinusitis is common. There may be a history of pertussis, measles, or other severe childhood pneumonia. Patients with cystic fibrosis may have a history of failure to thrive, meconium ileus, or a family history of same. Patients with immune disorders may have had recurrent nonpulmonary infections.

2. Pulmonary sequestration.   The history may be similar to that of bronchiectasis. In other instances, the patient may have been asymptomatic previously.

3. Idiopathic pulmonary hemosiderosis.   This condition usually occurs in children and young adults. Cough and hemoptysis are the usual symptoms. Anemia is a common accompaniment.

4. Goodpasture's syndrome.   The symptoms are similar to those in idiopathic pulmonary hemosiderosis, but in addition symptoms and signs of uremia may be present. The symptoms of renal disease may antedate those of pulmonary disease, or vice versa.

5. Coagulation disorders.   Patients with known coagulopathies or those on anticoagulant therapy may present with respiratory tract bleeding. Usually there is a history of bleeding from other sites (e.g., the skin, gastrointestinal tract, the nares).

6. Intracavitary fungus balls.   Aspergillomas are found only in patients with preexisting cavitary disease due to tuberculosis or other causes. They are more likely to be seen in older, debilitated patients.

7. Pulmonary arteriovenous malformations.   A family history of pulmonary arteriovenous malformations can be elicited in 60 percent of cases. Dyspnea is a common complaint. In addition to hemoptysis, the patient may have experienced epistaxis, hematemesis, or cerebral hemorrhage.

PHYSICAL EXAMINATION

1. Halitosis and clubbing are frequent in bronchiectasis. Examination of the chest may reveal signs of chronic airway obstruction, but the most consistent findings are coarse, "sticky" bibasilar rales. In localized bronchiectasis, the findings are confined to the area of involvement. Patients with Kartagener's syndrome have a triad of bronchiectasis, sinusitis, and situs inversus viscerum.

2. In pulmonary sequestration, there may be localized rales over the site of sequestration.

3. In idiopathic pulmonary hemosiderosis, diffuse or localized rales may be heard. Pallor secondary to anemia is common.

4. Patients with Goodpasture's syndrome demonstrate physical findings similar to those of idiopathic pulmonary hemosiderosis; signs of uremia may be present.

5. Coagulation disorders frequently show evidence of bleeding from multiple sites. Ecchymoses are quite common. Examination of the chest may reveal diffuse or localized rales.

6. An aspergilloma produces no characteristic physical findings, although findings of the preexisting condition (e.g., tuberculosis, lung abscess) may be present.

7. The physical findings associated with pulmonary arteriovenous malformations include clubbing, cyanosis, and telangiectasis in the skin and mucous membranes. On examination of the chest, continuous murmurs may be heard over the lesion.

ROENTGENOGRAPHIC FINDINGS

1. In bronchiectasis, the chest roentgenogram may be normal, or evidence of basilar fibrosis, with or without cystic changes, may be noted. In more severe cases, the fibrotic and cystic changes may be more diffuse. Cavity formation with air-fluid levels may be present. Situs inversus viscerum is evident in Kartagener's syndrome.

2. Pulmonary sequestration presents radiographically as a circumscribed shadow, usually in the left lower lobe and contiguous with the diaphragm.

3. In idiopathic pulmonary hemosiderosis, during the acute phase, evidence of diffuse or localized acinar-filling process may be seen. There may be resolution of these abnormalities or progression to an interstitial fibrotic pattern.

4. The roentgenographic findings in Goodpasture's syndrome are similar to those of idiopathic pulmonary hemosiderosis. The "butterfly" pattern of uremic pulmonary edema may be seen if the renal disease is severe.

5. The roentgenogram in hemoptysis due to coagulation disorders is similar to that of idiopathic pulmonary hemosiderosis and Goodpasture's syndrome.

6. An aspergilloma typically presents a mass within a cavity. When the patient is placed in the lateral decubitus position, movement of the mass may be noted.

7. A pulmonary arteriovenous malformation presents radiographically as a sharply defined, round or oval, homogeneous mass 1 to 5 cm in di-

ameter. It is usually in the lower lobes, and vascular structures may appear to be continuous with the mass.

LABORATORY DATA

1. **CBC.**   Iron deficiency anemia is normally seen in idiopathic pulmonary hemosiderosis and in Goodpasture's syndrome. Pulmonary arteriovenous malformations may have iron deficiency anemia secondary to recurrent bleeding, but more commonly, erythrocytosis secondary to chronic hypoxemia is seen. Rarely, massive hemoptysis may produce the picture of anemia due to acute blood loss.

2. Urinalysis.   Urinalysis is usually helpful in the diagnosis of Goodpasture's syndrome and may demonstrate evidence of nephritis.

3. Blood chemistries.   Laboratory findings of uremia may be present in Goodpasture's syndrome.

4. Examination of the sputum.   Patients with Goodpasture's syndrome or idiopathic pulmonary hemosiderosis show hemosiderin-laden macrophages in their sputum.

5. Electrocardiogram.   If pulmonary hypertension is present, there may be evidence of right axis deviation, right ventricular hypertrophy, and P pulmonale.

6. Other diagnostic procedures.
   a. Pulmonary function tests are of little value in differentiating between the various disorders. However, in bronchiectasis there may be evidence of obstruction to air flow. A patient with idiopathic pulmonary hemosiderosis or Goodpasture's syndrome may have a restrictive defect and reduction of the diffusing capacity.
   b. Bronchograms are diagnostic in saccular bronchiectasis.
   c. Arteriography.   In a patient with suspected pulmonary sequestration, aortography should be done.
   d. Biopsy.   In patients with suspected Goodpasture's syndrome, a lung or renal biopsy should be performed, with immunofluorescent staining of the tissue. Patients with suspected idiopathic pulmonary hemosiderosis should have a lung biopsy.
   e. Serologic tests.   Precipitating antibodies may be present in aspergillosis.
   f. Coagulation screening should be performed when coagulopathies are suspected.
   g. Miscellaneous studies.   Sweat chlorides are elevated in cystic fibrosis. Increased fecal excretion of fat may be noted in cases of untreated cystic fibrosis and in some immune disorders. Serum globulins are usually abnormal in immunologic diseases.

h. Bronchoscopy should be performed when it is necessary to rule out intraluminal disease.

Cyanosis

Marvin I. Schwarz
Paul M. Cox

DEFINITION

Cyanosis is a bluish color of the skin and mucous membranes, usually due to the presence of at least 5 gm of reduced hemoglobin in the circulating blood. Although cyanosis frequently indicates arterial oxygen unsaturation, it reflects the degree of hypoxemia imperfectly. Not all cyanosis is related to the presence of increased amounts of reduced hemoglobin in the blood. Severe cyanosis, for example, may be due to the presence of abnormal pigments (methemoglobin or sulfhemoglobin) within the red blood cells.

ETIOLOGY

Cyanosis may be classified as central or peripheral. *Central cyanosis* usually results from arterial hypoxemia caused by right-to-left cardiac shunts, pulmonary arteriovenous fistula, or acute or chronic pulmonary disease. It may occur in polycythemia vera in the absence of arterial oxygen unsaturation because of the presence of an increased amount of reduced hemoglobin in the blood. In central cyanosis, both the skin and the mucous membranes are blue. Polycythemia and digital clubbing are commonly present when cyanosis is severe. *Peripheral cyanosis* is caused by stagnant circulation through the peripheral vascular beds. Arterial oxygen saturation is normal unless cardiopulmonary disease is also present. The cyanosis primarily affects the exposed portions of the body, such as the hands, ears, nose, cheeks, and feet. Peripheral cyanosis may be generalized or localized. Peripheral cyanosis may be caused by exposure to cold, nervous tension, reduced cardiac output, or vascular obstruction.

In the adult, pulmonary disease, especially chronic obstructive airway disease, is the most common cause of central cyanosis. Intracardiac right-to-left shunts are less common causes. Peripheral cyanosis is most commonly due to exposure to cold or emotional tension.

Central Cyanosis

1. Cyanotic congenital heart disease (e.g., tetralogy of Fallot, Eisenmenger's syndrome, trilogy of Fallot, tricuspid atresia, Ebstein's anomaly, transposition of the great vessels, pulmonary arteriovenous fistula).

2. Pulmonary disease.
   a. Acute (e.g., pneumonia, pulmonary embolism, atelectasis).
   b. Chronic.
      (1) Obstructive airway disease.
      (2) Restrictive lung diseases.

3. Hemoglobin abnormalities (methemoglobinemia, sulfhemoglobinemia).
   a. Congenital.
   b. Acquired.

Peripheral Cyanosis

1. Reduced cardiac output (e.g., congestive heart failure, mitral stenosis).
2. Exposure to cold, including Raynaud's phenomenon.
3. Arterial obstruction.
4. Venous obstruction.

HISTORY

Central Cyanosis

1. Cyanotic congenital heart disease.   There may be a history of cyanosis, dyspnea, a heart murmur, syncope, squatting, congestive heart failure, or other cardiac symptoms dating from birth or childhood.

2. Pulmonary disease.   The most common presenting symptoms are dyspnea, cough, sputum production, wheezing, hemoptysis, and recurrent pulmonary infections.

3. Hemoglobin abnormalities.
   a. Congenital (deficiency of NADH diaphorase; hemoglobin M disease): A history of cyanosis from birth may be elicited in these types of methemoglobinemia.
   b. Acquired (methemoglobinemia; sulfhemoglobinemia): A history of exposure to chemicals or drugs may be obtained. The chief offenders are nitrates, nitrites, chlorates, quinones, certain aniline dyes, acetanilid, sulfonamides, and phenacetin.

Peripheral Cyanosis

1. Decreased cardiac output.   A history of mitral stenosis, myocardial infarction, or other etiologic types of heart disease usually can be elicited. In cases due to shock, evidence of hemorrhage, gram-negative sepsis, or other underlying disease may be obtained.

2. Exposure to cold (including Raynaud's phenomenon): A history of exposure to cold is usually obvious. In Raynaud's phenomenon, paroxysmal pain, pallor, and cyanosis followed by redness, usually involving the fingers, occur upon exposure to cold or emotional stress.

3. Arterial obstruction.   A history of antecedent intermittent claudication if often obtainable from patients with arterial occlusion. Diabetes predisposes individuals to arterial insufficiency. When arterial obstruction is embolic, the source is often a mural thrombus from mitral stenosis or myocardial infarction, or a bacterial vegetation in infective endocarditis.

4. Venous obstruction.   There may be a long history of varicose veins, thrombophlebitis, edema, previous leg trauma, or immobilization.

PHYSICAL EXAMINATION

Central Cyanosis

There is bluish discoloration of the skin and mucous membranes.

1. Right-to-left shunt.   Cardiac murmur(s) and evidence of right-sided cardiac enlargement are present.

2. Pulmonary disease.   See the section Dyspnea, earlier in the chapter.

3. Clubbing is common in severe central cyanosis but is absent in cyanosis due to hemoglobin abnormalities.

Peripheral Cyanosis

There is discoloration of only the distal extremities or nail beds.

1. Decreased cardiac output.   Hypertension, tachycardia, cold moist extremities, decreased urinary output, and mental confusion are common. Signs of shock may be noted. Evidence of underlying heart disease may be present.

2. Raynaud's phenomenon.   Evidence of underlying disease such as scleroderma, systemic lupus erythematosus, and the cryoglobulinemias may be noted unless the condition is idiopathic (Raynaud's disease).

3. Arterial obstruction.   Signs of arterial occlusion are present.

4. Venous obstruction.   Signs of venous disease such as varicose veins, edema, ulceration, and increased pigmentation of the skin may be noted.

CHEST ROENTGENOGRAPHIC FINDINGS

Characteristic roentgenographic findings may be noted in certain types of heart disease and in pulmonary disease. Otherwise, chest films are of little or no diagnostic help in the evaluation of cyanosis.

LABORATORY DATA

1. **CBC.** Erythrocytosis may be seen in right-to-left shunts and in chronic pulmonary disease.

2. **Urinalysis.** The urinalysis may be abnormal in Raynaud's phenomenon associated with connective tissue disease and renal involvement. The abnormal findings include proteinuria, hematuria, and cylindruria.

3. **Serum electrolytes.** The serum bicarbonate level may be elevated in any patient with chronic alveolar hypoventilation. The BUN may be elevated in circulatory collapse and decreased cardiac output, and in patients with renal hypoperfusion. Acute hepatic injury may be reflected in abnormal liver function tests in patients with circulatory collapse. Liver function tests may also be abnormal in patients with cor pulmonale and chronic passive congestion of the liver. Serum levels of LDH, SGOT, and CPK may be elevated in patients with arterial and venous obstruction because of skeletal muscle damage. In these patients, the serum bilirubin, serum proteins, and prothrombin time usually are normal.

4. **Electrocardiogram.** In patients with right-to-left shunt, the electrocardiogram may show findings related to the underlying disease. In patients with pulmonary disease, there may be evidence suggestive of chronic obstructive pulmonary disease with or without cor pulmonale. The electrocardiogram is usually normal in patients with Raynaud's phenomenon, but in those with connective tissue disease, evidence of pericardial or myocardial involvement may be noted. In patients with circulatory collapse, a pattern simulating myocardial infarction is sometimes seen.

5. **Arterial blood gases.** Hypoxemia will be seen in all conditions causing central cyanosis. Usually the arterial tension is normal in patients with peripheral cyanosis. Determination of pO_2 is thus useful in differentiating between central and peripheral causes of cyanosis. The arterial pCO_2 level is usually elevated in patients who are cyanotic from chronic alveolar hypoventilation.

6. **Ventilatory function tests.** Ventilatory function tests demonstrate a characteristic obstructive pattern in patients with chronic obstructive pulmonary disease. A restricted pattern is observed in patients with interstitial fibrosing diseases of the lung. A restrictive or obstructive pattern, or both, may be seen in patients with left ventricular failure.

7. **Other procedures.**
   a. Arterial blood gases drawn while the patient is breathing 100 percent oxygen often show large alveolar-arterial gradients (greater than 100 mm Hg) in patients with right-to-left shunts and pulmonary arteriovenous fistulas. Large alveolar-arterial gradients may also be seen in advanced obstructive or restrictive pulmonary dis-

ease. These are easily differentiated from shunts by the association of markedly abnormal ventilatory function tests.

b. Cardiac catheterization and pulmonary angiography may be indicated for the diagnosis of congenital cyanotic heart disease and pulmonary arteriovenous fistulas.

c. Mass spectroscopy of a hemoglobin sample is employed to confirm the diagnosis of methemoglobinemia or sulfhemoglobinemia.

Acute Pulmonary Radiographic Abnormalities

William C. Earley

Acute pulmonary lesions often pose problems in differential diagnosis. Pneumonia, pulmonary edema, pulmonary infarction, atelectasis, and pulmonary embolism are the entities usually involved.

ACUTE PARENCHYMAL INFILTRATES

Excluding neoplasm, parenchymal infiltrates are of three basic types: alveolar, interstitial, and mixed. This differentiation is frequently of considerable help in determining the etiology of an infiltrate. On chest films, interstitial infiltrates are linear, linear-nodular, or nodular, with the nodules generally less than 5 mm in diameter. Alveolar infiltrates tend to be fluffy in appearance, with poorly defined borders, they commonly involve segments of lobes or entire lobes, and they frequently demonstrate air bronchograms.

PNEUMONIA

Although the radiographic patterns are quite variable and nonspecific, the following points may prove helpful in the diagnosis of pneumonia. Pneumonia due to aspiration may involve any or all segments of both lungs but is more generally seen in the most dependent portions of the lung. Thus, with the patient lying supine, the most dependent parts of the lung are the posterior segments of the upper lobes. Bacterial pneumonia is likely to present an alveolar pattern and involve segments of the lungs asymmetrically. Viral pneumonia tends to be interstitial in pattern and more symmetrical and diffuse in distribution. It should be emphasized that these are generalities and that overlapping of patterns and exceptions may occur.

PULMONARY EDEMA

Pulmonary edema is most commonly caused by left-sided heart failure, but it may also be the result of other conditions, such as iatrogenic fluid overloading, an allergic reaction to medications (particularly blood transfusions), or the acute adult respiratory distress syndrome.

The lung changes in left-sided heart failure usually include the following: (1) pulmonary congestion, manifested by distended upper lobe veins, (2) interstitial edema, demonstrable primarily as narrow, linear strands perpendicular to the nearest pleural surface in the lower lobes, lamellar markings in the upper lobes, a hilar or a peripheral haze or both, and at times thickened interlobar fissures, and (3) alveolar edema, appearing typically as a fluffy infiltrate that tends to involve both lungs symmetrically but is nonetheless quite variable in appearance.

ATELECTASIS

Atelectasis, or consolidation collapse of the lung, is discussed separately in the next section. However, it is important to realize that atelectasis is the most common postoperative respiratory complication. Plate, disc, or focal atelectasis is the variety most commonly encountered. The appearance of plate atelectasis is that of a rather thin, streaky density, usually located toward the lung bases. These densities are approximately perpendicular to the long axis of the body, but considerable variation is seen. Parenchymal scars from previous inflammatory disease or infarcts are the major differential possibilities. Large areas of atelectasis involving segments, lobes, or entire lungs are seen less frequently, but it is important to recognize them because they may represent serious disease. The major condition to be differentiated from lobar collapse, particularly in the lower lobes, is an encapsulated pleural effusion. The differentiation may be difficult or impossible, but two points may be helpful: (1) Signs of lobar collapse are usually not associated with encapsulated effusions. (2) Decubitus films may occasionally demonstrate fluid shifts with a change in body position.

PULMONARY EMBOLISM WITH INFARCTION

Pulmonary embolism that goes on to infarction may show an area of alveolar infiltrate near a pleural surface. Sometimes an infarct may be seen as a homogeneous density with its base adjacent to a pleural surface and its convexity directed toward the hilum. A resolving infarct may appear as a rather broad, streaky density, much like an area of plate atelectasis. The roentgenographic findings in infarction and infection may be identical, and the differentiation between the two entities cannot be made on the basis of chest films alone.

PULMONARY EMBOLISM WITHOUT INFARCTION

Pulmonary embolism without infarction frequently shows little or no abnormality in chest roentgenograms. Plain films may show pleural effusion, decreased vascularity of a lobe or a segment of a lobe, serial changes in the main pulmonary arteries due to alterations of blood flow, or a parenchymal infiltrate. None of these findings is specific for embolism.

Pulmonary angiography, although it is an accurate method for the diagnosis of pulmonary embolism, is not completely free of hazard and is difficult to perform in an emergency. Its major drawback diagnostically is its frequent failure to demonstrate small peripheral emboli satisfactorily.

Lung scans are often of value in the diagnosis of pulmonary embolism. The commonly performed perfusion scan consists of the intravenous injection of myriads of tiny particles labeled with a radioisotope to permit detection of their distribution. The particles act like microemboli that ultimately lodge in the capillaries and precapillary arterioles. Although the procedure is safe and there are no contraindications to its use, abnormal perfusion scans are not specific for embolism. Such conditions as pneumonia, chronic bronchitis, emphysematous bullae, asthma, neoplasm, pleural effusion, and congestive heart failure may also produce abnormal scans. When interpreting lung scans, it is imperative to have a current chest film available for comparison. The perfusion scan is most useful when the chest film is normal or, if abnormal, when no lesion is demonstrable at the site of the abnormal scan.

Even in patients with normal chest films and abnormal perfusion scans, it is not always possible to be certain of the diagnosis of embolism because of the presence of preexisting or coexisting disease. In such cases, a ventilation lung scan may be helpful. In this procedure, the patient inhales a radioactively labeled gas, usually xenon, and its distribution in the lungs (ventilation pattern) is recorded. Rapid sequence images are then made serially during quiet respiration to reveal the pattern and rapidity of washout of the gas. Normally, most of the xenon is gone from the lungs in about 1 minute. Chronic obstructive pulmonary disease characteristically shows a slight delay in ventilation but a marked delay in the washout from involved areas. As with perfusion scans, ventilation scans may be abnormal in the presence of a parenchymal infiltrate.

An abnormal perfusion scan in association with a normal ventilation scan is considered diagnostic of pulmonary embolism. In pulmonary embolism with infarction, both perfusion scans and ventilation scans are abnormal.

Table 4-1 lists the results of perfusion and ventilation scans in commonly occurring disease entities.

TABLE 4-1.   Perfusion and Ventilation Scans in the Differential Diagnosis of Pulmonary Lesions

Disease	Perfusion Scan	Ventilation Scan
Embolism without infarction	No perfusion	Normal ventilation
Pneumonia	No perfusion	No ventilation
Embolism with infarction (infiltrate in lungs)	No perfusion	Decreased to no ventilation
Emphysematous bullae	No perfusion	Delayed ventilation; delayed washout
Chronic bronchitis	Decreased perfusion	Normal to delayed ventilation; delayed washout

Consolidation Collapse of the Lung

Stanley B. Reich

DEFINITION

Occasionally, patients present with consolidation collapse, or atelectasis, of the lung on routine chest roentgenograms. This loss of volume of a segment, a lobe, or the whole lung is shown primarily by increased density of the area because of replacement of the air by fluid and displacement of the fissures because of the volume loss. Secondary changes include elevation of the diaphragm, shift of the mediastinum, approximation of the ribs, and overinflation of the remainder of the lung, shown by alteration of vascular shadows. This condition is also called atelectasis, but consolidation collapse is a more precise and descriptive term.

ETIOLOGY

1. The most serious cause is an endobronchial lesion, such as bronchogenic carcinoma, which causes absorption of air and collection of secretions. The symptoms and signs of infection or irritation may or may not be present.

2. Another cause is passive collapse secondary to adjacent disease, such as pleural effusion, pneumothorax, or thoracoplasty. These conditions usually can be easily identified on the roentgenogram.

3. Adhesive collapse occurs in conditions in which surfactant is diminished, as in the acute respiratory distress syndrome of infants or adults, or following cardiac bypass surgery. These entities usually can be recognized clinically, but radiographic studies are useful in following the progress of the disease.

4. Cicatrization as a result of prior infection and fibrosis may also cause this radiographic appearance. Patients may be asymptomatic at the time of examination but may recall the previous infection responsible for the condition.

5. Occasionally an acute or subacute inflammatory lesion or a pulmonary embolus may cause consolidation and loss of volume of a lung. Improvement and ultimate clearing of the involved lung may take a period of time varying from days to months.

DIAGNOSTIC APPROACH

1. As a first step, all prior films should be obtained if they are available. This may help in determining the time of onset of the disease process.

2. If the changes were present previously and are slowly progressive, a neoplasm must be excluded by bronchoscopy or bronchial brushing, or both.

3. If the lesion was present previously but has remained unchanged for a period of 6 months to 1 year, bronchoscopy, brushing for cytologic and bacteriologic study, and probably bronchography are indicated to exclude an indolent neoplasm or a chronic inflammatory lesion with fibrotic changes.

4. If the lesion was present previously but has remained unchanged for a year or two, further observation with films taken at 2- to 3-month intervals is probably warranted. During this time noninterventional investigation can be carried out (e.g., sputum cytologic and bacteriologic studies).

5. If the lesion was not present previously, it may be observed for a 2- to 3-week period while the usual clinical noninterventional investigation is pursued. If the lesion clears completely in that period, no further studies may be necessary except for follow-up films in approximately 3 months. If a residual infiltrate remains or if symptoms persist, it becomes necessary to do bronchoscopy and bronchial brushing because neoplasms may show temporary improvement with clearing of an associated inflammatory reaction.

6. If pulmonary embolism is suspected, a lung perfusion scan should be done to look for other areas of decreased vascular perfusion. If they are found, a radioactively labeled xenon inhalation scan can help exclude other lung diseases (see p. 164).

Coin Lesions of the Lung
Alan D. Rothberg

DEFINITION

Solitary nodules of the lung discovered on chest films, called coin lesions, are a frequent diagnostic dilemma. Coin lesions are usually defined as discrete intrapulmonary lesions under 6 cm in size. They may be of any shape but are usually somewhat rounded.

ETIOLOGY

Numerous conditions can produce coin lesions in the lung. The most common causes are healed granulomas from tuberculosis or fungus disease, primary pulmonary malignancies, pulmonary metastases, arteriovenous malformations, and pulmonary hamartomas. Less common causes are parasitic infestations, bronchial adenomas, multiple myeloma, rheumatoid nodules, and amyloidosis.

DIAGNOSTIC APPROACH

1. The primary problem confronting the physician is to determine whether or not the lesion is malignant. If calcification can be demonstrated within the lesion, it almost certainly is either a pulmonary harmartoma or a healed granuloma. Therefore, the initial studies in these patients are directed at determining whether or not calcification is present.

2. Examination of the initial films is most helpful. Calcification within the lesion can often be determined by this study alone, and if this is the case, further work-up is generally not needed.

3. When calcification is not demonstrable in conventional films, coned views of the lesion may be extremely helpful in bringing out calcification. Frequently, a coned grid film will demonstrate fine calcifications that are not visible in plain films.

4. If coned films do not help, tomography should be performed. It will not only demonstrate smaller calcifications but will clearly determine whether the calcifications are within the lesion. Tomograms are also helpful in the diagnosis of arteriovenous malformations, since they will often demonstrate the draining veins and feeding arteries. Furthermore, tomograms can verify that a nodule is within the lung and not outside of it.

5. Irregular calcification within a lesion, resembling popcorn in appearance, is almost pathognomonic of pulmonary hamartomas.

6. When the entire lesion is calcified, it is sometimes difficult to appreciate the calcification. The nodule then presents a homogeneous density much like uncalcified nodules. The difference is only in density, and recognition of somewhat increased density in a nodule is sometimes the only clue to the diagnosis. Comparison with rib density is often helpful.

7. Certain specific aids are helpful in occasional cases. Patients with neurocutaneous syndromes (e.g., the Sturge-Weber syndrome) often have pulmonary nodules that are arteriovenous malformations. When feeding arteries and draining veins are not demonstrable on conventional films or tomograms, pulmonary angiography will clearly identify the lesion.

8. If calcium cannot be demonstrated in a solitary nodule, and previous studies either are not available for comparison or yield negative findings, there is about a 50 percent chance that the lesion is malignant even if located peripherally. Peripheral malignancies account for ap-

proximately 60 percent of all lung cancers. The presence of a scar in the region of the nodule is not helpful in excluding malignancy since about 20 percent of all pulmonary carcinomas occur in scarred areas.

9. Opinions differ as to how to proceed with uncalcified solitary pulmonary nodules. The following guidelines are recommended:

   a. In the asymptomatic patient, radiographic studies should be repeated 1 month later, proceeding in the meantime with sputum cultures and other appropriate studies for the diagnosis of tuberculosis and fungus disease. If evidence of active tuberculosis is discovered, treatment should be instituted and the nodule followed radiographically at monthly intervals for an additional 2- to 3-month period. If the lesion remains unchanged in size or enlarges during this period of time, it should be excised.

   b. Immediate surgical resection is also indicated if after 1 month of study the cause of the nodule is still undetermined and the lesion either has remained unchanged in size or grown larger.

   c. On the other hand, if the lesion becomes smaller during the 1-month observation period, it is likely that the nodule represents an atypical inflammatory or embolic lesion rather than a neoplasm. Under these circumstances, a more conservative approach is probably warranted. It is then appropriate to continue taking chest films monthly for an additional 3-month period, and once the lesion has stabilized, at intervals of 6 months or longer.

   d. Some authorities recommend percutaneous lung biopsy and bronchial brushing prior to surgical exploration for uncalcified coin lesions. These procedures are of greatest value in patients who are poor operative risks since negative results do not exclude malignancy.

Mediastinal Masses
John C. Riley

THE MEDIASTINUM

The mediastinum is the extrapleural space within the thorax lying between the lungs. It is bounded by the sternum anteriorly, the paravertebral regions posteriorly, the thoracic inlet superiorly, and the diaphragm inferiorly. The aerated lungs outline the structures within the mediastinum.

The mediastinum may be divided into three compartments: anterior, middle, and posterior. The anterior mediastinum contains the thymus, trachea, ascending aorta, caval vessels, and pericardium. The middle mediastinum contains the hilar regions, including the lymph nodes, bifurcation of the trachea, arch of the aorta, and the heart. The posterior mediastinum, lying behind the heart, contains the descending aorta, the lower portion of the esophagus, and part of the sympathetic chain.

TABLE 4-2. Sites of Predilection of Mediastinal Masses

Anterior Mediastinum	Middle Mediastinum	Posterior Mediastinum
Lymphoma	Bronchogenic cysts	Neurogenic tumors
Thymoma	Lymph node disease	Meningocele
Substernal goiter	Lymphoma	Aneurysm of the aorta
Teratoma	Pericardial cysts	Abscess
Parathyroid adenoma	Neural tumors (vagus)	Hematoma
Vascular abnormalities	Tracheal tumors	Extramedullary
Pericardial cysts and tumors	Vascular abnormalities	hematopoiesis
Mesothelioma	Esophageal lesions	
Hematoma	Hematoma	
Hernias (Morgagni)	Hiatal hernia	
Aneurysm of the ascending aorta	Bronchogenic carcinomas	

ETIOLOGY

Each type of mediastinal tumor has a predilection for one of the three mediastinal compartments. Table 4-2 lists the common causes of mediastinal masses according to the region in the mediastinum where they are most likely to be found. About 55 percent of mediastinal tumors occur in the anterior mediastinum, 30 percent in the middle mediastinum, and 15 percent in the posterior mediastinum. Approximately 50 percent of all mediastinal tumors are malignant.

The masses found most commonly in the anterior mediastinum include thymomas, aneurysms of the ascending aorta, teratomas, substernal goiters, and lymphomas. In the middle mediastinum, bronchogenic carcinomas, lymphomas, and bronchogenic cysts occur most frequently. In the posterior mediastinum, most masses are of neurogenic origin, but aneurysms of the descending aorta often masquerade as posterior mediastinal neoplasms.

It is important to note that about 90 percent of middle mediastinal lesions are either primary or metastatic malignancies. Bilateral hilar lymph node enlargement is usually due to lymphoma but may occasionally be due to sarcoidosis. Unilateral lymphadenopathy is usually caused by a central or peripheral lesion of the lung, such as bronchogenic carcinoma or infection.

DIAGNOSTIC APPROACH

1. The history and physical examination are usually of little value in the diagnosis of mediastinal tumors. Usually the diagnosis is established by routine chest roentgenograms. Symptoms such as cough, dyspnea, hemoptysis, and chest pain may be noted, but they are nonspecific. The occurrence of facial edema, hoarseness, nonpulsatile distention of the neck veins, or Horner's syndrome may suggest compression or displacement due to mediastinal structures. A history of anorexia,

weakness, fever, and weight loss in association with generalized lymph-adenopathy suggests lymphoma, Hodgkin's disease, or leukemia.

2. Routine PA and lateral chest films may be adequate for the detection and localization of mediastinal masses. More commonly, overpene-trated or high-kilovoltage AP and oblique supine Bucky films are necessary for this purpose. They are invaluable in determining the position, configuration, density, and content of mediastinal masses, as well as their relationship to the surrounding structures.

3. Observation of the barium-filled esophagus with both films and fluo-roscopy, in addition to detecting hiatal hernia, may give important information concerning mediastinal abnormalities. Its most important purpose is to distinguish between extrinsic and intrinsic lesions of the esophagus.

4. Fluoroscopy of the chest may also be of value. If a lesion moves with respiration, it is more likely to be in the lung than in the mediastinum.

5. When it is difficult, on the basis of PA, lateral, or overpenetrated films, to establish whether a mass is mediastinal or parenchymal, to-mography will usually reveal the anatomic location of the lesion. Moreover, if the tomograms show an air bronchogram within the lesion, the lesion is much more likely to be parenchymal than extra-pleural.

6. Certain radiologic signs may provide clues to the causes of mediastinal tumors. These are discussed below.

   a. Content of the lesion.   The presence of fat in the lesion suggests mediastinal teratoma, lipoma, fat pad, omental hernia, or hiber-noma. Curvilinear calcifications suggest a cyst or an aneurysm, but they may also be seen in thymomas or thyroid adenomas. An anterior calcified mass in a patient with myasthenia gravis is al-most certainly a thymoma. A tooth is a sign of teratoma; and a phlebolith, of a hemangioma. Gas in the mediastinum may occur in hiatal hernia, ruptured esophagus, or pneumomediastinum. Usually, these conditions can be easily differentiated from one another.

   b. Configuration of the mass.   The configuration of mediastinal masses may have diagnostic significance. A huge esophagus, di-lated from stricture, achalasia, or tumor, is likely to be long and broad, and to contain an air-fluid level. Benign pericardial cysts, which are inseparable from the cardiac silhouette and occur most frequently in the anterior cardiophrenic angle, typically appear as sharply defined lesions of soft-tissue density. They may or may not transmit the cardiac pulsations. Thymic tumors in adults are irregular but smoothly outlined anterior mediastinal masses. Tera-tomas are usually well-defined structures containing hair, bone, or teeth. Substernal goiters merge with the soft tissues of the neck, move with swallowing, and tend to displace the trachea. Lymphomas may occur as frequently in the anterior as in the middle mediastinum and usually appear as dense, rounded masses. Bronchogenic cysts usually present as oval, sharply demarcated, soft-tissue densities that compress adjacent structures. Neural tumors in the posterior mediastinum may have a dumbbell or hourglass configuration.

c. Change in size. The rapidity of growth of a mass is of limited diagnostic value because benign lesions may grow quickly and malignant ones slowly.

d. Evidence of disease in other locations. It is almost certain that a mediastinal mass is metastatic in a young male with a testicular carcinoma. Enlarged mediastinal nodes are frequently found in lymphomas, leukemia, Hodgkin's disease, tuberculosis, and sarcoidosis. Paraspinal widening in a young child strongly suggests abdominal neuroblastoma.

7. In the presence of lymphadenopathy, skin tests for tuberculosis, histoplasmosis, coccidioidomycosis, and sarcoidosis may be indicated. Bone marrow examination and scalene or other lymph node biopsy may also be advisable.

8. Sputum cultures should be performed if tuberculosis or fungus disease is suspected.

9. If the diagnosis cannot be established on the basis of the foregoing studies, or if confirmation of a presumptive diagnosis is necessary, one or more of the following procedures may be indicated.

10. Angiography is an accurate method of diagnosing vascular lesions of the mediastinum and determining their nature, extent, and resectability. Thoracic aortography is useful in demonstrating aneurysms, malformations of the aorta, and vascular tumors. Angiocardiography is helpful in establishing the presence of a ventricular aneurysm and distinguishing it from pericardial cysts or mediastinal tumors. Pericardial effusions may also be evaluated in this manner, although echocardiography and radioisotope scans are more practical and less hazardous for this purpose. Venography is useful when searching for anomalies or obstruction of the superior vena cava. Selective arteriography is of help in studying parathyroid adenomas and thymomas.

11. Substernal goiters are easily demonstrated on scans following the administration of radioactive iodine. Cardiac isotope scanning may help in the diagnosis of pericardial effusion.

12. Bronchoscopy and bronchography may be of value in delineating displacement of the trachea or bronchi or for the detection of endobronchial lesions (e.g., bronchogenic carcinoma).

13. Myelography is employed to determine involvement of the spinal canal by posterior neural tumors and may be important in the diagnosis of anterior meningoceles.

14. Ultrasound is often valuable in the diagnosis of pericardial effusion and other cardiac abnormalities. It may also be helpful in the evaluation of aneurysms and in differentiating between cystic and solid masses.

15. Pneumomediastinography has been of value in the past in the diagnosis of mediastinal tumors. It is rarely used nowadays.

16. The final step in any approach to mediastinal tumors, unless the diagnosis has been established by other means, is a biopsy of the lesion by either thoracotomy or mediastinoscopy.

17. It is dangerous and inadvisable to "treat" a mediastinal tumor by observation. Every effort must be made to establish a diagnosis promptly to insure proper treatment. If the lesion is malignant, it may be curable by surgery even though the resectability rate is low. An aggressive approach is also warranted in the diagnosis of benign lesions of the mediastinum because life-threatening complications may ensue if the lesion is not treated appropriately.

Differential Diagnosis of Pleural Effusion

Marvin I. Schwarz
Paul M. Cox

The diagnostic features of pleural effusions are shown in Table 4-3. In the evaluation of a pleural effusion, it is important first to determine whether it is an exudate or a transudate. If it is believed to be an exudate, additional diagnostic studies (e.g., cytologic study, culture, biopsy) must be undertaken. If the fluid is a transudate, attention should be directed to the underlying cause of the effusion (e.g., congestive heart failure, cirrhosis of the liver, nephrotic syndrome, hypoproteinemia). Exudates are characterized by one or more of the following features: a pleural fluid-to-serum protein ratio greater than 0.5, a pleural fluid lactic dehydrogenase (LDH) greater than 200 IU, and a pleural fluid-to-serum LDH ratio greater than 0.6. Transudates exhibit none of these abnormalities.

TABLE 4-3. Differential Diagnosis of Pleural Effusion

Etiology	Characteristics of Effusion	Clinical Findings	Laboratory Findings and Diagnostic Procedures
Transudates: Protein less than 3 gm/100 ml with normal serum protein concentration			
Congestive heart failure	Usually right-sided, but may be bilateral; may be localized to an interlobar fissure	Orthopnea, paroxysmal nocturnal dyspnea, tachycardia, cardiomegaly, gallop rhythm, murmurs, rales, peripheral edema	Chest films; electrocardiogram
Cirrhosis	Right-sided, occasionally left-sided or bilateral	Ascites, peripheral edema, physical signs of cirrhosis	Liver function tests; liver biopsy
Nephrotic syndrome	Bilateral or unilateral	Generalized edema; periorbital edema is characteristic; pallor	Cylindruria and proteinuria, hypoalbuminemia, hyperlipidemia
Meigs' syndrome	Usually right-sided, occasionally left-sided or bilateral; rarely, effusion is bloody; no malignant cells present	Benign or malignant ovarian tumor, rarely uterine fibroma; ascites always present	Removal of the tumor resolves the effusion and ascites
Exudates: Protein greater than 3 gm/100 ml with normal serum protein concentration			
Bacterial or viral pneumonia	Same side as infiltrate; polymorphonuclear leukocytes; **no** organisms seen; may be loculated	Pleuritic pain; friction rub may be present; may see recurrence of fever	Precedes clinical picture of pneumonia; usually reabsorbed within 2 weeks
Pulmonary infarction	May be serosanguinous; polymorphonuclear leukocytes	Pleuritic pain, friction rub, fever; right ventricular heave; murmur of pulmonary insufficiency; increased P₂, right-sided S₁ or S₃	Positive radioisotope scans; pulmonary angiography may also be diagnostic
Tuberculosis	Lymphocytic pleural effusion; may be serosanguinous; acid-fast organisms rarely seen; increased cholesterol content if chronic	Usually pleuritic pain and fever in young adults; frequently asymptomatic	Positive skin test; pleural biopsy with histopathologic and bacteriologic studies

TABLE 4-3. (*Continued*)

Etiology	Characteristics of Effusion	Clinical Findings	Laboratory Findings and Diagnostic Procedures
Rheumatoid arthritis	Polymorphonuclear leukocytes; glucose low; cholesterol may be elevated; rheumatoid factor may be positive in high titers, but this is nonspecific; LDH elevated	More common in males; other systemic rheumatoid involvement (e.g., arthritis, subcutaneous nodules)	Positive serum rheumatoid factor; biopsy of subcutaneous nodule or synovium rarely indicated
Lupus erythematosus	Polymorphonuclear leukocytes; fluid glucose equals blood glucose; may be transudate if associated with heart failure or the nephrotic syndrome	Arthritis, skin rash, renal disease; superficial thrombophlebitis	Positive serologic results; urinary sediment abnormalities; renal or skin biopsy
Lymphoproliferative disorders	Polymorphonuclear leukocytes, lymphocytes, rarely eosinophils; occasionally transudate; rarely chylothorax	Night sweats, fever, pruritus; adenopathy; hepatosplenomegaly; chest roentgenogram may reveal hilar and mediastinal lymphadenopathy or parenchymal nodules or infiltrates	Lymph node, skin, pleural, liver, or bone marrow biopsy diagnostic
Primary lymphedema	No specific characteristics	Yellow fingernails, peripheral lymphedema; may follow upper respiratory illness	Normal cardiac, renal, and liver function
Myxedema	Frequently bilateral; may be transudate if associated with myocardial or pericardial disease	Clinical findings of myxedema; large heart on x-ray	Abnormal thyroid function tests
Subphrenic abscess	Polymorphonuclear leukocytes occasionally a transudate ("sympathetic" effusion)	May follow ruptured viscus, amebic abscess, complication of abdominal surgery	Liver-lung radioisotope scan
Peritoneal dialysis	No specific characteristics	Clinical picture is evident	Disappears following drainage of peritoneal cavity
Hydronephrosis	No specific characteristics	Picture of urinary obstruction	Disappears with relief of obstruction

Leakage through a subclavian vein catheter	Reflects characteristics of the intravenous fluid; may be transudate		
Malignancy	Malignant cells; lymphocytes or polymorphonuclear leukocytes; major cause of hemorrhagic pleural effusions	History and physical findings of a primary or metastatic cancer; history of asbestos exposure in suspected mesothelioma	Pleural biopsy frequently positive
Pancreatitis	Polymorphonuclear leukocytes; high amylase; usually on left, but may be bilateral; occasionally it is transudate	Severe abdominal pain with radiation to back	Elevated serum and urine amylase
Pneumothorax	May contain inflammatory cells	Sudden onset of pain, dyspnea, cough; chest radiogram demonstrates an air-fluid level	
Chest trauma	May contain inflammatory cells; frequently hemorrhagic	May be closed or open; chest x-ray may demonstrate fractured ribs or a pulmonary contusion	

Chylothorax

Chest trauma; lymphoma; postsurgical complication	Milky fluid; normal cholesterol; increased lipid content	Recent trauma or chest surgery; findings of lymphomatous disease	Positive Sudan III stain

Empyema

Bacterial, fungal, or tuberculous pneumonia; chest trauma; thoracic surgery; mediastinitis; lung abscess; ruptured subdiaphragmatic abscess	Polymorphonuclear leukocytes; may be lymphocytic in tuberculosis; organisms may be seen by gram stain; may be loculated	Fever, pleuritic chest pain, and findings associated with underlying etiology	Fluid culture positive (fungus, tuberculous, aerobic, or anaerobic cultures); blood cultures occasionally positive

5.

Gastrointestinal Problems

Heartburn (Pyrosis)

Barry W. Frank

DEFINITION

Heartburn, or pyrosis, is a painful or burning sensation located retrosternally or in the subxiphoid region. The discomfort may radiate to the lateral anterior chest, jaws, and arms. Heartburn is frequently worse after meals and aggravated by recumbency or bending forward. It is almost always relieved within 15 minutes by the ingestion of an antacid.

MECHANISM

Heartburn arises from alterations in the esophageal epithelium induced by the reflux of acid and pepsin, or bile and pancreatic juice, or both. Motor abnormalities of the esophagus may contribute significantly to its production. However, since pyrosis may be experienced when esophageal motility is normal, it seems likely that chemical stimulation from esophageal reflux is the most important factor in its pathogenesis.

GASTROESOPHAGEAL REFLUX

The primary determinant of gastroesophageal reflux is the tone of the lower esophageal sphincter (LES). Although the LES cannot be identified anatomically, its presence can be verified by physiologic means. Modern manometric methods have established that the LES possesses a resting tone that causes the intraluminal esophageal pressure to exceed that in the stomach.

Thus, in the normal individual, an intact LES prevents the reflux of gastric contents into the esophagus, even when stomach pressures are high. The following are some of the complications of gastroesophageal reflux:

1. Esophagitis (histologic alteration of the esophageal mucosa).
    a. With bleeding.
    b. With ulceration.
    c. With stricture.

2. Tracheal aspiration with chronic cough, pneumonitis, and fibrosis.

ETIOLOGY

1. Gastroesophageal reflux due to an incompetent sphincter, with or without hiatal hernia.

2. Diffuse esophageal spasm.

3. Medications.

4. Scleroderma, with involvement of the lower esophageal sphincter.

5. Barrett syndrome (lower esophagus lined by columnar epithelium with ulceration at the transitional zone).

6. Tumor, by affecting sphincter function or altering motility.

DIAGNOSTIC APPROACH

Initial Evaluation

1. Upper GI series should be performed to detect intrinsic lesions of the esophagus and stomach. Unfortunately, reflux cannot be detected by this method in more than 20 to 25 percent of patients with heartburn.

2. Esophageal cineradiography with neutral barium swallow. With cineradiography it is possible to follow the passage of swallowed barium through the esophagus. The patient should be examined in both the upright and the supine positions. Esophageal motility can be visualized, reflux observed, and small mucosal defects detected.

3. If the preceding studies show reflux without evidence of intrinsic esophageal disease, further tests are usually not necessary and treatment may be instituted.

4. If the aforementioned studies are negative, the additional procedures listed below are indicated.

5. If x-ray studies show stricture, tumor, or an abnormal mucosal pattern, esophagoscopy and biopsy should be performed.

6. In the presence of persistent pyrosis unresponsive to treatment, further investigation is warranted.

Subsequent Evaluation

1. Esophageal cineradiography with acid barium swallow. Following baseline observations with neutral barium, barium to which hydrochloric acid has been added (to a pH of 1.0 to 1.5) is administered. If the acid-containing barium creates a motility disturbance not observed with neutral barium, the presence of significant reflux and esophagitis may be inferred, particularly if the patient experiences pyrosis during the procedure.

2. Esophageal acid perfusion test (Bernstein test). The acid perfusion test determines whether the esophagus is sensitive to acid but does not necessarily prove that reflux is present. It is designed to reproduce the symptoms created by acid reflux. A nasogastric tube is passed into the midesophagus and positioned by fluoroscopy. With the patient seated upright, normal saline is administered via the nasogastric tube at a rate of 6 to 7.5 ml per minute. Then, without the patient's knowledge, 0.1 N HCl is substituted for the saline. This is perfused at the same rate until pain is produced or until 15 minutes have elapsed. The solutions are again interchanged without notifying the patient. The test is considered to give a positive result if heartburn is elicited by acid perfusion but not by saline. A high incidence of false-positive and false-negative results, ranging between 5 and 15 percent, makes it necessary to interpret the results with caution.

3. Esophagoscopy and biopsy. The newer, flexible endoscopes permit biopsy, suction, insufflation of air and fluid, and photography of the mucosa. The entire esophagus can be visualized. Endoscopy and biopsy make possible confirmation of tumors, strictures, or other lesions observed by x-ray. Esophagoscopy is also invaluable when radiologic studies are negative, because less evident lesions (e.g., esophagitis) may be detectable by this technique. It is ordinarily unnecessary to biopsy the esophagus in the presence of esophagitis. However, biopsy may be useful in revealing esophagitis when the mucosa is grossly normal in appearance.

4. Esophageal motility studies and measurement of the intraesophageal pH. Gastroesophageal reflux is demonstrated best by measurement of the intraluminal pH combined with simultaneous measurement of the intraesophageal pressure. To perform the test the patient swallows an assembly consisting of a pH electrode and three manometric catheters whose tips are placed 5 cm apart. The LES is located and its pressure characteristics noted. The motility of the esophagus is then recorded, and the reflux is measured by the pH electrode.

Dysphagia

Barry W. Frank

DEFINITION

Dysphagia is nonpainful difficulty in swallowing. It is a subjective sensation experienced during the act of deglutition. There is usually a sticking sensation retrosternally as the bolus descends. In most instances, dysphagia is experienced at the same level as the lesion or above it, but not below it. *Odynophagia* is the term applied to painful swallowing. Dysphagia is a highly specific and significant symptom of organic disease. It should never be considered functional without an exhaustive evaluation. Dysphagia can be differentiated by a careful history from globus hystericus, which is a functional complaint. Globus hystericus is a sensation of a "lump in the throat." It is not necessarily associated with deglutition. The symptom is intermittent. It is not associated with regurgitation. Foods and liquids can be swallowed without difficulty.

ETIOLOGY
Oropharyngeal Dysphagia

1. Loss of tongue function (myasthenia gravis, myotonia dystrophica).

2. Pharyngeal dysfunction (myasthenia gravis, vascular brainstem disease, dermatomyositis, hyperthyroidism).

3. Mechanical obstruction.
   a. Zenker's diverticulum.
   b. Tumor.
   c. Inflammatory stricture.

Esophageal Dysphagia

1. Intraluminal obstruction.
   a. Esophageal webs.
   b. Lower esophageal ring (Schatzki's ring).
   c. Tumor.
   d. Lower esophageal sphincter spasm (hypertensive sphincter).
   e. Inflammatory stricture.
   f. Caustic stricture.
   g. Foreign body.

2. Extraluminal obstruction.
   a. Compression by tumors, enlarged lymph nodes, or substernal thyroid gland.

b. Vascular abnormalities (aortic aneurysm, aberrant right subclavian artery).

3. Motility disorders.
  a. Achalasia.
  b. Scleroderma.
  c. Diabetic neuropathy.
  d. Diffuse esophageal spasm.
  e. Amyloidosis.

4. Miscellaneous causes.
  a. Infections (candidiasis).
  b. Regional enteritis.

SYMPTOMS

1. A detailed history may provide a significant clue to the etiology of dysphagia and hence aid in its evaluation.

2. Dysphagia of oropharyngeal disease is characterized by difficulty in moving a bolus of food from the mouth to the pharynx. There may be instant regurgitation of food through the nares, choking, and repetitive swallowing, particularly in neuromuscular disorders.

3. Esophageal dysphagia usually presents as a sticking sensation. It may be intermittent, as in the case of a lower esophageal ring, or progressive, as in the presence of a tumor. Regurgitation of undigested food may occur minutes to hours after a meal. Patients find that they must chew their foods thoroughly and that fluids may be required to "wash the food down." The time taken to eat frequently is prolonged.

4. The presence of weight loss suggests marked obstruction due to benign disease or a malignancy.

5. Respiratory symptoms, most often nocturnal, may occur from tracheal aspiration of esophageal contents.

6. Heartburn suggests an inflammatory stricture or disease that involves the lower esophageal sphincter.

7. Raynaud's phenomenon suggests a connective tissue disease as the cause of dysphagia, which in turn is due to a motility disorder.

PHYSICAL EXAMINATION

The physical examination is of little value in the diagnosis of dysphagia except in the presence of neuromuscular disorders, scleroderma, diabetes mellitus, cervical lymphadenopathy, or malnutrition.

DIAGNOSTIC APPROACH

1. X-ray examination.
   a. A barium swallow is the most valuable procedure.
   b. Cineradiography with barium, as described in the preceding section, Heartburn, is helpful in motility disorders.
   c. The addition of a marshmallow or a barium-soaked cotton ball is useful in an attempt to reproduce the dysphagia or define more precisely the location, type, and degree of obstruction.

2. Esophagoscopy and biopsy are most valuable in the diagnosis of esophagitis, strictures, and tumors.

3. When properly performed, exfoliative *cytologic studies* may be expected to yield the correct diagnosis in 95 percent of patients with esophageal carcinoma.

4. Esophageal motility study is, as described in the preceding section, Heartburn, essential to the diagnosis of motility disorders. It is the only technique that elucidates the status of the lower esophageal sphincter as well as the overall motility of the esophagus.

5. The esophageal acid perfusion test (Bernstein test) if of little value in the evaluation of dysphagia except when esophageal reflux is suspected.

Hematemesis and Melena

A. J. Kauvar

DEFINITION

Hematemesis is the vomiting of gross blood. The blood may be bright red when fresh or black when digested in the presence of hydrochloric acid. *Melena* refers to the passage of stools that are black and tarry from blood that has been digested and converted to acid hematin.

GENERAL CONSIDERATIONS

Hematemesis and melena result from hemorrhage into the esophagus, stomach, or small intestine. Hematemesis and melena sometimes result from swallowed blood of nasopharyngeal or respiratory tract origin. It is generally but not always true that hematemesis without melena is usually due to lesions proximal to the pylorus, and melena without hematemesis is usually due to lesions between the pylorus and jejunum. For example, the former may be seen with bleeding duodenal ulcers, and the latter from lesions as far down as the ileocecal valve or just distal to it. Blood from the upper gastrointestinal tract ordinarily must be retained in the bowel for at least 6 to 8 hours in order to produce melena.

Tarry stools may result from the ingestion of as little as 60 cc of blood. Stools may remain tarry for a 48- to 72-hour period after bleeding has stopped. This means that the passage of tarry stools is no proof that bleeding is continuing. Occult blood may be present in the stool for as long as 7 to 10 days after a single bleeding episode. Bright red blood in the stool usually arises from a bleeding site in the rectosigmoid or colon. However, in the presence of intestinal hypermotility, significant upper GI bleeding may also result in bright red blood in the stool. The color of the stool, whether red, dark brown, or tarry, depends more on the amount and rapidity of bleeding and the speed of intestinal transport than on the level at which bleeding occurs. The guaiac test differentiates between blood and other substances that either darken the stool (e.g., iron) or make it red (e.g., the ingestion of beets).

Hematemesis and melena should be regarded as symptoms of a disease process that is potentially serious and life-threatening.

ETIOLOGY

The causes of hematemesis and melena are listed in Table 5-1. The more important conditions are considered below. About 55 to 75 percent of cases of massive upper GI hemorrhage are due to peptic ulcer of the duodenum or stomach. Gastritis, esophagitis, and esophagogastritis are responsible for about 15 percent, and varices for about 10 percent. Gastric carcinoma, hiatal hernia, the Mallory-Weiss syndrome, and miscellaneous or undetermined causes account for the remainder.

1. Varices. Esophageal and gastric varices occur in patients with cirrhosis of the liver and portal hypertension. Ruptured varices are the usual source of hemorrhage in this disease. However, in the 15 percent of cirrhotics who have concomitant peptic disease, an ulcer must be considered in the differential diagnosis of GI hemorrhage.

2. Esophagitis, gastritis, and esophagogastritis.
   a. Esophagitis may be due to such causes as trauma, repeated vomiting, foreign bodies, achalasia, or the ingestion of caustic substances.
   b. Peptic ulceration occurs less frequently in the esophagus than in the stomach or duodenum.
   c. Acute or chronic gastritis may cause slight or massive bleeding from shallow ulcerations or erosions.
   d. Atrophic gastritis is usually not associated with bleeding.
   e. Alcohol, sepsis, or uremia may cause gastritis with bleeding. Other, less common forms of gastritis, such as stomal and eosinophilic gastritis, may also bleed.

TABLE 5-1.   Causes of Hematemesis and Melena

1. Diseases of the esophagus
   a. Varices secondary to portal hypertension
   b. Esophagitis and esophageal peptic ulcer
   c. Benign and malignant tumors
   d. Mallory-Weiss syndrome
   e. Barrett syndrome
2. Diseases of the stomach and duodenum
   a. Peptic ulcer (including anastomotic and drug-induced)
   b. Gastritis and erosions of the stomach
   c. Benign and malignant tumors of the stomach
   d. Carcinoma of duodenum or of ampulla of Vater
   e. Miscellaneous (ruptured sclerotic vessel, diverticulum, syphilis, tuberculosis, heterotopic pancreatic tissue)
3. Disease of the small intestine
   a. Benign and malignant tumors
   b. Peutz-Jeghers syndrome
   c. Meckel's diverticulum
4. Disease of the proximal colon
   a. Benign and malignant tumors
   b. Diverticulosis
   c. Ulcerative or granulomatous colitis
   d. Tuberculosis
   e. Amebic dysentery
   f. Miscellaneous (telangiectasis, cirsoid aneurysm)
5. Bleeding disorders: polycythemia vera, lymphoma, leukemia, pernicious anemia, purpura, hemophilia, hypoprothrombinemia, myeloma, Christmas disease, etc.
6. Disease of the blood vessels
   a. Hereditary hemorrhagic telangiectasia
   b. Cavernous hemangioma
7. Systemic disease: amyloidosis, sarcoidosis, connective tissue diseases, uremia, etc.

   3. Mallory-Weiss syndrome.
      a. Violent vomiting may cause perforation of the mucosal and submucosal layers of the esophagus, with subsequent bleeding from the submucosal arteries. Although this syndrome is most common in alcoholics, it may occur whenever there is severe or protracted vomiting or retching. It is not a common cause of GI bleeding.
      b. The lesions are difficult to identify by x-ray examination. Endoscopy is usually helpful, but oftentimes the lesions are discovered only at the time of surgery.

   4. Peptic ulcer.
      a. Peptic ulcer is the most common cause of hematemesis and melena.
      b. Hematemesis and melena may occur together, but each may occur alone with either gastric or duodenal ulcer.
      c. Melena occurs more frequently than hematemesis alone because of the greater incidence of duodenal as compared to gastric ulcer (4:1).

d. Gastric ulcers are likely to bleed more frequently and more severely than duodenal ulcers. Anastomotic and postbulbar ulcers are more likely to bleed than either of the foregoing.

e. Hemorrhage may be the first symptom of peptic ulcer in 10 percent of patients with this disease.

f. The sudden cessation of ulcer distress in patients with acute peptic disease may herald a bleeding episode.

g. Ulcer pain may disappear for long periods following hemorrhage. The cause of this phenomenon is unknown.

h. The persistence of pain following hemorrhage may be indicative of continued bleeding, failure of the ulcer to heal, or perforation.

i. Stress ulcers and ulcers secondary to burns are also subject to hemorrhage.

j. Anticoagulants may be responsible for precipitating hemorrhage in patients with known or silent peptic ulcer disease.

k. Some drugs may be ulcerogenic or may aggravate a preexisting ulcer. Salicylates, ACTH, steroids, phenylbutazone, indomethacin, and reserpine are the more common offenders.

5. Hiatal hernia.   In hiatal hernia, GI bleeding is likely to be chronic and intermittent rather than massive. The bleeding is apparently due to congestion of the herniated portion of the stomach in association with either ulceration or peptic esophagitis.

6. Carcinoma of the stomach.   Carcinoma of the stomach is an uncommon cause of GI hemorrhage. Bleeding is due to ulceration or necrosis of the tumor. Massive hemorrhage may be the first manifestation of gastric carcinoma.

7. Benign tumors of the stomach.   Benign tumors of the stomach, such as leiomyoma, adenoma, polyp, and neurofibroma, are infrequent causes of GI hemorrhage because they are relatively rare. However, bleeding is one of the most common symptoms of benign gastric neoplasms.

8. Diseases of the colon.   Bright red blood in the stool is the usual finding in disease of the colon, whether it be due to neoplasm, infection, or hematologic disorder. Melena is rarely produced by lesions of the colon.

9. Miscellaneous causes.

a. Blood dyscrasias, mesenteric thrombosis, connective tissue diseases, the Peutz-Jeghers syndrome, uremia, Meckel's diverticulum, and neoplasms of the GI tract other than gastric carcinoma are important but much less frequent causes of GI bleeding.

b. Hemorrhage into the bile ducts, or hemobilia, is an interesting but rare cause of GI hemorrhage. It is usually associated with liver trauma or rupture of the hepatic artery or one of its branches. The clue to the diagnosis is a combination of biliary colic and GI hemorrhage.

DIAGNOSTIC APPROACH

Hospitalization of patients with massive GI hemorrhage is obligatory and is almost mandatory in any patient with hematemesis or melena. The treatment or prevention of shock has priority over diagnostic investigations.

History

1. When a patient with a known peptic ulcer has GI bleeding, the ulcer is the most likely source. Even in the absence of an ulcer history, the likelihood of ulcer is high, but other conditions, particularly gastritis, must also be considered.

2. A history of bleeding tendencies should suggest blood dyscrasia.

3. A family history of GI bleeding is usually associated with hemophilia or hereditary hemorrhagic telangiectasia.

4. A history of alcoholism implicates varices or gastritis as possible causes.

5. Specific inquiry should be made concerning the use of potentially ulcerogenic drugs such as salicylates, steroids, phenylbutazone, and indomethacin, since these can induce bleeding.

6. A patient who reports black stools should be questioned about the use of medications that change the color of the stool (such as iron and bismuth compounds, licorice, and beets), particularly if the patient is otherwise asymptomatic.

7. A history of severe vomiting and retching, particularly in an alcoholic, merits consideration of the Mallory-Weiss syndrome.

8. A hiatal hernia is suggested when the patient complains of long-standing heartburn, belching, and substernal or epigastric discomfort, particularly on recumbency.

9. A history of anorexia, weakness, weight loss, and digestive symptoms, particularly in the elderly, points to malignancy.

10. The usual mode of onset of significant hemorrhage is a sudden desire for defecation accompanied by weakness, faintness, lightheadedness, sweating, or nausea, followed by the evacuation of tarry stools. Similar symptoms may also be associated with hematemesis.

Physical Examination

1. The initial examination of patients with massive hemorrhage usually has to be limited. Unnecessary manipulations should be avoided until the patient is out of danger.

2. Primary attention should be directed to the vital signs, which should be checked frequently.

3. The skin should be examined for vascular spiders, which direct attention to liver disease, particularly if jaundice is present. The presence of brown, freckle-like spots on the skin of the face and the buccal mucosa suggests the Peutz-Jeghers syndrome. Telangiectatic lesions that pulsate are indicative of hereditary hemorrhagic telangiectasia. Stigmata of pseudoxanthoma elasticum in the skin and ocular fundi should be sought. Purpura and enlarged lymph nodes should raise suspicion of a blood dyscrasia.

4. A palpable liver and spleen, ascites, vascular spiders, distended veins over the chest and abdomen, and jaundice are virtually diagnostic of cirrhosis. An abdominal mass suggests carcinoma.

5. Gastric malignancy may be revealed by the presence of a left supraclavicular node or a rectal shelf.

6. Fever is common in patients with GI hemorrhage. It usually appears within a day of the onset and may last from a few days to a week or slightly longer. The fever is usually low-grade, but the temperature may be as high as 103° F.

Estimation of Blood Loss

1. Of paramount importance is the estimation of the severity of the hemorrhage. However, it is often difficult to assess accurately the amount of blood loss.

2. It is generally accepted that the presence of hypovolemic shock in a patient with a hemoglobin value of 8.0 gm or less, or a red cell mass that is depleted by 40 percent, is indicative of massive hemorrhage.

3. The determination of hemoglobin and hematocrit values is important. However, they may sometimes be misleading: early, because of hemoconcentration; and later, because of hemodilution. Serial determinations are of much greater value than isolated, randomly performed hemograms. Blood volume determinations are more accurate than blood counts in estimating blood loss.

4. The effect of transfusions in correcting blood values and improving the clinical state is a valuable method for estimating the degree of blood loss and the presence of continued bleeding.

Laboratory Procedures

The following baseline studies are recommended, and they should be repeated as often as warranted by the circumstances:

1. CBC and hematocrit reading.

2. Blood typing and cross-matching for blood transfusion.

3. **BUN.** Azotemia is common following GI hemorrhage. The degree of azotemia depends on the quantity of blood lost, the duration of bleeding, and the integrity of renal function. Azotemia occurs irrespective of the cause of bleeding. The BUN has prognostic importance: A maximum BUN of 30 mg/100 ml suggests a favorable outlook. A level of 50 to 70 mg/100 ml is associated with a mortality rate of about 33 percent. Values above 70 mg/100 ml portend a fatal outcome in two cases out of three.

4. **Serum bilirubin.** Hyperbilirubinemia is common 3 to 4 days after massive hemorrhage. An initial determination is useful in evaluating subsequent changes.

5. **Serum electrolytes.** Hypochloremic alkalosis on admission to the hospital suggests that gastric retention may have preceded the bleeding episode or that vomiting has been substantial.

6. **Blood volume** determinations, as indicated previously, are useful in establishing the amount of blood loss.

7. Blood NH_3 determination is indicated in cirrhotics. Rising levels may herald hepatic coma.

Diagnostic Studies

1. A Levine or similar tube should be passed to empty the stomach, to determine whether the bleeding is in the upper GI tract, and to ascertain whether pyloric obstruction is present.

2. The stomach may be lavaged with iced water or saline in order to slow or halt the bleeding, pending further studies.

3. A fluorescein string test is sometimes helpful in determining the bleeding site.

4. As soon as the patient's condition is stable, x-ray examination of the GI tract or endoscopy, or both should be performed.

5. If the diagnosis of esophageal varices is suspected, it may be advisable, when bleeding is uncontrollable, to produce esophageal tamponade by means of a Sengstaken-Blakemore or Nachlas tube before proceeding with further investigations.

6. Esophageal varices may be demonstrated by esophagoscopy or barium study of the esophagus. They may also be demonstrated by percutaneous splenoportal venography.

7. Abdominal arteriography is sometimes helpful in localizing the bleeding site, especially when the patient is bleeding actively. It may also be useful in detection of the lesion producing hemorrhage.

Diarrhea

Barry W. Frank

DEFINITION

Diarrhea may be defined as the frequent passage of unformed stools. Whether acute or chronic, it results from, or is associated with water and electrolyte malabsorption. There are four basic pathophysiologic mechanisms involved in the production of diarrhea. One or more of these factors may play a significant role in any given diarrheal state. They include the following: (1) abnormal intestinal motility, (2) increased vascular or mucosal permeability, resulting in fluid and electrolyte exsorption, (3) impaired intestinal absorption, and (4) intraluminal nonabsorbable osmotically active solutes.

ACUTE DIARRHEA

Acute diarrhea is usually of abrupt onset and short duration.

Etiology

1. Infectious diarrhea.
   a. Bacterial: *Salmonella, Shigella, Vibrio cholerae*, enteropathogenic *Escherichia coli, Clostridium, Neisseria gonorrhoeae*.
   b. Viral: enterovirus, adenovirus, hepatitis-associated virus.
   c. Fungal: *Candida, Actinomyces, Histoplasma*.
   d. Protozoal: *Giardia lamblia, Endamoeba histolytica*.
   e. Helminthic: *Ascaris lumbricoides, Ancylostoma duodenale, Necator americanus, Trichuris trichiura, Strongyloides stercoralis*.

2. Toxic diarrhea.
   a. Bacterial toxins (food poisoning): staphylococcus, *Clostridium welchii, E. coli, Clostridium botulinum*.
   b. Chemical poisons: arsenic, lead, mercury, mushrooms.

3. Dietary causes.   Irritating foods, alcohol, drugs, food allergies.

4. Miscellaneous causes.   Appendicitis, diverticulitis, GI hemorrhage, Schönlein-Henoch's purpura, Stevens-Johnson syndrome, pseudomembranous enterocolitis, fecal impaction, ischemic colitis.

Symptoms

The symptoms are usually abdominal cramps, urgency, tenesmus, nausea and vomiting, and watery stools with or without blood and mucus. Systemic symptoms, particularly fever and myalgias, may be present.

Signs

The signs vary with the etiology and severity of the disease, but diffuse abdominal tenderness and active bowel sounds are usually present. The temperature may be elevated. Involuntary guarding and rebound tenderness of the abdomen are rare.

Diagnostic Approach

Acute diarrhea frequently is self-limiting. The etiology is generally established by the history and physical examination. However, immediate evaluation is necessary in the presence of severe abdominal pain, systemic symptoms, dehydration, bloody stools, or when symptoms persist beyond 24 hours. Under these circumstances, the following studies should be performed:

1. CBC.

2. Rectal swab for bacterial culture and sensitivity studies.

3. Immediate examination of a freshly passed stool for ova and parasites.

4. Serum electrolytes to aid in the diagnosis and management of dehydration.

5. Sigmoidoscopic examination, which is helpful in the diagnosis of shigellosis, amebic colitis, and acute ulcerative colitis. It should be performed as a part of the immediate evaluation on any patient with bloody diarrhea.

6. A three-way abdominal x-ray examination should be obtained if there is bloating, severe abdominal pain, or obstructive-type bowel sounds upon auscultation, or if obstruction or perforation is suspected.

CHRONIC DIARRHEA

Etiology

Table 5-2 lists the many causes of chronic diarrhea. Cases of diarrhea seen in office practice are caused most often by the following conditions: (1) functional disorders (irritable colon, mucous colitis, emotional diarrhea), (2) disease of the colon (diverticulitis, ulcerative colitis, carcinoma), (3) disease of the small intestine (regional enteritis malabsorption syndromes), (4) diarrhea secondary to laxative abuse, and (5) gastrogenic diarrhea, including the postgastrectomy and postvagotomy syndromes. Other diseases are encountered less frequently. It is beyond the scope of this text to consider but a few of these conditions.

Functional Enterocolonopathies

Patients with functional enterocolonopathies are ordinarily young, neurotic individuals with a long history of intermittent or chronic diarrhea. Exacerbations usually are precipitated by emotional stress and anxiety. Diarrhea is

TABLE 5-2.   Etiology of Chronic Diarrhea

A. Disease of the stomach
   1. Postgastrectomy (dumping syndromes)
   2. Postvagotomy
   3. Hypertrophic atrophic gastritis (Menetrier's disease with hypoalbu-
      minemia)
   4. Pernicious anemia with associated megalocytosis of the intestinal
      mucosal cells
   5. Zollinger-Ellison syndrome

B. Disease of the small intestine
   1. Inflammatory disease
      a. Regional enteritis
      b. Radiation enteritis
      c. Whipple's disease
      d. Collagen disease (polyarteritis, systemic lupus erythematosus, scle-
         roderma)
   2. Malabsorption diarrhea
      a. Gluten-sensitive enteropathy (sprue)
      b. Disaccharidase deficiency
      c. Intestinal lymphoma
      d. Intestinal amyloidosis
      e. Intestinal scleroderma
      f. Hypogammaglobulinemia
      g. Intestinal lymphangiectasia
      h. Pancreatic insufficiency
      i. Diarrhea of intestinal stasis (blind loop syndrome, small bowel
         diverticula, postgastrectomy steatorrhea)
      j. Small bowel resection with loss of absorptive surface
      k. Malabsorption associated with chronic skin disease (dermatitis
         herpetiformis, atopic dermatitis)
      l. Chronic giardiasis

C. Disease of the colon
   1. Ulcerative colitis
   2. Granulomatous colitis
   3. Ulcerative proctitis
   4. Diverticulitis
   5. Colonic carcinoma
   6. Villous adenoma

D. Miscellaneous causes
   1. Superior mesenteric artery insufficiency
   2. Addison's disease
   3. Diabetes mellitus associated with visceral neuropathy
   4. Postvagotomy diarrhea
   5. Endocrine tumors (carcinoid tumor, Zollinger-Ellison syndrome,
      nonbeta islet cell tumor of the pancreas with watery diarrhea, hy-
      pokalemia and hypochlorhydria, medullary thyroid carcinoma)
   6. Hyperthyroidism
   7. Drugs
   8. Functional bowel syndromes (irritable colon, mucous colitis)
   9. Small bowel tumors
   10. Eosinophilic gastroenteritis
   11. Parathyroid disease

most likely to occur in the morning or after meals. The stools may be large or small, semiformed or liquid, and mucus- or nonmucus-containing. Blood is not found in the stool unless produced by a complicating anorectal lesion. Systemic symptoms are absent, and nutrition is usually good. The diagnosis is made by history and by exclusion. The findings on physical examination, study of the feces, proctosigmoidoscopy, and barium enema are negative.

Diseases of the Colon and the Small Intestine

1. **Diverticulitis.** Diverticula of the colon occur more frequently with advancing age; they are usually asymptomatic unless complicated by inflammatory disease. The resulting diverticulitis may be manifested by acute attacks of left lower quadrant pain, tenderness, and fever. A palpable tender mass may be present. Constipation is usual but diarrhea may occur, with bloody stools. Symptoms may disappear after the acute episode subsides. In patients with low-grade inflammation, diarrhea is likely to occur intermittently, although it may be chronic. Crampy lower-abdomen pain is often a feature. In many patients, constipation alternates with diarrhea. The diagnosis is usually established by barium enema.

2. **Ulcerative colitis.** Ulcerative colitis is primarily a disease of youth, although it may occur at any age. Its course is characterized by remissions and exacerbations. During the acute phase, the diarrhea may be quite severe, with daily passage of as many as thirty or more bloody, mucus-, and pus-containing stools. Fever, weight loss, abdominal griping, and tenesmus are common accompaniments. Complications include pericolitis, perforation of the bowel, malignant transformation, perianal disorders, nutritional deficiencies, arthritis, spondylitis, iritis, pericholangitis, pyoderma gangrenosum, and other conditions. The diagnosis in over 90 percent of cases can be established by sigmoidoscopy and confirmed by rectal biopsy and barium studies. The sigmoidoscopic findings may be positive even when the contrast examination is negative.

3. Regional enteritis and enterocolitis (Crohn's disease). Regional enteritis or enterocolitis is a disorder that occurs most frequently in adolescence and early adult life. Like ulcerative colitis, its course is marked by remissions and exacerbations. During acute attacks, there may be right lower quadrant pain, diarrhea, low-grade fever, and weight loss. The clinical picture of acute appendicitis is simulated in some patients. During periods of remission, constipation may be present but with normal function. Fistula formation and intestinal obstruction are common sequelae. Nutritional deficiency and malabsorption are less frequent complications. The diagnosis is usually established by x-ray. Abnormality of the terminal ileum and skipped areas of involvement are typical. At times the clinical picture is indistinguishable from that of ulcerative colitis. Differentiating features that are helpful when present include sharp demarcation between diseased and healthy areas of bowel, absence of rectal and sigmoidal lesions in early cases, and evidence of involvement of all layers of the bowel wall.

4. Malabsorption.   Diarrhea manifested by the passage of pale, bulky, greasy, frothy, foul-smelling stools, in association with evidence of nutritional deficiency and weight loss, suggests malabsorption. Fever, hypermetabolism, and significant loss of appetite do not occur. The diarrhea can usually be made to disappear in a 1- to 2-day period if oral feedings are withheld. The laboratory studies most useful in the diagnosis of malabsorption are listed below. Evidence of increased fecal excretion of fat is the most important test in establishing the presence of steatorrhea. The differential diagnosis of various causes of malabsorption is beyond the scope of this discussion.

Diagnostic Approach

History
The history may provide clues to the etiology of the diarrhea and the localization of the disease process.

1. Age.   Diarrhea beginning in adolescence or early adult life suggests diseases such as ulcerative colitis, regional enteritis, tuberculosis, and functional disorders. In middle age and in the elderly, carcinoma of the colon, diverticulitis, laxative abuse, and pancreatic disease are among the more common causes.

2. Diarrhea patterns.   Diarrhea alternating with constipation suggests consideration of carcinoma of the colon, diverticulitis, functional enterocolonopathies, excessive use of laxatives, and gastric disorders. Continuous diarrhea may be seen in ulcerative colitis, regional enteritis, abdominal fistulas, laxative abuse, and gastric disease. Intermittent diarrhea is a common feature of functional disorders, diverticulitis, allergies, and malabsorption.

Relief of abdominal cramping by defecation suggests colonic disease; persistence after bowel movements suggests disease of the small intestine. Large-stool diarrhea suggests disease of the small bowel or proximal colon; small-stool diarrhea, involvement of the distal colon. Diarrhea with rectal tenesmus suggests inflammatory disease of the bowel combined with anorectal lesions. Diarrhea associated with abdominal distention should raise the possibility of partial obstruction, but it may be due to other causes.

3. Diurnal variations and relationship to meals.   Diarrhea occurring primarily in the morning and after meals is found in gastric conditions, emotional disorders, regional enteritis, enterocolitis, and ulcerative colitis. Diarrhea that is not related to normal diurnal variations in colonic activity is often found in infectious disease. Nocturnal diarrhea is characteristic of diabetic neuropathy but is not specific for this diagnosis. When inflammatory disease of the bowel is severe, diarrhea may occur at night as well as during the day. Nocturnal diarrhea should always suggest an organic cause.

4. Weight loss.   Weight loss in the presence of undiminished appetite suggests hyperthyroidism or malabsorption. Weight loss in association with fever and other systemic symptoms implies inflammatory disease of the bowel. Weight loss preceding the onset of diarrhea suggests carcinoma of the pancreas or other malignancy, tuberculosis, diabetes, hyperthyroidism, or malabsorption. Weight loss is uncommon in carcinoma of the colon until late in the course of the disease. Diarrhea without weight loss or other systemic manifestations is often functional in origin.

5. Characteristics of the stools.   Watery stools with little fecal material occur commonly in psychophysiologic disturbances, severe inflammatory disease of the bowel, internal fistulas, and shortened intestines (after surgery). Semiformed, bulky, pale, foul-smelling, frothy, greasy stools bespeak malabsorption. Chronic bloody diarrhea with griping abdominal pain and rectal tenesmus may result from amebic or bacillary dysentery, ulcerative colitis, regional enteritis, and, less often, other conditions. It should be remembered that in any diarrhea, bloody rectal discharge may occur from an associated proctitis or anusitis. Frequent, soft, nonfatty stools should suggest gastrogenic diarrhea. Stools that contain large amounts of mucus without pus or blood are a feature of functional bowel disorders. Semiformed or liquid stools with a greenish color because of excessive amounts of bile may result from excessive use of cathartics or from an infection.

Physical Examination
There are few signs that have specific diagnostic value in chronic diarrhea. Evidence of weight loss, malnutrition, dehydration, and anemia point to disease of a serious nature. The physical examination may provide clues to specific diseases: reddish-purple flushing of the skin suggests metastatic carcinoid tumor; mucocutaneous pigmentation—Addison's disease or the Peutz-Jeghers syndrome; ecchymosis—malabsorption or Schönlein-Henoch's purpura; erythema nodosum or pyoderma gangrenosum—ulcerative colitis; Argyll Robertson pupils in the absence of lues—diabetic neuropathy; exophthalmos—Graves' disease; macroglossia—amyloidosis; lymphadenopathy— lymphoma, tuberculosis, metastatic carcinoma, or Whipple's disease; lymphedema—lymphangiectasia; peripheral arthritis or spondylitis—ulcerative colitis, regional enteritis, or Whipple's disease; uremic breath—renal failure; and clubbing—sprue or ulcerative colitis. In the abdominal and rectal examination, special attention should be paid to tenderness, masses, gaseous distention, bowel sounds, organomegaly, anal fistulae, and the presence of a rectal shelf or frozen pelvis. A palpable mass in the left lower quadrant should arouse suspicion of carcinoma or diverticulitis; on the right side of the abdomen, carcinoma, regional enteritis, and granulomatous enterocolitis. A palpable, stiff descending colon is common in ulcerative colitis and diverticulitis, but this may result from spasm.

Proctosigmoidoscopy
This procedure is indicated in all patients to detect rectal and colonic inflammatory disease, neoplasm, and parasitic disease.

Radiologic Studies
Roentgenographic examination is warranted in all patients. It should include plain abdominal films as well as a barium enema, upper GI series, and small

bowel study. The routine abdominal films may reveal visceromegaly, partial obstruction, pancreatic calcification, and postoperative foreign bodies.

Laboratory Procedures

1. CBC to screen for anemia that may suggest blood loss, malabsorption, infection, or neoplasia. Eosinophilia suggests parasitic disease, an allergic reaction, eosinophilic gastroenteritis, or neoplasia.

2. Stool, examined immediately for culture, ova and parasites, and occult blood.

3. Serum electrolytes and BUN electrolyte disturbances or uremia.

4. Serum protein electrophoresis to detect GI protein loss, evidence of chronic inflammation, or hypogammaglobulinemia.

5. Serum carotene to screen for fat malabsorption. The results may be invalid if the patient has had either a limited or an excessive intake of vegetables.

6. Serum calcium, phosphorus, and alkaline phosphatase to detect parathyroid disease.

7. Thyroid function tests (T_4, T_3 resin uptake) to detect hyperthyroidism.

8. Fasting or 2-hour postprandial blood sugar tests to detect diabetes.

9. Serum folate level to detect deficiency that may be due to malabsorption.

Specialized Tests in the Evaluation of Chronic Diarrhea

The initial evaluation may well provide the proper diagnosis so that treatment can be instituted. Often, however, the initial evaluation will only suggest the cause or the anatomic site of the lesion. More specialized procedures, such as those that follow, are then required.

1. Gastric analysis with histolog stimulation. A nonbeta islet cell tumor of the pancreas should be suspected when diarrhea is associated with chronic peptic ulcer disease. In this entity, there is hypersecretion of hydrochloric acid resulting from the excessive production of gastrin. Gastric analysis should be performed before and after the intramuscular injection of Histolog (100 mg, or 1.5 mg per kilogram of body weight). The Zollinger-Ellison syndrome is usually associated with a baseline hydrochloric acid secretion above 15 mEq per hour and a ratio of basal to post-Histolog secretion of 60 percent or more. The diagnosis of nonbeta islet cell tumor is further supported by high serum gastrin levels.

2. Serum level of vitamin B_{12} and a Schilling test may identify pernicious anemia associated with chronic diarrhea.

3. Seventy-two-hour fecal fat test.   This test, although time-consuming, is invaluable in documenting a malabsorption problem as a cause of diarrhea. The patient must be on a diet containing a minimum of 80 gm of fat per day. All feces excreted during a 72-hour period are collected and analyzed for lipid content. A normal individual should excrete no more than 5 to 7 gm of fat every 24 hours. Increased fecal excretion of fat indicates only a significant abnormality in fat absorption. Additional studies are necessary to establish its cause.

4. D-Xylose absorption.   D-Xylose (25 gm dissolved in 250 ml of water) is administered orally. The ability of the small intestine to absorb this carbohydrate is measured by determining the amount of xylose excreted in a 5-hour period. An abnormally low excretion of xylose (less than 5 gm in 5 hours) suggests jejunal mucosal disease.

5. Lactose tolerance test.   This test is indicated when the history suggests that the diarrhea is related to milk intolerance. Following oral administration of lactose (100 gm, or 1.75 gm per kilogram of body weight for patients weighing less than 100 lb.), patients with lactase deficiency will show a rise in blood sugar to a peak of less than 30 mg/100 ml (expressed as glucose) associated with bloating, flatulence, cramps, and diarrhea.

6. Intraduodenal secretin test.   This test is of value when chronic diarrhea is thought to be secondary to pancreatic exocrine insufficiency. A double-lumen tube is passed to the ligament of Treitz, and its position is verified by fluoroscopy: the proximal lumen is in the stomach, and the distal lumen in the duodenum. Constant suction insures separation of gastric and duodenal fluids. After a 20-minute control sample is obtained from the duodenal tube, secretin (1 unit per kilogram of body weight) is injected intravenously, and three consecutive 20-minute specimens of duodenal fluid are collected and measured both for volume and for concentration of bicarbonate. Pancreatic exocrine insufficiency is likely if the total fluid output is less than 2.42 ml per kilogram of body weight and the bicarbonate concentration does not exceed 80 mEq per liter in any one specimen. The pH should be alkaline in all collected specimens.

7. Small bowel culture.   A number of derangements of the gastrointestinal tract, such as multiple strictures, surgical blind loops, afferent loop partial obstruction, multiple jejunal diverticula, diabetic neuropathy, and scleroderma, may give rise to the intestinal stasis syndrome. The common feature is massive bacterial proliferation in the proximal small bowel. A sterile tube is passed into the stomach or the small intestine, and the aspirate is cultured on appropriate aerobic and anaerobic media. Cultures showing greater than 1 million colonies per milliliter of intestinal fluid should be regarded as abnormal.

8. Peroral small bowel biopsy.   Many types of suction and hydraulic biopsy instruments are now available for procuring mucosal specimens

to demonstrate histological abnormalities peculiar to certain diseases. Extreme care must be taken to ensure proper orientation and process- ing of the biopsy material.

9. Dye-marker transit time. The time required for ingested food to be eliminated in the stool may at times be useful in correlating the symptoms with the laboratory evaluation. Ingestion of an intense dye (50 mg brilliant blue mixed with 350 mg methylcellulose) along with a regular meal provides a means of measuring the mouth-to-anus transit time.

10. Arteriography. Judicious use of celiac arteriography may be helpful in the diagnosis of arterial insufficiency, suspected tumors, or obscure submucosal abnormalities on routine barium studies.

11. Colonofiberoscopy. With the development of fiberoptic colono- scopes, endoscopic examination of the colon beyond the range of the rigid proctosigmoidoscope has become a reality. It may be decisive in establishing a correct diagnosis of colonic diarrhea in patients whose barium enema study is questionable and inconclusive.

Constipation

H. Harold Friedman

DEFINITION

Constipation may be defined as the abnormal retention of fecal material or a delay in the passage of feces through the bowel. When a patient complains of constipation, it is well to ask him what he means by the term, because the symptom may be imagined. For example, patients who equate good health with regularity of bowel movements often believe they are constipated even when the stools are normal. Most patients, however, consider them- selves constipated if they have hard stools, infrequent bowel movements, or stools that are difficult to expel.

ETIOLOGY

Chronic Constipation

1. Chronic habitual constipation with the passage of hard or infrequent stools is usually caused by improper eating habits, poor bowel habits, inadequate fluid intake, lack of exercise, medications, laxatives, or a combination of these factors. It may also occur in patients with func- tional enterocolonopathies, who often complain of alternating con- stipation and diarrhea, abdominal distress, and the passage of scybalous stools that may or may not contain mucus. Constipation is sometimes the manifestation of an obsessive-compulsive neurosis or a psychotic depressed reaction. In all of the foregoing conditions, the gastrointestinal findings are negative. The diagnosis is made by exclusion.

2. Chronic constipation may be due to rectal insensitivity, which in many cases appears to be the result of persistent suppression of the urge to defecate or laxative abuse. In such individuals, the desire for bowel movement often is lacking even when the rectum is filled with feces.

3. Chronic constipation may be associated with anorectal disease, such as fissures, ulcers, or hemorrhoids. The diagnosis is usually evident from the history, examination, and proctosigmoidoscopy.

4. Lifelong obstipation (severe refractory constipation) is sometimes due to megacolon.

Acute Constipation

1. Constipation of fairly recent onset in a previously healthy individual, particularly if progressive, may be indicative of a serious disorder.

2. The most common cause of acute constipation, particularly in the elderly, is fecal impaction. The clinical setting is usually that of a feeble, weak, or debilitated individual, lying in bed and receiving frequent doses of sedatives or narcotics. Soiling and involuntary passage of stools around the impaction may be interpreted erroneously as diarrhea. Rectal discomfort may be severe. The diagnosis is made by rectal examination.

3. Other causes of constipation of recent or acute onset are neoplasm of the large bowel, mesenteric vascular occlusion, painful anorectal lesions, drugs, intestinal obstruction, urinary tract disease, and neurologic disorders.

DIAGNOSTIC APPROACH

1. Habitual constipation of long duration does not require extensive workup if the patient is otherwise in good health. The diagnosis of its cause may be apparent from the history. The physical findings are negative, as are those of rectal and stool examinations. Proctosigmoidoscopy and barium enema should probably be done once to exclude organic disease.

2. When constipation is of recent origin, a thorough investigation is warranted after fecal impaction is excluded. If rectal findings fail to explain the constipation, stool examination, proctosigmoidoscopy, and flat abdominal films, followed by barium enema and an upper GI series, are indicated. Systemic causes must be excluded by appropriate means.

Indigestion and Flatulence

H. Harold Friedman

DEFINITION

Indigestion is a nonspecific term used by patients to describe a variety of symptoms. In approaching the patient with indigestion, it is important, therefore, to have him describe his complaint fully. Most patients mean by indigestion such symptoms as "gas," belching, bloating, abdominal fullness, and flatulence. It is these symptoms that will be considered in this section.

ETIOLOGY

Flatulence is related to the presence of excessive quantities of gas in the gastrointestinal tract; it is believed to be the result of a functional disturbance in bowel motility. The major sources of intraluminal gas are swallowed air and gas produced by bacterial fermentation. Food intolerance appears to play a role in the genesis of flatulence and indigestion. Milk products may cause bloating, flatulence, and diarrhea in patients with lactase deficiency. Gluten-containing foods exacerbate the symptoms of nontropical sprue. Some food intolerances are undoubtedly allergic in origin, but in the majority of cases the mechanism is not understood. Reflex disturbance in bowel motility undoubtedly plays a role in at least some cases of abdominal distention and bloating (e.g., reflex ileus). Flatulence is often a noteworthy but never the sole symptom of malabsorptive states or intestinal disease.

SYMPTOMS

1. Aerophagia is the excessive swallowing of air. Aerophagia is usually associated with abdominal fullness, gaseous eructations, and the presence of a large air bubble in the fundus of the stomach. Belching ordinarily relieves the discomfort. Pain is uncommon but when present may mimic coronary artery disease. Aerophagia is usually a habit, although it may be associated with organic disease. Many aerophagics are not aware that they are air-swallowers.

2. Swallowed air that is not eructed passes down to the small bowel and colon. Should the air become trapped in the splenic flexure, left upper quadrant discomfort, which radiates to the left chest, left shoulder, and sometimes the left arm, may occur. This is the splenic flexure syndrome. Relief of the pain is characteristically obtained by defecation. The diagnosis is established by demonstrating large amounts of air in the splenic flexure either by percussion or on x-ray films. The important conditions to be differentiated are coronary artery disease and pulmonary disease.

DIAGNOSTIC APPROACH

1. A careful history and physical examination should be performed, with special reference to the nutritional status of the patient and the presence of psychologic disturbances, systemic disorders, or disease of the pancreas, biliary, and intestinal tracts.

2. Analysis of abdominal pain and associated symptoms, when present, may provide important clues to the diagnosis.

3. X-ray studies should include contrast studies of the esophagus, stomach, small intestine, and colon. A gallbladder series may also be indicated.

4. Stool examination should be performed.

5. Proctosigmoidoscopy, esophagoscopy, and gastroscopy may be indicated in selected cases.

6. In patients with both flatulence and diarrhea, special studies may be indicated. The reader is referred to the section Diarrhea, earlier in the chapter, for further details.

Abdominal Distention and Ascites

Barry W. Frank

ABDOMINAL DISTENTION

Definition

Abdominal distention may be defined as a sudden or gradual increase in the size of the abdomen. Distention may be persistent or intermittent.

Symptoms

Abdominal distention may be entirely asymptomatic. More often, however, there is a sensation of fullness or pressure. Pain of varying severity may be noted. Other symptoms, such as vomiting, gaseous eructations, expulsion of flatus, postprandial discomfort, constipation, localized pain, back pain, weight gain, shortness of breath, and edema, if present, may be clues to the etiology of the distention.

Physical Examination

Detailed examination of the abdomen is essential and should begin with inspection. The presence and location of abdominal scars, the abdominal venous pattern, and the contour of the abdomen should be noted. Examination for flank fullness, shifting dullness, and a fluid wave should be made.

Percussion aids in localizing abnormal areas of dullness, tympany, and resistance. Palpation defines enlarged organs, masses, areas of tenderness, and herniae. Auscultation reveals liver rubs, abnormal bowel sounds, and bruits. Pelvic and rectal examinations are essential to rule out pelvic disease.

Etiology

Localized
1. Upper abdomen.
   a. Hepatomegaly.
   b. Splenomegaly.
   c. Renal enlargement by mass or cyst.
   d. Gastric distention secondary to mechanical or functional obstruction.
   e. Inflammatory mass.
   f. Abdominal wall hernia.
   g. Aortic aneurysm.

2. Lower abdomen.
   a. Uterine enlargement.
   b. Ovarian mass or cyst.
   c. Distention of the urinary bladder.
   d. Inflammatory mass arising from the sigmoid colon, cecum, or ileum.
   e. Abdominal wall hernia.

Generalized
1. Ascites (discussed later in the section, p. 203).

2. Intestinal obstruction.
   a. Adynamic ileus.
   b. Mechanical obstruction (colonic obstruction tends to cause diffuse abdominal distention, whereas small bowel obstruction tends to affect primarily the lower abdomen).

3. Large intraabdominal cyst.

4. Diffuse peritonitis from any cause.

5. Extreme constipation with fecal impaction.

6. Neurogenic obstruction (Hirschsprung's disease).

Diagnostic Approach

1. *Initial procedures.* In addition to the history and physical examination, a hemogram, urinalysis, liver function tests, and serum and urinary amylase determinations should be performed on every patient.

2. X-ray studies.

    a. Four-way abdominal films.   Such films are indicated in virtually all cases, especially if intestinal obstruction is suspected. With this procedure, evaluation of the size of the liver is inaccurate, but splenomegaly can be recognized. The kidneys are usually seen as well-defined shadows on each side of the spine at approximately the level of the third lumbar vertebra. The psoas shadows extend obliquely and laterally toward the pelvis. Distortion of these shadows suggests retroperitoneal disease. A clearly defined line in the flank represents the translucent area occupied by the properitoneal fat; this line is obliterated in the presence of abscess or infection. It is important to note the character of the gas patterns in the intestinal tract. Fluid levels, abnormal calcium deposition, intraperitoneal air and organ displacement are also important. The nature and diagnostic implications of the many abnormalities that can occur are beyond the scope of this text, but proper interpretation is essential to accurate diagnosis.

    b. Barium studies of the GI tract.   When intestinal obstruction is suspected, regardless of its cause, barium x-ray studies should not be performed without consultation with the radiologist and not without detailed consideration of the clinical problem. Barium should not be used orally when perforation is suspected, when intestinal obstruction is complete, or when vomiting is persistent. Water-soluble contrast material, such as gastrografin, should be used cautiously in patients susceptible to aspiration to avoid pulmonary edema. In the hands of a skilled radiologist, barium enemas can be of great value in the diagnosis of colonic obstruction. If obstruction is not present, barium x-rays are indicated to look for intrinsic lesions or for displacement or alterations produced by extrinsic lesions. Unless the clinical history and physical examination strongly suggest the upper or lower GI tract, a barium enema should be obtained first because it makes subsequent preparation for upper GI and small bowel series easier for the patient.

    c. Intravenous pyelogram.   Retroperitoneal abnormalities often will not produce alterations of the barium x-rays. An intravenous pyelogram may be of value in defining renal pathology as well as disease in the retroperitoneum.

3. Liver scan.   When distention occurs in the upper abdomen or when a right upper quadrant mass is present, a liver scan may be helpful in delineating the size and contour of the liver, or in revealing intrahepatic defects due to abscesses, cysts, or neoplasms.

4. Abdominal angiography.   This diagnostic procedure may be of assistance in the diagnosis of suspected masses. Vascular abnormalities of significance include vascular occlusion, vessel displacement or straightening, and the presence of a vascular blush.

5. Ultrasonic scanning.   Although still in its infancy and not available in many hospitals, ultrasonic scanning may be helpful in the diagnosis of intraabdominal and retroperitoneal cysts, pancreatic pseudocysts, and aortic aneurysms or other fluid-filled lesions. The procedure has little value in the evaluation of solid tumors within the abdomen.

6. Laparoscopy. This relatively safe, simple procedure is being used more frequently as a method for internal inspection of the upper and lower abdomen. The technique involves three basic steps: induction of a pneumoperitoneum, insertion of the instrument, and inspection of the superficial structures of the abdominal cavity. Best seen are significant portions of the liver, the peritoneum, the anterior wall of the stomach, the uterus, and the ovaries. The ability to obtain biopsies is an added diagnostic dimension that may save the patient from the need for surgical laparotomy.

7. Paracentesis.   See page 204.

ASCITES

Definition

Ascites may be defined as an accumulation of fluid in the peritoneal cavity. The fluid is most often serous in nature.

Symptoms and Physical Examination

See the section Abdominal Distention, earlier in the chapter.

Etiology

The most common causes of ascites are cirrhosis of the liver and congestive heart failure. Ascitic fluid may be a transudate or an exudate, or it may be chylous. The causes are listed below.

Transudative Ascites
1. Prehepatic causes.
   a. Right-sided heart failure.
   b. Constrictive pericarditis.
   c. Venous occlusion.
      (1) Supradiaphragmatic occlusion of the inferior vena cava.
      (2) Budd-Chiari syndrome (hepatic vein occlusion due to thrombosis, tumor, or venous web).
      (3) Veno-occlusive disease secondary to hepatotoxins (e.g., seneciosis).

2. Hepatic causes.
   a. Cirrhosis of the liver.
      (1) Micronodular.
      (2) Macronodular.
      (3) Cardiac.
   b. Tumors of the liver (occasionally).

Exudative Ascites
  1. Peritonitis.
     a. Ruptured viscus.
     b. Tuberculosis.
     c. Pancreatitis.
     d. Bile peritonitis.

  2. Tumors.   Metastatic to the liver or peritoneum, or both.

Chylous Ascites
  1. Trauma to the cysterna chyli in the abdomen.
  2. Tuberculosis (occasionally).
  3. Cirrhosis of the liver (occasionally).
  4. Chronic inflammation, fibrosis, or hyperplasia of the major intestinal lymphatics.
  5. Tumor involving the major intestinal lymphatics.

Miscellaneous Causes
  1. Meigs' syndrome (ovarian fibroma).
  2. Myxedema.
  3. Endometriosis.
  4. Pseudomyxoma peritoneii.
  5. Anasarca with hypoalbuminemia.

Diagnostic Approach

  1. Liver function tests.   Since the most common cause of ascites is liver disease, the initial laboratory tests should include a serum bilirubin, alkaline phosphatase, glutamic oxaloacetic transaminase (SGOT), isocitric dehydrogenase (ICD), prothrombin time, and protein electrophoresis. Bromsulphalein (BSP) excretion studies should be done only if the bilirubin level is normal and the other liver function findings are either normal or nondiagnostic. If acute or chronic hepatitis is suspected, the serum should be examined for the presence of hepatitis-associated antigen.

  2. Diagnostic paracentesis.   Diagnostic paracentesis is a valuable procedure in ascites because the character of the fluid is often helpful diagnostically. The procedure should be performed under sterile conditions. Ordinarily, 100 to 200 ml of fluid is adequate for the studies outlined below.
     a. Appearance of the fluid.   Clear, straw-colored fluid is usually seen in liver disease or prehepatic obstruction. Bloody fluid suggests malignancy but may occur in nonmalignant liver disease. Turbid fluid implies infection or inflammation. Milky fluid is virtually pathognomonic of chylous ascites.
     b. Specific gravity.   Ascitic fluid with a specific gravity greater than 1.017 is indicative of an exudative process.

c. Protein content. Fluid with a protein content greater than 3.0 gm/100 ml is found in exudates. When the protein content exceeds 4.0 gm/100 ml, tuberculous ascites should be suspected.

d. White cell count. White counts are often variable. However, when the count is greater than 10,000 per cubic millimeter, peritonitis is possible. A predominance of lymphocytes suggests tuberculosis.

e. Amylase. Amylase levels above 500 units suggest pancreatitis or pancreatic ascites.

f. Serum electrolytes. Electrolyte determinations are of little diagnostic value.

g. Stains and cultures for bacteria. A gram stain should be performed routinely to detect suspected or unsuspected infection of the peritoneum. Routine cultures for aerobic and anaerobic organisms, acid-fast bacilli, and fungi are advisable.

h. Triglycerides. Although frank chylous ascites is detectable by the naked eye, a slightly turbid fluid may pose a diagnostic problem. The presence of chylous ascites is confirmed by finding elevated triglyceride levels in the fluid.

i. Cytologic study. When intraabdominal malignancy presents with "studding" of the peritoneum by tumor nodules and ascites, confirmation of the diagnosis can be obtained by histologic study of smears prepared from a centrifuged specimen of ascitic fluid.

3. Barium studies of the gastrointestinal tract. Contrast examinations are often necessary in the patient with ascites of unknown cause. In addition to disclosing intrinsic disease of the gastrointestinal tract and varices, displacement of the gut by extrinsic lesions may be revealed.

4. Liver scan. This test is most helpful in the diagnosis of space-occupying lesions of the liver and least helpful in determining liver size or liver function.

5. Needle biopsy of the liver. Percutaneous liver biopsy should be considered in most cases when liver abnormality is suspected as the cause of ascites. It is useful in establishing the histologic diagnosis in primary disease of the liver, in detecting malignancy, and in revealing hepatic manifestations of systemic disease (e.g., tuberculosis).

6. Selective angiography and retrograde venous catheterization. Selective arteriography of the hepatic and splenic arteries with delayed films to visualize the portal vein may be helpful in ascites of obscure cause. Retrograde venous catheterization may be useful in the diagnosis of cardiac and pericardial disease.

7. Peritoneoscopy. The introduction of pneumoperitoneum, insertion of a laparoscope, and inspection of the abdominal contents are useful for the direct visualization of the liver, gallbladder, pelvic organs, omentum, and peritoneal surfaces. Biopsies can be taken for histologic examination and culture. This procedure should be strongly considered when ascites is associated with a pelvic tumor, positive cytologic examination result, or suspected tuberculous peritonitis. With some exceptions, it should not be performed if the patient has undergone previous intraabdominal surgery.

8. Exploratory laparotomy. In the vast majority of cases, it is possible to discover the cause of ascites by means of the foregoing procedures. However, should the etiology remain undetermined after adequate study, exploratory laparotomy may be necessary to establish a correct diagnosis.

Hepatomegaly
Solomon Papper

DEFINITION

Hepatomegaly is defined as an enlarged liver. Liver size is best measured by the distance between the upper border of dullness and the palpable or lower percussable edge of the liver in the midclavicular line. Normal values depend on body habitus, but in the adult male, the liver span is 12 ± 2 cm. Measuring only the distance below the costal margin is inadequate, since a low diaphragm, as in chronic obstructive lung disease, will displace the liver downward without its being enlarged.

ETIOLOGY

1. Congestive heart failure.

2. Inflammatory disease: hepatitis.
  a. Bacterial hepatitis (e.g., septicemia).
  b. Viral hepatitis.
  c. Parasitic (e.g., amebiasis).
  d. Leptospiral hepatitis.
  e. Toxic hepatitis (e.g., carbon tetrachloride).

3. Alcoholic liver disease.
  a. Acute alcoholic hepatitis.
  b. Chronic cirrhosis.

4. Cirrhosis of nonalcoholic etiology.

5. Infiltrative disease.
  a. Tumors.

   b. Amyloid.

   c. Lymphoma and leukemia.

   d. Extramedullary hematopoiesis.

   e. Glycogen storage disease.

   6. Biliary tract obstruction.

DIAGNOSTIC APPROACH

History

A history of heart failure, acute febrile illness, alcoholism, past evidence of liver disease, or general symptoms of malignant disease are especially helpful.

Physical Examination

1. Tenderness of the liver is indicative of acute enlargement of the liver and capsular stretching (e.g., heart failure, acute hepatitis of any cause). Chronic processes are less likely to be associated with tenderness.

2. With acute engorgement or inflammation, the liver has no nodularity and has a soft consistency. With chronic infiltration or scar tissue, there may be some fine nodularity, and the liver feels firm.

3. Large nodules or masses suggest tumor.

4. Ascites is more likely in the chronic conditions.

Laboratory Data

See the next section, Jaundice.

1. Any of the conditions listed above (see Etiology) may be associated with jaundice, and the bilirubin is present in the serum in conjugated or unconjugated forms, or both.

2. Serum albumin is more likely to be reduced in chronic conditions.

3. The hepatocellular enzyme levels (e.g., SGOT) may be elevated in any of the conditions, but the highest levels are found in the acute inflammatory state.

4. Serum alkaline phosphatase levels are highest in the infiltrative processes but may also be somewhat elevated in heart failure and the inflammatory states.

5. Liver biopsy may be required when diagnosis remains uncertain.

Jaundice
Solomon Papper

DEFINITION

Jaundice, or icterus, refers to yellow color of the skin and mucous membranes due to an excess of bile pigments. (A laboratory definition might be a serum bilirubin concentration in excess of 1.2 mg/100 ml even in the absence of clinically detectable yellow coloration.) Jaundice may be hemolytic, hepato-cellular, or obstructive.

HISTORY

1. A family history of jaundice suggests Gilbert's disease, Dubin-Johnson syndrome, hereditary spherocytosis, or Wilson's disease.

2. A history of hepatotoxic exposure may be very helpful whether the disease produced is primarily hepatocellular or cholestatic in type. Such hepatotoxic exposures include but are not limited to ethyl alcohol, carbon tetrachloride, phenothiazines, methyltestosterone, oral contra-ceptives, monamine oxidase inhibitors, needle punctures, and contact with jaundiced patients. For any jaundiced patient a complete list of every drug used by the patient and its possible hepatotoxicity should be prepared.

3. Viral hepatitis is most frequently seen in young adults, while gall-bladder disease is predominantly a disease of middle life, especially in women.

4. The history of associated symptoms may be extremely useful. Vague gastrointestinal complaints, anorexia, nausea, vomiting, fever, and mal-aise prior to the onset of jaundice suggest viral hepatitis. A long history of fatty food intolerance and postprandial bloating support considera-tion of gallbladder disease. Chills and fever suggest possible cholangitis. Severe debility and weight loss are consistent with malignancy. Pruritus suggests obstruction or cholestatic drug reaction.

5. Patients with viral hepatitis are more likely to have a heavy feeling than true pain in the epigastrium and right upper quadrant. However, pain occurs and may be referred to the umbilicus. The nature of the pain provides important clues. Gallstone pain is likely to have occurred before and tends to have a sharper quality and to be localized in the right upper quadrant. Any new pain of mild to moderate degree in an elderly person suggests pancreatic carcinoma. The pain may go through to the back and be aggravated in the supine position.

6. A history of dark urine and light stools indicates obstruction, whether intrahepatic or posthepatic in origin.

PHYSICAL EXAMINATION

1. An enlarged liver generally indicates disease. Tenderness suggests recent distention of the capsule, as in hepatitis or congestive heart failure. If the liver is large and not tender, it may be infiltrated with malignancy; this is especially likely if large nodular masses are felt. Postnecrotic (or macronodular) cirrhosis also produces this picture.

2. The presence of spider nevi, gynecomastia, palmar erythema, loss of axillary hair, parotid gland enlargement, Dupuytren's contracture, prominent abdominal wall veins, or ascites suggests parenchymal liver disease, most commonly cirrhosis. However, ascites may be due to peritoneal tuberculosis or tumor implantation.

3. A large gallbladder in a jaundiced patient is most consistent with carcinomatous obstruction of the common duct.

4. A palpable spleen indicates parenchymal liver disease or hemolytic jaundice.

5. A friction rub over the liver suggests tumor.

6. Physical findings of other disease that might involve the liver secondarily should be sought (e.g., lymphomatous adenopathy).

LIVER TESTS

1. Hemolytic jaundice is characterized by a high (>50 percent) indirect (unconjugated) bilirubin fraction, normally pigmented stool, absence of bile in the urine, and presence of urinary urobilinogen. There will also be other evidence of hemolysis (e.g., anemia, distorted red blood cells, reticulocytosis, and often splenomegaly).

2. Hepatocellular jaundice (e.g., viral and alcoholic hepatitis) may have an initial "obstructive phase" characterized by bile in the urine, acholic stools, and a high direct (conjugated) bilirubin fraction; these tend to improve fairly rapidly. In any event, serum alkaline phosphatase is generally less than 10 Bodansky units, while a moderate to marked elevation in SGOT (over 300 units) is the rule.

3. Obstructive jaundice (e.g., drug-induced cholestasis, stones, carcinoma) is characterized by bile in the urine, acholic stools, high direct bilirubin fraction, and serum alkaline phosphatase above 10 Bodansky units, with SGOT below 300 units.

OTHER PROCEDURES

1. Upper GI series may be very helpful to detect enlargement of the head of the pancreas by carcinoma.

2. Oral gallbladder series may be helpful if the serum bilirubin level is below 3 to 4 mg/100 ml; intravenous cholangiogram may be indicated if the serum bilirubin level is below 7 to 8 mg/100 ml; above these levels, visualization is most unlikely.

3. Liver scan may reveal large tumor masses or liver abscess.

4. Liver biopsy may be extremely helpful but is contraindicated in *obstructive* jaundice because of possible bile peritonitis.

5. Celiac axis angiography may reveal pancreatic carcinoma.

6. Surgical exploration may be required.

DIAGNOSTIC APPROACH

1. Hemolytic jaundice usually is readily identified by the means described. The major clinical question usually is, Does the patient need to be operated on?

2. Careful history and physical examination usually lead one in the correct direction, which is then confirmed by laboratory evaluation. A careful history includes all drugs and medications.

3. In the laboratory, the SGOT is especially helpful: values over 300 favor nonsurgical jaundice and those above 1000 virtually exclude surgery. Other tests, such as serum alkaline phosphatase, are less likely to be helpful. Abnormal prothrombin time readily corrected with parenteral vitamin K suggests extrahepatic obstruction.

4. Upper GI series, liver scan, and gallbladder series (when possible) are the next steps.

5. If diagnosis remains unclear, liver biopsy may be a valuable procedure to do next.

6. If diagnosis remains elusive, exploration is indicated.

6.

Hematologic Problems

Anemia
Robert G. Chapman

DEFINITION

1. Anemia is a subnormal total red cell volume. The normal volume in males is 32 ± 3.5 ml per kilogram and in females, 25 ± 3.5 ml per kilogram. Persons living at elevations higher than 8000 to 9000 feet above sea level have an increased total red cell volume. Below this altitude, normal increases are of smaller magnitude and difficult to detect.

2. The total red cell volume can be measured with ^{51}Cr- or ^{32}P-labeled red cells or it can be calculated from the measured plasma volume and hematocrit reading. Simple tests measuring red cell concentration (hemoglobin and hematocrit values, red cell count) are usually used in place of the expensive and time-consuming total volume determinations. A normal plasma volume is assumed in evaluating the results.

NORMAL VALUES

1. The normal hemoglobin concentration in males is not less than 14 gm per 100 ml; in females, it is not less than 12 gm per 100 ml. The normal hematocrit value in males is not less than 42 percent; in females, not less than 36 percent. The normal red cell count in males is not less than 4 million per cubic millimeter; in females, not less than 3.3 million per cubic millimeter. Of these, the red cell count is the least reliable. Automated determinations calculate the hematocrit

value from the red cell count and the average individual red cell volume. Hematocrit readings done by this method are not as reliable as those measured directly by centrifugation. The ratio of hematocrit value to hemoglobin value is close to 3:1. Significant deviations from this ratio on automated counts should be questioned.

2. Dehydration, such as occurs in vomiting and diarrhea, may deplete the plasma volume and produce a rise in hemoglobin or hematocrit value without changing the total red cell volume. Pregnancy and congestive heart failure, on the other hand, have the opposite effect. When there is a rapid loss of blood, the hemoglobin and hematocrit values do not reflect the degree of blood loss until readjustment of the plasma volume has taken place. Therefore, under all of the foregoing circumstances, caution must be employed in using the hemoglobin and hematocrit values as indicators of the red cell volume.

DIAGNOSTIC APPROACH

1. In order to arrive quickly and efficiently at a correct diagnosis of the kind of anemia, a logical, stepwise procedure should be followed.
   a. Study the history and physical findings.
   b. Attempt to classify the anemia into hemolytic, blood loss, or bone marrow failure types, based on the pathophysiologic mechanism responsible for the red cell deficit.
   c. Perform more detailed tests and, at times, institute a therapeutic trial to determine the specific cause.

2. Anemia may also be approached on the basis of the size and color of the red cells, although this method does not lend itself to a logical, easily remembered scheme. Its major virtue is that it leads from the initial data on the red cell size and chromaticity to a consideration of the most likely causes. Macrocytic anemias are generally associated with vitamin B_{12} or folic acid deficiency, hypothyroidism (marrow failure type), liver disease, or hemolysis (elevated reticulocyte count). Microcytic anemias, which usually are also hypochromic, as a rule are associated with iron deficiency, thalassemia (marrow failure type), or hemolysis (red cell fragmentation). Most varieties of anemia are normocytic and normochromic. Use of this morphological classification requires memorizing the appropriate association and selecting tests to determine the specific cause.

3. Anemia results from the inadequate formation of red cells, excessive blood loss, or increased destruction of red cells, or a combination of these factors. Determination of the reticulocyte count and the serum bilirubin level, together with an assessment of the rate of development of the anemia, suggests the mechanism in most cases.

4. The reticulocyte count, better expressed as number per cubic millimeter (normal is 30,000 to 80,000 per cubic millimeter) than simply

as a percentage, indicates the rate of red cell formation. It is elevated by a premature release of reticulocytes from the marrow as well as by increased red cell formation. A high count, especially if there is no improvement in the anemia over a week or more, is good evidence for excessive red cell loss. A low count, especially in the face of anemia to which a normal marrow should respond, is very good evidence for bone marrow failure. It should be noted, however, that it takes 5 to 7 days after sudden hemorrhage or hemolysis before reticulocytosis occurs. The marrow response to a hemolytic anemia may be blocked temporarily by any inflammatory process, resulting in a temporary depression of the reticulocyte count and a rapid worsening of the anemia.

5. The serum bilirubin (unconjugated) level, which normally does not exceed 0.8 mg per 100 ml, is an indicator of red cell destruction. It is also affected by liver function. Increased red cell destruction (hemolysis) may raise the bilirubin level to 2 or perhaps 3 mg per 100 ml but not higher unless liver function is also impaired. Mild hemolysis may not elevate the serum bilirubin at all. Hemoglobin loss from the body by hemorrhage or hemoglobinuria, of course, will not result in increased production of bile pigments. It should be remembered that anemia without increased hemolysis produces less than normal quantities of bilirubin. Hence, serum bilirubin levels in nonhemolytic anemias should be below 0.8 mg per 100 ml.

6. Mild hemolytic disease with a normally functioning bone marrow may not cause anemia. This so-called compensated hemolysis may produce a reticulocytosis and possibly an elevated serum bilirubin level.

7. In the acutely ill patient who must be treated before an etiology for anemia can be established, it is important to draw blood samples before therapy is begun. In all cases, the reticulocyte count and the serum bilirubin should be determined at the time of the initial hemogram. Blood samples should also be retained for the following tests: (a) serum iron and iron-binding capacity, (b) serum haptoglobin, (c) serum folate and vitamin B_{12} levels, (d) serum protein electrophoresis, and (e) hemoglobin electrophoresis. Because other red cell studies (e.g., fragility, autohemolysis, enzyme activity) require relatively fresh samples of blood, it is impractical to save blood for them. The first three tests listed are markedly affected by transfusion and by treatment with vitamin B_{12} or folic acid. It is therefore essential to hold the pretreatment blood samples until it is decided whether these tests should be performed.

INITIAL EVALUATION

History

Many facets of the history and physical examination are potentially helpful in the evaluation of anemia. Only the most important and useful ones are given here.

1. Any past anemia, the therapy employed, and the response to treatment should be reviewed in order to ascertain whether the present and the previous anemia are related. Chronic anemia or recurrent episodes of anemia over a period of years suggests a hereditary disease, whereas anemia of recent onset suggests an acquired disorder. Acceptance of any explanation for prior anemia must be predicated on objective evidence of an adequate response to specific measures. Anemia that is insidious in onset and gradual in development suggests bone marrow failure. Because of the relatively long life span of the red cell (4 months), failure of effective erythropoiesis will take some time to become apparent. Anemia that is rapid in its onset suggests either bleeding or hemolysis as a probable cause.

2. Inquiries should be made concerning diet, alcohol intake, medications used by the patient, and possible blood loss. An inadequate diet and excessive use of alcohol suggest possible folic acid deficiency. A review of the patient's medications is important because some drugs may cause hemolysis, and others, bone marrow depression. Questions related to bleeding are especially important. Black stools, especially if they are foul-smelling and sticky, may indicate intestinal bleeding, unless the patient is taking iron. Previous subtotal gastrectomy, often for bleeding ulcer, is frequently associated with continued iron deficiency anemia due to either iron malabsorption or persistent bleeding. In women, menorrhagia may be responsible for excessive iron loss. This symptom is difficult to evaluate because many women do not know what "normal" bleeding is. As a rule of thumb, the use of one box (10) of napkins or tampons per period may be considered average; more than that probably represents excessive bleeding. Large menstrual blood losses may result in iron deficiency anemia. Measurements have shown that women who bleed heavily may lose about 1 pint of blood with each period, representing a loss of about 200 mg of iron.

3. The family history is important in the hereditary anemias, especially in those with an autosomal dominant or sex-linked pattern. Inquiry should be made about anemia, jaundice, gallbladder disease, and splenectomy in blood relatives.

Symptoms

1. Dyspnea, palpitation, and fatigue are common complaints, but they are not specific.

2. Pallor may be noted by the patient or his family, but frequently this is missed by both.

3. Jaundice, similarly, may be present but overlooked.

4. Symptoms of postural hypotension are likely to occur when whole blood is lost rapidly.

5. Lifelong hemolysis may be asymptomatic except for the development of cholelithiasis at an early age and the occurrence of crises of abdominal pain or jaundice and weakness, or both.

Physical Examination

The physical examination may be helpful in detecting anemia, bleeding, jaundice, or hemolysis, and perhaps its cause. Most often, however, the cause of the anemia is left unresolved by examination. Marked postural changes in pulse and blood pressure usually indicate rapid loss of whole blood. These signs may occur before changes in hemoglobin or hematocrit values become apparent. Estimation of the patient's state of hydration is necessary for the proper evaluation of these parameters. Pallor, of course, suggests anemia; when associated with jaundice, it may be indicative of hemolysis. Petechiae or purpura suggest the presence of a disorder that is also thrombocytopenic. Hemorrhages in the eyegrounds may occur in severe anemia from any cause. Glossitis is often seen in pernicious anemia or severe iron deficiency. Hemic murmurs are commonly heard in many severe anemias. Careful palpation for splenomegaly is important in all patients with anemia. Splenomegaly may be due to congestion (e.g., cirrhosis of the liver), hemolytic disorders, infections, connective tissue disease, and infiltrative or neoplastic disorders. The presence of lymphadenopathy suggests the possibility of infectious disease, connective tissue disorders, or infiltrative lesions. Assessment of proprioception, best determined by position sense in the toes, may provide a clue to spinal cord involvement in vitamin B_{12} deficiency. Examination of the stool for occult blood is mandatory. A negative result, however, does not exclude the possibility of slight or intermittent bleeding. Iron therapy makes the stools black but does not invalidate the test for blood.

ANEMIA RESULTING FROM BONE MARROW FAILURE

Etiology

1. Lack of an essential nutrient (e.g., vitamin B_{12}, folic acid, iron).
2. Injury to the marrow (e.g., ionizing radiation).
3. Marrow inhibition (e.g., drug, immunologic agent).
4. Marrow replacement (e.g., neoplasm, fibrosis).
5. Hereditary defect.
6. Endocrine deficiency (e.g., hypothyroidism, hypopituitarism, renal failure).
7. Idiopathic ("refractory").

Diagnostic Approach

Peripheral Blood Count and Smear

1. Abnormality of peripheral blood cells other than red cells indicates a widespread marrow disorder. Vitamin B_{12} deficiency and folic acid deficiency both produce thrombocytopenia and neutropenia. Hypersegmented neutrophils with more than five nuclear lobes occur com-

monly in both conditions. Pancytopenia may also occur in bone marrow injury or marrow replacement. The peripheral blood smear may also be helpful in differentiating between leukemia and neoplasm metastatic to the marrow. Although there are exceptions, the presence of immature white cells in the smear suggests leukemia, whereas a normal white cell structure favors metastatic malignancy.

2. The red cell structure is not always abnormal in marrow failure anemia. Thus, in the anemia of renal disease, the red cells look normal, but there is a lack of polychromatophilic cells (reticulocytes on Wright's stain). Hypochromia indicates hemoglobin deficiency, not iron deficiency. Its most common causes are iron deficiency and thalassemia. The presence of basophilic stippling in the large polychromatophilic red cells strongly favors the diagnosis of thalassemia over that of iron deficiency. The finding of similar blood smears in the patient's blood relatives, together with the demonstration of increased hemoglobin A_2 or F on hemoglobin electrophoresis, helps to establish the diagnosis of β thalassemia. A mixed population of normal and hypochromic red cells is sometimes seen in untreated patients with poorly defined refractory anemias, some of which may terminate in acute granulocytic leukemia. Anisocytosis (abnormal variation in red cell size) is not a common feature of marrow failure anemia unless there is considerable poikilocytosis (abnormal variation in red cell shape). Marked poikilocytosis is a feature of thalassemia and, to a lesser degree, of iron deficiency. It may also be seen in severe vitamin B_{12} or folic acid deficiency and in the hemoglobinuric hemolytic diseases (artificial heart valve induced, paroxysmal nocturnal hemoglobinuria, hemolytic uremic syndrome), especially if iron deficiency becomes a secondary effect.

Bone Marrow Biopsy

Bone marrow biopsy is a most important procedure in the diagnosis of marrow failure anemia. Although marrow smears are useful in detecting the abnormal megaloblastic maturation of vitamin B_{12} or folic acid deficiency, histologic sections of the marrow, obtained preferably by core biopsy rather than by aspiration, are of much greater value. Sectioned material is the only reliable method for evaluating general marrow cellularity and the distribution of cell types. Fibrosis and the serous fat atrophy of malnutrition or hypothyroidism can be detected only in sections. Packed tumor cells, which may not aspirate for smearing, are readily identified. Moreover, the reticulum cells, in which hemosiderin is stored, do not appear readily in aspirates. Thus, it is essential to have sectioned material, stained with Prussian blue, for the evaluation of iron stores. The bone marrow findings in various types of marrow failure anemia are as follows:

1. Generalized hypocellularity suggests a toxic injury to the marrow by drugs, chemicals, or ionizing radiation. It may also be seen in hypothyroidism or malnutrition.

2. Normal cellularity, except for a lack of erythroid tissue, suggests an immunologic cause, as may occur occasionally in thymoma; it may also be drug related.

3. Any cellularity with a lack of hemosiderin establishes the diagnosis of iron deficiency.

4. General hypercellularity of all marrow elements is seen in vitamin B_{12} and folic acid deficiency. Patchy hypercellularity is also a finding in marrow fibrosis.

5. Hypercellularity with large numbers of abnormal cells is found in acute leukemia, lymphoma, multiple myeloma, and metastatic malignancy.

6. Hypercellularity due to increased erythroid tissue is observed in thalassemia and is often striking in the idiopathic refractory marrow failure anemias.

Routine Laboratory Tests
1. Most important are renal function tests (BUN or serum creatinine). Marrow suppression, with its concomitant anemia, is a common occurrence in renal failure. Sometimes the anemia is severe before other symptoms of renal insufficiency are evident.

2. Mild anemia resulting from marrow suppression is also a frequent finding in chronic illness, such as rheumatoid arthritis or infectious disease. An increased sedimentation rate and varying degrees of diffuse hypergammaglobulinemia frequently are associated findings.

Special Laboratory Tests
1. Decreased blood levels of vitamin B_{12} and folic acid may indicate which substance is lacking in a megaloblastic anemia. The normal values for vitamin B_{12} and folate exceed 180 pg per milliliter and 6.5 ng per milliliter, respectively.

2. The serum iron and iron-binding capacity, from which the saturation of the iron-binding globulin is calculated, may help demonstrate inadequate iron stores. Saturation less than 16 percent is seen in iron deficiency anemia, especially when the hemoglobin is under 8 gm per 100 ml. Similar desaturation may also occur in a wide variety of inflammatory conditions (e.g., rheumatoid arthritis, infections). In any case, bone marrow sections stained for hemosiderin are more reliable indicators of iron deficiency than are the serum iron levels.

X-ray Examination
The demonstration of metastases suggests neoplastic marrow replacement as the cause of anemia. The finding of increased density of all bones is indicative of myelosclerosis, a condition in which fibrous tissue replaces the marrow. Chest films may show evidence of a thymoma, a tumor often associated with a lack of erythroid tissue in the marrow, resulting presumably from the effects of thymic humoral factors on red cell formation. The anemia is cured or relieved by removal of the tumor.

Therapeutic Trials
Diagnosis by a well-designed therapeutic trial is appropriate in selected instances. In all trials, one agent at a time should be used. A rise in the hemo-

globin and hematocrit values or an increase in the reticulocyte count is indicative of a positive response. When reticulocytosis is too slight to be detected, as may occur when the anemia is mild, one must rely on a rise in the hemoglobin and hematocrit values. Such changes are usually evident by the end of 2 weeks of treatment. A negative response does not necessarily preclude the possibility that the patient is deficient in the substance tested. For example, a patient with iron deficiency anemia may not respond to orally administered iron because of intestinal malabsorption or because a concomitant inflammatory process interferes with the marrow response to iron.

1. Therapeutic trials with vitamin B_{12} or folic acid should employ very small doses (1 and 200 μg per day, respectively, administered parenterally) to avoid the cross-responsiveness of the marrow to these agents. However, when the patient is severely anemic, it is impractical to wait 1 or 2 weeks to observe the response to either folic acid or vitamin B_{12}. Therefore, large doses of both substances are often used simultaneously while waiting for the results of the serum folate and B_{12} levels to be reported.

2. Some cases of refractory marrow failure anemia, with increased iron stores and significant numbers of ring sideroblasts in the marrow, may respond slowly to large doses of pyridoxine. Since no laboratory test is currently available to predict pyridoxine responsiveness, an empiric trial of this vitamin (daily oral dosage of 200 mg) is worthwhile in this type of anemia.

3. There are also other refractory anemias, presumably based on an immune mechanism, with a predominant incidence in older women, that respond to treatment with corticosteroids. A trial with steroid therapy is probably warranted in otherwise unresponsive refractory anemias.

Specific Etiology
Once a diagnosis of a specific deficiency anemia is made, the cause of the deficiency must be sought.

1. Folic acid deficiency may be the result of decreased intake, increased requirements, or interference with the metabolic activity of folic acid. It is usually the result of an insufficient intake of dietary sources (fresh green vegetables) because of either a poor diet, alcoholism, or intestinal malabsorption. Increased requirements of folic acid occur during pregnancy, and if intake is inadequate, a megaloblastic anemia may occur. Chronic hemolysis may also exhaust folic acid stores. Folic acid metabolism may be impaired by drugs such as diphenylhydantoin and methotrexate. In such cases, the megaloblastic anemia generally improves when the drug is stopped.

2. Dietary deficiency of vitamin B_{12} occurs rarely. Although decreased intake may occur from intestinal disease or from competition for B_{12} by intestinal organisms and parasites, it is usually caused by a lack of the gastric intrinsic factor that is essential for the absorption of the vitamin. This absorptive defect is demonstrable with the Schilling test.

A small dose of cobalt 60-labeled vitamin B_{12} is given orally; this is followed by the parenteral administration of a large amount of non-radioactive vitamin B_{12}. The urine is collected for 24 hours. Kidney function must be normal. If excretion of the labeled substance is normal, there is no indication for vitamin B_{12} therapy. If excretion is low, the test should be repeated with the addition of intrinsic factor given orally. If the poor excretion in the first test is due to intrinsic factor deficiency, the result of the second test should be normal; if it is abnormal, other causes must be found for the malabsorption of the vitamin.

3. Iron deficiency in adults is rarely due to dietary deficiency alone. Intestinal malabsorption of iron is also an uncommon cause of iron deficiency except in malabsorption syndromes or after gastrointestinal surgery. Bleeding is by far the most common cause of iron deficiency in adult men and postmenopausal women. In adult women, iron deficiency is most commonly due to unreplaced iron losses from menstruation or repeated pregnancies. When bleeding is occult, it is usually of gastrointestinal origin. Every effort must be made to demonstrate the source of the bleeding. Stools should be examined repeatedly for occult blood. Proctosigmoidoscopy and radiologic examination of the gastrointestinal tract are also indicated.

ANEMIA DUE TO BLEEDING

1. Bleeding may be rapid and massive, slow and hidden, internal or external. Bleeding is most commonly external, arising from the gastrointestinal or genitourinary tracts or from sites of trauma. When hemorrhage takes place internally into the body tissues, the red cell iron is usually recovered and used again in hemoglobin synthesis. The degradation of heme leads to increased bile pigment production and hyperbilirubinemia.

2. Routine blood counts may fail to indicate the degree of blood loss when hemorrhage occurs rapidly, because cells and plasma are lost together. Significant blood loss (over 500 ml) is suggested by symptoms and signs of postural hypotension or shock. Direct measurement of the total plasma or red cell volume provides the only accurate assessment of anemia in such cases.

3. Recovery from bleeding can occur when the bleeding is slow or controlled and tissue stores of iron are adequate. During recovery, a reticulocytosis is seen. The hemoglobin may rise as much as 1 gm per 100 ml per week.

4. Protracted bleeding results in exhaustion of the iron stores. Reticulocytosis then stops, and iron deficiency anemia develops. Hemosiderin is absent from marrow sections and serum transferrin iron saturation falls. Typical peripheral blood cell and serum iron changes may not be evident unless the anemia is severe (hemoglobin 8 gm per 100 ml).

5. Frequent testing of stools for occult blood is an excellent way to detect mild bleeding, but negative results do not rule out intermittent or a very slow rate of bleeding (less than 4 ml of blood loss per day).

6. Aspirin ingestion is a frequent cause of low-grade bleeding. If continued long enough, iron deficiency anemia may result.

7. Menstrual blood loss is seldom rapid enough to cause either hypovolemia or acute anemia, but it may result in iron deficiency anemia, as mentioned previously.

ANEMIA RESULTING FROM HEMOLYSIS

Definition and Etiology

Human red blood cells have a normal life span of 120 days. A decrease in this life span for any reason other than bleeding is termed *hemolysis*. If the bone marrow is normal, it can compensate for a fourfold to sixfold decrease in the red cell life span and prevent anemia, producing what is called *compensated* hemolytic disease.

There are many causes of hemolysis. It is convenient to consider them in two categories: (1) intracorpuscular defects, nearly always hereditary, in which the red cell is abnormal from the time it is formed in the marrow, and (2) extracorpuscular defects, nearly always acquired after birth, in which the red cell is formed normally in the marrow but is injured by something in the circulation in which it lives.

The presence of an *intracorpuscular hemolytic disorder* is suggested by:

1. Evidence of a similar hemolytic disorder in a blood relative.

2. A history of lifelong anemia, recurring jaundice, or the development of gallstones before the age of 30 years.

3. A negative Coombs' test result.

4. Ancestry that is Jewish, Negro, Mediterranean, or Southeast Asian, because of the higher incidence of sickle hemoglobin, thalassemia, and glucose 6-phosphate dehydrogenase (G-6-PD) deficiency in these populations.

Hereditary hemolytic disease may not be discovered until later in life, either because it is episodic (e.g., the drug-induced group with G-6-PD deficiency) or because it is well compensated until the vicissitudes of age compromise the marrow's ability to maintain compensation (e.g., hereditary spherocytosis).

Extracorpuscular hemolytic disease is frequently associated with an anti-erythrocytic antibody that is demonstrable by the direct Coombs' test. A positive Coombs' test result means only that the red cells are coated with gamma globulin; it does not necessarily imply that hemolysis is present.

A seldom used but very sensitive method for distinguishing intracorpuscular from extracorpuscular defects is the measurement of the survival of

⁵¹Cr-tagged compatible normal red cells in the patient. The life span of the donor cells is normal in patients with intracorpuscular defects but is shortened in those with extracorpuscular disorders.

Hemolytic Anemia Due to Intracorpuscular Defects

Etiology
Intracorpuscular hemolytic disorders have the following causes:

1. Abnormal hemoglobin (S, C, D, E, unstable).
2. Defective globin synthesis (thalassemia).
3. Defective heme synthesis (porphyria).
4. Defective carbohydrate enzyme (G-6-PD, pyruvate kinase).
5. Possible membrane defect (hereditary spherocytosis, elliptocytosis).
6. Paroxysmal nocturnal hemoglobinuria (the one acquired red cell defect in this group).

Laboratory Tests
1. Peripheral blood smear.
2. Sickle cell preparation.
3. Hemoglobin electrophoresis for abnormal hemoglobin and for measurement of A_2 and F hemoglobins.
4. Incubated sample for Heinz body formation or precipitation of unstable hemoglobin.
5. Screening for heat-unstable hemoglobin.
6. Autohemolysis test and perhaps osmotic fragility.
7. Enzyme screening for G-6-PD and pyruvate kinase (PK) deficiency.
8. Urinary hemosiderin; if positive, perhaps also an acid hemolysis test.

All of these tests should not be performed at once, because some, such as the acid hemolysis and osmotic fragility tests, are time-consuming and expensive. The peripheral smear should be examined carefully first, since it may provide excellent clues to the cause.

Interpretation of Findings
1. Increased numbers of spherocytes with only mild to moderate anisocytosis suggest hereditary spherocytosis. In most instances, blood smears of parents and siblings will detect at least one other, similar case.

2. Basophilic stippling, best detected at a high magnification in the large polychromatophilic red cells, suggests abnormal RNA. This phenomenon is common in thalassemia and helps greatly to distinguish this disease from iron deficiency anemia, which produces an otherwise similar smear.

3. Sickling of the red cells may occasionally be seen in the smear, indicating the need for a sickle cell preparation and hemoglobin electrophoresis.

4. The presence of many target cells with little or no anemia, although not highly specific, suggests hemoglobin C abnormality, a condition in which mild hemolysis may occur.

5. Neutropenia occurs in the later stages of paroxysmal nocturnal hemoglobinuria (PNH). In addition, the continued loss of iron because of the hemoglobinuria may lead to iron deficiency and to changes in the peripheral smear due to this type of anemia.

6. Howell-Jolly bodies in the red cells occur in the absence of splenic function, most often the result of previous splenectomy. However, they may also be seen late in the course of sickle cell disease when "autosplenectomy" has taken place because of repeated splenic infarctions.

7. Other red cell inclusions, some evident only with vital staining (methylene blue), may be seen in patients with abnormal unstable hemoglobins (e.g., Zürich, Köln).

8. If the peripheral smear suggests a specific disease, additional tests to support that diagnosis should be made:

   a. The autohemolysis test is indicated for the diagnosis of hereditary spherocytosis or enzyme deficiency. Increased hemolysis is almost always observed, but the addition of glucose before incubation does not always prevent it.

   b. Hemoglobin electrophoresis is performed for the measurement of A_2 and F hemoglobins in suspected thalassemia. Elevations of one or both of these hemoglobins may be seen in this disease. However, failure to find them increased does not exclude the possibility of thalassemia.

   c. A sickle cell preparation and hemoglobin electrophoresis are done for the diagnosis of sickle cell disease.

   d. Hemoglobin electrophoresis is required for the diagnosis of hemoglobin C disease.

   e. If PNH is suspected, the first test should be an examination of the urine for hemoglobin and of its sediment for hemosiderin. Hemoglobinuria in PNH is intermittent, but, as in any condition with recurring hemoglobinuria, hemosiderin is present at all times in the shed cells of the urinary sediment. If the hemosiderin test result is positive, the diagnosis of PNH should be confirmed by a carefully performed Ham's acid hemolysis test.

   f. The suspicion of an unstable hemoglobin may be confirmed by the examination of a heated (50°C) hemolysate for a precipitate or by incubating a methylene blue–stained red cell suspension to search for Heinz bodies or precipitated hemoglobin.

9. Red cell enzyme deficiencies do not produce any characteristic morphologic abnormalities in the peripheral smear. Those described so far

are classified as hereditary nonspherocytic hemolytic anemia. An enzyme deficiency should be suspected if the problem appears to be intracorpuscular and no other causes of intracorpuscular hemolytic disorders are found. Although most frequently associated only with episodic hemolysis related to drug exposure or infection, some variants of red cell G-6-PD deficiency found in non-Mediterranean Caucasians may produce chronic hemolysis in the absence of exogenous factors. Because of its sex-linked inheritance, G-6-PD disease is expressed mainly in males. Screening tests for G-6-PD deficiency are available, but unfortunately they may be normal during the hemolytic episodes when many young red cells are present. Under such circumstances, the test should be repeated several months after recovery to confirm the diagnosis. Much rarer is the autosomally recessive red cell pyruvate kinase (PK) deficiency. Enzyme assays for red cell PK for the confirmation of this diagnosis are becoming more readily available.

10. The most common cause of intracorpuscular hemolytic anemia is hereditary spherocytosis (HS). Because of a membrane defect, the red cells in this disorder have a decreased surface area. The spherocytosis is the result of a decreased surface-to-volume ratio. The mean red cell diameter (not the volume) is decreased, and the mean corpuscular hemoglobin concentration is increased. Autohemolysis and osmotic fragility of the red cells, especially after incubation, are increased. No test is absolutely pathognomonic for the diagnosis of HS, but the demonstration of similar changes in a parent or sibling provides adequate proof in most cases. If splenectomy fails to eliminate evidence of hemolysis, the correctness of a diagnosis of HS should be seriously questioned.

Hemolytic Anemia Due to Extracorpuscular Defects

Etiology
Extracorpuscular hemolytic anemias have the following causes:

1. Primary or idiopathic (i.e., no underlying disease is detectable), associated with a strongly positive Coombs' test result.

2. Secondary.
   a. Physical agents (water, burns, artificial heart valves, fibrin in small vessels).
   b. Chemical agents (venom, drugs).
   c. Infections (e.g., malaria, Welch's bacillus sepsis, infectious mononucleosis, granuloma).
   d. Neoplasm (especially lymphoma and leukemia).
   e. Connective tissue disease (systemic lupus erythematosus, rheumatoid arthritis).
   f. Splenomegaly from any cause.
   g. Isosensitization (transfusion, newborn).
   h. Paroxysmal cold hemoglobinuria.

Laboratory Tests

1. Laboratory procedures that are useful in the evaluation of these disorders include the following:
    a. Peripheral blood smear.
    b. Plasma haptoglobin and perhaps plasma hemoglobin.
    c. Urine hemosiderin.
    d. Fibrinogen and fibrin split products, if the latter test is available.
    e. LE test, RA factor, ANA test.
    f. Immunohematology tests in addition to the Coombs' test.
    g. Donath-Landsteiner test and serologic test for syphilis.
    h. Various additional studies needed to detect underlying infections, neoplasm, etc.

2. The choice of tests for the evaluation of extracorpuscular disease depends to some extent on the clinical features. The history and physical examination are likely to be more helpful in evaluating these disorders than the hereditary diseases. A disease associated with acquired hemolysis may be evident before anemia becomes a problem. On the other hand, hemolysis may present a problem well in advance of other manifestations of the disease (e.g., systemic lupus erythematosus).
    a. The peripheral smear may be very helpful. Abnormalities of white cells and platelets may indicate the presence of another condition, such as leukemia or disseminated intravascular coagulation. The latter diagnosis is suggested by the occurrence of red cell fragmentation in the smear. Fragmentation is also seen in other conditions characterized by mechanical damage to the cell (e.g., abnormally functioning artificial aortic heart valves). Spherocytosis of the red cells suggests coating of the cells by antibody, but it may also result from thermal injury in burned patients. Spherocytosis, neutropenia, and varying degrees of thrombocytopenia may occur in systemic lupus erythematosus or in any condition in which the spleen is large enough to trap and destroy blood cells. In malaria, the parasites are seen within the affected red cells.
    b. When intravascular hemolysis is suspected because of red cell fragmentation in the peripheral blood or because of the occurrence of hemoglobinuria without hematuria, absence of haptoglobin and elevation of free hemoglobin levels in the plasma confirm the diagnosis. Plasma haptoglobin tends to be diminished in other hemolytic processes, but its complete absence in these conditions is rare. Significant intravascular hemolysis can often be detected by simple visual inspection of the patient's plasma for red hemoglobin or brown methemoglobin. As mentioned previously, the urine sediment contains hemosiderin in cases of recurrent hemoglobinuria. The loss of iron in the urine may be sufficient to cause the superimposition of iron deficiency on the original anemia. Intravascular hemolysis is accompanied by an elevation of the serum bilirubin, LDH, and SGOT levels. These findings may lead to confusion with liver disease.

c. When intravascular coagulation is suspected, fibrinogen levels and fibrin degradation products should be assayed. The finding of fibrinogen levels and thrombocytopenia in association with red cell fragmentation is most suggestive of this disorder. An increase in fibrin split products helps to confirm the diagnosis. Other clotting factors also tend to be at low levels; these may be measured for confirmation if available. Prompt diagnosis and anticoagulant therapy are often needed to save the patient suffering from disseminated intravascular coagulation.

d. Connective tissue diseases, particularly systemic lupus erythematosus and less frequently rheumatoid arthritis, are commonly associated with the presence of antibodies against the patient's own red cells and thus with a positive Coombs' test result. Because of this association, LE cell preparations and tests for antinuclear antibody and rheumatoid factor should be performed on every patient with a Coombs'-positive hemolytic anemia. Negative test results do not rule out the possibility of SLE, because the hemolytic disease may develop long before other manifestations of the disease appear.

e. In addition to the Coombs' test, other immunologic studies can be done to characterize the protein coating of the damaged red cells.

(1) The thermal characteristic of the antibody is important. The cold agglutinins found in infectious mononucleosis and mycoplasma pneumonia may cause hemolysis. Although warm agglutinins are more common, they are less specific.

(2) All Coombs'-positive hemolytic disorders may be classified into cold and warm agglutinin types. Unfortunately, this classification is often of little help in determining the cause of the autoantibody or in predicting the outcome of the illness.

(3) An unusual but specific disease picture occurs in paroxysmal cold hemoglobinuria. This illness, which at times is associated with syphilis and diagnosed by the Donath-Landsteiner test, is characterized by episodes of brisk intravascular hemolysis and hemoglobinuria following exposure to cold.

f. No attempt is made here to describe additional tests and procedures that might be helpful in establishing the cause of an acquired hemolytic anemia. Suffice it to say that a careful search for underlying disease is indicated in all such patients.

3. Coombs'-positive hemolytic anemias are regarded as primary or idiopathic if no evidence of an underlying disease can be found. The diagnosis of idiopathic acquired hemolytic disease is thus made by exclusion. However, such a diagnosis should remain tentative for at least a year or two because many such cases eventually turn up with a systemic disease such as systemic lupus erythematosus or a lymphoma.

Polycythemia

H. Harold Friedman

DEFINITION

The terms *polycythemia* and *erythrocytosis* refer to a blood picture characterized by an increase in the number of circulating red cells accompanied
by a corresponding increase in the hemoglobin and hematocrit values. In
uncomplicated polycythemia, the total red cell count regularly exceeds 6
million per cubic millimeter, the hemoglobin value is more than 18 gm/
100 ml, and the hematocrit value is greater than 54 percent. Absolute polycythemia is erythrocytosis in which the red cell mass per unit of body weight
is increased. Relative polycythemia, also called stress erythrocytosis, is a
condition in which the red count and hemoglobin and hematocrit values are
elevated but the red cell mass is normal.

CLASSIFICATION

1. Absolute polycythemia.
   a. Primary polycythemia or polycythemia vera.
   b. Benign familial erythrocytosis.
   c. Secondary polycythemia.
      (1) With low arterial oxygen saturation.
         (a) Pulmonary disease due to ventilation-perfusion imbalance,
             impaired diffusion, or alveolar hyperventilation (e.g.,
             chronic obstructive pulmonary disease, diffuse pulmonary
             fibrosis, Pickwickian syndrome).
         (b) Right-to-left shunts (e.g., various types of cyanotic con-
             genital heart disease).
         (c) Exposure to high altitude.
      (2) With normal arterial oxygen saturation.
         (a) Congestive heart failure (some cases).
         (b) Hemoglobinopathies with familial polycythemia (e.g., M
             hemoglobin).
      (3) With inappropriate erythropoietin production.
         (a) Renal lesions (e.g., cysts, hydronephrosis, hypernephroma).
         (b) Nonrenal lesions (e.g., cerebellar hemangioblastoma, hepa-
             toma, uterine myomata).
         (c) Androgen administration.

2. Relative polycythemia.
   a. Hemoconcentration.
   b. Gaisböck's syndrome.

CLINICAL FEATURES

Polycythemia Vera

1. Polycythemia vera is a myeloproliferative disorder characterized by panmyelosis.

2. The symptoms and signs are related to the pathophysiologic disturbances:
   a. Increased blood volume and hyperviscosity of the blood (headache, fullness in the head, dizziness, lethargy, fatigue, dyspnea, epigastric distress, paresthesias).
   b. Hypermetabolism (weight loss, night sweats).
   c. Thrombocytosis and vascular disease (thromboses, angina, cerebrovascular insufficiency, intermittent claudication, thrombophlebitis).
   d. Basophilia (pruritus).
   ?e. Increased urate production and hyperuricemia (secondary gout).
   f. Myeloid metaplasia (splenomegaly and hepatomegaly).

3. Physical findings include a plethoric appearance, venous engorgement, splenomegaly (almost 100 percent of cases), hepatomegaly (50 percent of cases), and nonspecific cutaneous lesions. Cyanosis and clubbing do not occur. Thrombosis and abnormal bleeding are commonly observed.

4. Laboratory abnormalities include panhyperplasia of the bone marrow, an elevated red count, leukocytosis, basophilia, thrombocytosis, increased urate excretion and hyperuricemia, normal arterial oxygen saturation, a high leukocyte alkaline phosphatase score, high serum B_{12} levels and elevated B_{12}-binding capacity of the serum, and increased blood histamine levels.

Benign Familial Erythrocytosis

Benign familial erythrocytosis is a heritable, familial disorder characterized by an increased total red cell volume with normal white cell and platelet counts. The only bone marrow abnormality is erythroid hyperplasia. Splenomegaly usually does not occur.

Secondary Polycythemia

With Low Arterial Oxygen Saturation

1. This type of polycythemia is most commonly due to chronic pulmonary disease or cyanotic congenital heart disease. Evidence of the underlying disease is usually obvious.

2. Cyanosis, clubbing, and arterial oxygen unsaturation (below 90 percent) are observed commonly. Hepatosplenomegaly is absent unless due to associated disease.

3. Aside from the polycythemia and hypoxemia, the laboratory findings are essentially negative. The white cell and platelet counts are normal. The bone marrow examination shows only erythroid hyperplasia. Occasionally, hyperuricemia is present, but it does not reach the high levels found in polycythemia vera. Erythropoietin production is increased.

With Normal Arterial Oxygen Saturation

The conditions in this category are uncommon causes of polycythemia.

1. Decreased arterial blood flow without a change in oxygen content may occur in congestive heart failure associated with a low cardiac output. Evidence of the primary disease is usually overt, and correction of the decompensated state is associated with the return of red cell values to normal.

2. Polycythemia is sometimes due to familial disorders in which the transport or release of oxygen is interfered with because of an abnormal hemoglobin. Hemoglobin electrophoresis and determination of the oxygen dissociation curve of the patient's hemoglobin are necessary to establish the diagnosis of such a hemoglobinopathy.

3. Polycythemia may sometimes result from erythropoietin-producing lesions or tumors, or from the administration of drugs such as androgens.

Relative Polycythemia

1. Loss of fluids and electrolytes, as in dehydration, burns, adrenocortical insufficiency, or after strenuous diuretic therapy, may cause spurious polycythemia because of hemoconcentration.

2. Gaisböck's syndrome is a disorder seen primarily in middle-aged, obese, tense, or anxious males. It is often associated with mild or moderate hypertension. The spleen is not enlarged. Although the red cell count and hemoglobin and hematocrit values are elevated, the red cell mass is normal. This finding distinguishes relative polycythemia from both primary and secondary polycythemia. The white cell and platelet counts are normal, as is the bone marrow.

DIFFERENTIAL DIAGNOSIS

The differential diagnosis between polycythemia vera, secondary hypoxic polycythemia, and relative polycythemia (Gaisböck's syndrome) is considered in Table 6-1. Two points are worthy of special comment.

1. Primary and secondary polycythemia can almost always be distinguished on the basis of the bone marrow findings. In sections of an adequate bone marrow biopsy, the finding of a hypercellular marrow showing erythroid and granulocytic hyperplasia, together with megakaryocytosis

TABLE 6-1. Differential Diagnosis of Polycythemia Vera, Secondary (Hypoxic) Polycythemia, and Relative Polycythemia (Gaisböck's Syndrome)

Manifestation	Polycythemia Vera	Secondary Polycythemia	Relative Polycythemia
Central cyanosis	Absent	Frequently present	Rare
Cardiac or pulmonary disease	Absent	Present	Hypertension common
Splenomegaly	Present in over 95%	Absent	Absent
Hepatomegaly	Present in 50%	Absent	Absent
Red cell mass	Increased	Increased	Normal
White cell count	Increased in 95%; basophilia and eosinophilia common	Normal unless increased as a result of infection	Normal
Platelet count	Elevated in 50%	Normal	Normal
Bone marrow	Hypercellular; increased erythropoiesis and granuloporesis; megakaryocytosis; absence of stainable iron	Erythroid hyperplasia; other elements normal	Normal
Arterial oxygen saturation	Usually above 94%, sometimes lower	Usually below 90%, occasionally higher	Normal
24-Hour urinary urate excretion	Markedly increased	Slightly increased	Normal
Serum uric acid	Commonly elevated to high levels	Normal or slightly increased	Normal or slightly increased
Serum B_{12} level	Elevated	Normal	Normal
Serum B_{12}-binding capacity	Elevated in 75%	Normal	Normal
Leukocyte alkaline phosphatase	Elevated in 85 to 90%	Normal	Normal
Erythropoietin	Decreased or normal	Increased	Normal
Serum iron	Decreased	Normal	Normal
Blood histamine	Increased	Normal	Normal

Source: Reprinted with modifications from *Hematology* by W. C. Beck (Ed.) by permission of the M.I.T. Press, Cambridge, Massachusetts. Copyright © 1973 by The Massachusetts Institute of Technology.

and absence of stainable iron, is virtually diagnostic of polycythemia vera. In secondary erythrocytosis, the hyperplasia is limited to erythroid elements.

2. One should not rely too heavily on the arterial oxygen saturation in differentiating between polycythemia vera and secondary hypoxic polycythemia unless the value (under basal conditions) is above 94 percent or below 90 percent, the former indicating primary and the latter, secondary polycythemia. Values between 90 and 94 percent may be found in both conditions and thus have little discriminating value. Arterial oxygen analyses are helpful in the evaluation of polycythemia due to obscure lung disease or inapparent right-to-left shunts.

DIAGNOSTIC APPROACH

1. In the presence of chronic pulmonary disease or venoarterial shunts, especially when associated with cyanosis, clubbing, and hypoxemia, it may be assumed that the polycythemia is secondary to the underlying disorder. Further work-up for the polycythemia per se is then unnecessary.

2. When clinical evidence of the disorders listed in the preceding paragraph is lacking, the diagnostic possibilities include primary, secondary, and relative polycythemia.

3. If the patient has leukocytosis and thrombocytosis as well as splenomegaly, polycythemia vera is the most likely possibility. Sections of an adequate bone marrow biopsy (not smears) should be performed, and the arterial oxygen saturation should be determined. If the bone marrow findings are typical, and the arterial blood is fully saturated with oxygen, the diagnosis of primary polycythemia is virtually assured. Additional support for the diagnosis may be obtained by finding increased urate excretion, hyperuricemia, a high leukocyte alkaline phosphatase score, elevated serum B_{12} levels, and an increased serum B_{12}-binding capacity.

4. It is unnecessary to determine the total volume of circulating red cells if the hemoglobin value is greater than 20 gm/100 ml and the hematocrit value is over 60 percent, because such values are virtually diagnostic of absolute polycythemia in the absence of causes of acute plasma volume depletion. Measurement of the red cell mass is indicated when the hemoglobin value is between 16 and 20 gm/100 ml and the hematocrit value is between 45 and 60 percent, to help differentiate between absolute and relative polycythemia.

5. If the peripheral blood studies and bone marrow biopsy are not diagnostic, and the spleen is not palpable, the differential diagnosis usually rests between secondary and relative polycythemia. To distinguish between these possibilities, the following tests may be helpful:

   a. Measurement of the red cell mass to decide whether the polycythemia is absolute or relative.

b. Determination of the arterial oxygen saturation to diagnose inapparent secondary hypoxemic polycythemia.

c. An intravenous pyelogram to rule out renal lesions capable of causing polycythemia.

d. Hemoglobin electrophoresis and determination of the oxygen dissociation curve of the patient's hemoglobin to detect a hemoglobinopathy.

White Blood Cell Abnormalities
John H. Saiki

NEUTROPENIA
Definition

Neutropenia (and its near synonym granulocytopenia) is defined as an absolute neutrophil count of less than 1500 per cubic millimeter.

Clinical Significance

1. Host resistance is related to the degree of neutropenia.

   a. More than 1500 neutrophils per cubic millimeter is associated with normal host resistance.

   b. 1000 to 1500 neutrophils per cubic millimeter is associated with mildly impaired host resistance.

   c. 500 to 1000 neutrophils per cubic millimeter is associated with moderately impaired host resistance.

   d. Less than 500 neutrophils per cubic millimeter is associated with markedly impaired host resistance.

2. The major consequence of neutropenia is vulnerability to infection. The usual clinical manifestations of infection are often absent because of the lack of granulocytes. Thus, pneumonia may be present without a significant infiltrate, meningitis may occur without pleocytosis, and pyelonephritis may be found without pyuria.

Normal Granulocyte Kinetics

The highlights of granulocyte kinetics are illustrated in Figure 6-1. Granulocytes are produced and stored in the bone marrow from which they are discharged into the vascular compartment. The cells are about equally divided between the circulating and marginal pools. Granulocytes eventually make their way into the body tissues but once there do not reenter the bloodstream.

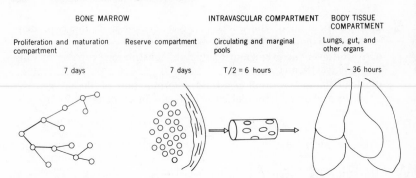

FIG. 6-1.   Normal granulocyte kinetics.

Mechanisms of Neutropenia

Neutropenia can result either from decreased production of neutrophils by the bone marrow or their accelerated removal from the blood by immune or nonimmune mechanisms. Transfer of neutrophils from the circulating to the marginal pool may also result in low white cell counts.

Etiology

1. Proliferation defects (hypoproliferation).
   a. Marrow injury (e.g., radiation, drugs).
   b. Marrow infiltration (e.g., leukemia, fibrosis, metastatic carcinoma).

2. Maturation defects (ineffective proliferation): vitamin B_{12} and folate deficiency.

3. Distribution abnormality (increased margination): endotoxin.

4. Survival defect.
   a. Accelerated consumption (e.g., infection).
   b. Accelerated destruction (e.g., immune mechanisms and hypersplenism).

Diagnostic Approach

See Table 6-2.

NEUTROPHILIA

Definition

Neutrophilia is defined as an absolute granulocyte count in excess of 7500 per cubic millimeter.

TABLE 6-2.   Diagnostic Features of Neutropenia of Various Origins

Disorder	Peripheral Blood Findings	Bone Marrow Findings
1. Proliferation defects		
a. Marrow injury	Pancytopenia; toxic changes in granulocytes; large reticulocytes	Hypocellularity; vacuolation of cytoplasm in precursor cells
b. Marrow infiltration	Pancytopenia; leukoerythroblastic reaction	Hypercellularity; reduced normal hematopoiesis; infiltration by fibrosis, tumor cells, or leukemia
2. Maturation defects	Macroovalocytes; Howell-Jolly bodies; hypersegmentation of granulocytes; pancytopenia	Hypercellularity; panhyperplasia; megaloblasts; giant metas and bands
3. Distribution abnormality	Pseudoneutropenia; normal smear	Normal
4. Survival defect		
a. Accelerated consumption (infection)	Left shift; toxic granulation; Döhle inclusion bodies	Increased granulocytic proliferation; depleted reserve compartment
b. Accelerated destruction (immune)	Left shift	Increased granulocytic proliferation; depleted reserve compartment

Clinical Significance

A neutrophilic leukocytosis most frequently is a nonspecific manifestation of inflammation. An absolute granulocytosis, when it manifests as a leukemoid reaction, must be differentiated from chronic granulocytic leukemia. A granulocytic leukemoid reaction may be defined as an elevated granulocyte count associated with the appearance of immature granulocytic precursors in peripheral blood (i.e., myelocytes, promyelocytes, and myeloblasts).

Etiology

1. Increased production of granulocytes.
   a. Reactive (e.g., infection, steroids, Hodgkin's disease).
   b. Myeloproliferative (e.g., chronic granulocytic leukemia).

2. Increased release of granulocytes from reserve compartment.
   a. Etiocholanolone.
   b. Endotoxin.

3. Decreased margination of granulocytes: epinephrine (endogenous or exogenous).

4. Decreased egress of granulocytes from the blood.
   a. Adrenal steroids.
   b. Prednisone.

Diagnostic Approach

In the clinical setting the practical problem is the differential diagnosis of reactive and malignant granulocytosis (see Table 6-3).

LYMPHOCYTOSIS

Definition

Lymphocytosis is defined as an absolute lymphocyte count in excess of 4500 per cubic millimeter.

TABLE 6-3.   Differential Diagnosis of Chronic Granulocytic Leukemia and Leukemoid Reaction

Parameter	Chronic Granulocytic Leukemia	Leukemoid Reaction
Clinical picture	Usually no symptoms, or symptoms related to splenomegaly	Often exhibit overt manifestations of underlying disease (e.g., carcinoma, infection)
Peripheral blood findings	Leukocytosis related to spleen size; few blasts common; giant platelets; basophils increased	Leukocytosis unrelated to spleen size; myeloblasts rarely present; platelets normal in appearance; basophils not increased
Bone marrow findings	Hypercellular; megakaryocytes increased (early); myeloid:erythroid = 10+:1; myelocyte dominates granulocytic series; basophils increased	Cellularity variable; megakaryocytes usually normal; myeloid:erythroid usually greater than normal; granulocytic "pyramid" intact; basophils not increased
Leukocyte alkaline phosphatase activity	Usually decreased	Usually increased
Serum B_{12}	Marked increase	Slight increase
Karyotype abnormality (Ph[1] anomaly)	Usually present	Absent

Clinical Significance

Lymphocytosis is most common in childhood and usually a nonspecific finding associated with viral infections. In the adult, lymphocytosis has greater specificity and therefore greater diagnostic value.

Etiology

1. The etiologic mechanisms of lymphocytosis are not well known. Significantly, not all cases are a result of increased proliferation. In pertussis, the mechanism is thought to be related to a blockade of lymphocyte entry into lymph nodes.

2. Causes of nonactivated lymphocytosis (normal inactive small lymphocytes).
   a. Infectious lymphocytosis.
   b. Mumps.
   c. Varicella.
   d. Rubeola.
   e. Herpes simplex.
   f. Influenza.
   g. Tuberculosis.
   h. Pertussis.
   i. Other causes; the most important is chronic lymphocytic leukemia.

3. Causes of activated lymphocytosis (atypical or "turned on" lymphocytes).
   a. Infectious mononucleosis.
   b. Infectious hepatitis.
   c. Toxoplasmosis.
   d. Cytomegalovirus.
   e. Posttransfusion syndrome.
   f. Drug-induced: para-aminosalicylic acid, diphenylhydantoin, mesantoin.

4. A middle-aged or older adult who presents with a nonactivated lymphocytosis almost invariably will prove to have chronic lymphocytic leukemia. The same blood picture in a child usually proves to be pertussis or a pertussis-like syndrome.

BASOPHILIA

Definition

Basophilia is defined as an absolute basophil count of more than 100 per cubic millimeter.

Clinical Significance

Basophilia of itself seldom presents as a clinical problem, but frequently may be a clue to diagnosis. Increases are particularly striking in the myeloproliferative disorders.

Associated Conditions

1. Hypersensitivity states.

2. Myxedema.

3. Ulcerative colitis.

4. Myeloproliferative disorders.
   a. Polycythemia vera.
   b. Chronic granulocytic leukemia.
   c. Essential thrombocythemia.
   d. Myelofibrosis with myeloid metaplasia.

EOSINOPHILIA

Definition

Eosinophilia is defined as an absolute eosinophil count of more than 500 per cubic millimeter.

Clinical Significance

Counts between 500 and 1000 per cubic millimeter are nonspecific and should not be pursued as a clinical problem. Counts greater than 4000 per cubic millimeter have specificity.

Associated Conditions

1. Allergic disorders (e.g., hay fever, bronchial asthma).

2. Parasitic infestation with tissue invasion (e.g., trichinosis).

3. Skin diseases (e.g., dermatitis herpetiformis).

4. Tumors (e.g., Hodgkin's disease).

5. Granulomatous disease (e.g., tuberculosis).

6. The hypereosinophilic syndromes.
   a. Eosinophilic leukemia.
   b. Fibroplastic endocarditis.
   c. Systemic vasculitis.
   d. Löffler's syndrome.
   e. Tropical eosinophilia.

Splenomegaly

John H. Saiki

DEFINITION

Clinically, a palpable spleen represents an enlarged spleen. Enlargement may also be identified by scan measurements.

CLINICAL SIGNIFICANCE

1. Splenomegaly may represent a manifestation of associated disease or may represent primary disease (lymphoma).

2. Impaired gastric filling with early satiety may lead to weight loss. There may be increased susceptibility to rupture from trauma because of lack of protection by the rib cage.

3. Hypersplenism with cytopenia (single or multiple) occasionally is associated with increased susceptibility to infection and hemorrhage.

ETIOLOGY

1. Congestion.
   a. Congestive heart failure.
   b. Portal hypertension.

2. Reactive hyperplasia.
   a. "Work hypertrophy" (e.g., hemolytic disease).
   b. Infections.
      (1) Bacterial (e.g., tuberculosis, infective endocarditis, brucellosis).
      (2) Viral (e.g., cytomegalovirus, infectious mononucleosis).
      (3) Fungal.
      (4) Parasitic (e.g., malaria, toxoplasmosis).
   c. Connective tissue diseases (e.g., SLE, RA).
   d. Serum sickness.

3. Infiltrative diseases.
   a. Nonneoplastic.
      (1) Lipidosis.
      (2) Sarcoidosis.
      (3) Amyloidosis.
   b. Neoplastic.

(1) Lymphoproliferative disorders (acute and chronic lymphocytic leukemia and lymphoma).

(2) Myeloproliferative disorders (polycythemia vera, chronic granulocytic leukemia, and myelofibrosis with myeloid metaplasia).

(3) Metastatic tumor is extremely rare.

DIAGNOSTIC APPROACH

1. History and physical examination.

2. Confirmation of splenomegaly by spleen scan.

3. Initial screening studies.
   a. CBC, reticulocyte count, and platelet count.
   b. Serum bilirubin (total and direct), alkaline phosphatase, SGPT, SGOT, LDH, serum electrophoresis, acid phosphatase.
   c. ANA and RF.
   d. Serologic tests for fungi and complement-fixation test for toxoplasmosis.
   e. X-rays: PA and lateral films of chest, flat plate of abdomen; barium swallow for evaluation of varices.
   f. Liver and spleen scan.
   g. Bone marrow for culture and cytologic and histologic evaluation, including staining for amyloid.

4. If the above studies are unremarkable and the etiology remains unknown, splenectomy should be performed because (a) tissue will be available for culture and definitive histologic diagnosis, and (b) primary lymphoma of the spleen does occur, and long-term benefits of splenectomy in this setting have been demonstrated. If cytopenias are pronounced from hypersplenism and risks of infection or hemorrhage are great, splenectomy will resolve this problem.

Lymphadenopathy
John H. Saiki

DEFINITION

Lymphadenopathy is an abnormal increase in size or altered consistency of lymph nodes. It is a clinical manifestation of regional or systemic disease and serves as an excellent clue to the underlying etiology.

ETIOLOGY

1. Reactive.
   a. Infectious.
      (1) Bacterial (e.g., pyogenic, tuberculosis).
      (2) Viral (e.g., cytomegalovirus, infectious mononucleosis).
      (3) Fungal (e.g., coccidioidomycosis).
      (4) Parasitic (e.g., toxoplasmosis).
   b. Noninfectious.
      (1) Sarcoidosis.
      (2) Connective tissue disease.
      (3) Dermatopathic.
      (4) Drug-induced (e.g., diphenylhydantoin).

2. Infiltrative.
   a. Benign (e.g., histiocytosis, lipidosis).
   b. Malignant (e.g., primary lymphoma, metastatic carcinoma).

DIAGNOSTIC APPROACH

Differential Diagnosis of Regional and Generalized Lymphadenopathy

Regional Lymphadenopathy
1. Cervical and supraclavicular regions (head and neck).
   a. Careful evaluation of oral, nasal, ear, pharyngeal, thyroid, and cutaneous regions.
   b. Etiologic considerations include pyogenic infection, tuberculosis, fungi, viral exanthems, infectious mononucleosis, and malignancy.

2. Hilar and superior mediastinal lymphadenopathy.
   a. Careful evaluation for primary lung disease.
   b. Etiologic considerations include tuberculosis, cryptococcosis, histoplasmosis, sarcoidosis, pneumoconiosis, and malignancy.

3. Axillary, inguinal, or femoral lymphadenopathy. Careful evaluation of the breast and skin of the upper extremity for axillary adenopathy and the genital region and skin of the lower extremity for inguinal and femoral lymphadenopathy.

Generalized Lymphadenopahy
1. Careful evaluation for systemic disease.

2. Etiologic considerations include tuberculosis, infectious mononucleosis, toxoplasmosis, serum sickness, connective tissue disease, diphenylhydantoin-induced hyperplasia, and the lymphoproliferative disorders (acute and chronic lymphocytic leukemia, and lymphoma).

Lymph Node Biopsy

A lymph node biopsy should be considered early in the evaluation of lymphadenopathy. In the case of infection, it will provide valuable culture material. When the diagnosis of lymphoma is made, an entirely new phase of evaluation is then carried out for clinical staging. If the histopathology is nonspecific, the pathologist can still give valuable clues for further evaluation. Selection of the node for biopsy is particularly important. The largest node and the supraclavicular region yield the best results. It should be emphasized that biopsy of localized cervical adenopathy should be performed only after a thorough ENT examination.

Bleeding and Clotting Disorders

Jerome S. Nosanchuk

DEFINITION AND CHARACTERISTICS

Bleeding is defined as a breakdown in hemostasis. Hemostasis depends upon the vascular integrity, the number and quality of platelets, and blood coagulation factors. Clotting requires the conversion of soluble plasma fibrinogen into an insoluble fibrin clot (Fig. 6-2). This conversion is mediated by a protease enzyme, thrombin; the end product, fibrin, is rendered stable by factor XIII (fibrin stabilizing factor). Thus, bleeding occurs when there is impairment of the hemostatic mechanism due to either defective synthesis or excessive utilization of clotting factors. Coagulation may also be impaired by circulating inhibitors of clotting factors or the proteolytic action of plas-

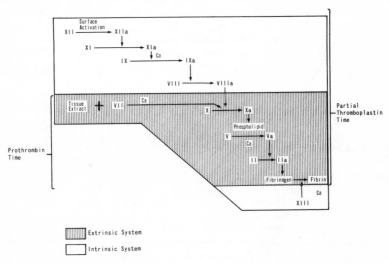

FIG. 6-2.   Clotting reaction.

TABLE 6-4. Characteristics of Bleeding in Hemorrhagic Disorders

Type of Bleed	Definition	Location	Cause
Petechia	Smallest; punctate; about 1 mm in diameter	On extremities; usually absent over pressure points	Vascular or platelet abnormality
Purpura	1 mm to 1 cm	Generally trunkal; occasionally extremities	Vascular abnormality
Ecchymosis	Larger bleed with local extravasation	Soft tissues, joints	Factor deficiency or open blood vessel
Generalized	Diffuse or generalized ecchymosis	Large areas, mucous membranes, wounds, etc.	Disseminated intravascular clotting or primary fibrinogenolysis

min. The degree of bleeding is related to both the nature and the severity of the deficiency. A thorough history and physical examination are adequate to identify most bleeding disorders. The characteristics of bleeding in hemorrhagic disorders are shown in Table 6-4.

Most operative and postoperative hemorrhage is due to inadequate surgical hemostasis. Patients with delayed bleeding or those whose bleeding is controlled initially but who bleed again subsequently are more likely to have intrinsic defects in coagulation factors than platelet abnormalities. This type of bleeding, especially if acquired, is more frequently due to multiple factors than to a single cause.

The final diagnosis of coagulation disorders rests heavily upon laboratory support (Fig. 6-2 and Table 6-5). Functional deficiency or inhibition of a factor in the intrinsic pathway is generally detected by the partial thromboplastin time (PTT). Factors involved in the extrinsic system are usually detected by measuring the one-stage prothrombin time (PT). Both these times are prolonged when fibrin formation is defective. Neither the PT nor the PTT necessarily detects abnormalities in factor XIII or platelets. It requires a significant reduction in any single factor to affect either the PT or the PTT. For example, pure factor VIII or IX deficiency must be reduced to a level that is 30 to 40 percent of normal before the PTT is prolonged. Paradoxically, severe deficiencies of factor II may not prolong the PT. However, a modest combination of multiple factor deficiencies usually prolongs clotting times. Consultation with the clinical laboratory director is not only advisable but often is mandatory for correct diagnosis and appropriate therapy.

EVALUATION OF THE PREOPERATIVE PATIENT

1. The most important initial step is to obtain an adequate history and physical examination. It is also important to ascertain whether the patient has experienced abnormal bleeding or bruising in the past. The site, extent, and duration of previous hemorrhagic phenomena and the

TABLE 6-5. Diagnosis of Clotting Factor Deficiencies

Deficient Factor	Prothrombin Time	Partial Thrombo-plastin Time	Platelet Count	Bleeding Time
I Fibrinogen	A	A	N	N
II Prothrombin	A	A	N	N or A
III Tissue thromboplastin	. . .	. . .	. . .	. . .
IV Calcium	. . .	. . .	. . .	. . .
V Labile factor	A	A	N	N or A
VI (Not assigned)	. . .	. . .	. . .	. . .
VII Stable factor	A	N	N	N
VIII Antihemophilic factor	N	A	N	N
IX Christmas factor	N	A	N	N
X Stuart-Prower factor	A	A	N	N or A
XI Plasma thromboplastin antecedent	N	A	N	N
XII Hageman factor	N	A	N	N
XIII Fibrin stabilizing factor	N	N	N	N
Von Willebrand's	N	N or A	N	N or A
thrombocytopenia	N	N	A	N or A

N = normal, A = abnormal

response to treatment may be helpful. The patient should also be questioned concerning the use of drugs that may interfere with hemostasis. A positive family history of bleeding suggests the presence of sex-linked or autosomal dominant disorders.

2. Knowledge of the patient's underlying disease may provide a clue to potential bleeding problems. Obviously, a patient with significant hepatic disease or uremia is a greater risk than a patient who is otherwise well.

3. The incidence of coagulation hazards is increased in some surgical operations. Cardiopulmonary bypass procedures and hypothermia may cause inactivation or destruction of clotting factors and platelets. Prostate surgery is associated with an increased frequency of fibrinolysis. The use of water rather than saline irrigation in bladder surgery can provoke hemolysis. Cardiovascular surgery, trauma, and other situations in which massive bleeding and replacement transfusion occur also have an increased potential for hemorrhage because of deficiencies in various clotting factors.

4. If, despite negative history and physical findings, a preoperative coagulation screen is still deemed necessary, the following studies are recommended. Negative findings with these tests virtually exclude the presence of a significant preexisting coagulopathy.

   a. Partial thromboplastin time (PTT).

   b. Prothrombin time (PT).
   c. Thrombin time.
   d. Platelet count.
   e. Bleeding time.

EVALUATION OF A BLEEDING PATIENT

The approach to the problem of a bleeding patient should be logical. A history and physical examination are, of course, mandatory. The following laboratory studies should detect the cause(s) and permit guidance in therapy for all but the rare coagulation defects (e.g., platelet factor 3 or factor XIII deficiency).

   1. PT.
   2. PTT.
   3. Platelet count.
   4. Fibrinogen level.
   5. Thrombin time.
   6. Bleeding time.
   7. Fibrin split products.
   8. Hemoglobin and hematocrit readings.
   9. Peripheral blood smear.
   10. Clot for blood typing and cross-matching, for packed cells or component therapy, or both.

   Most operative and postoperative bleeding is due to inadequate local control of a severed blood vessel. Once a patient begins to hemorrhage, it is mandatory to stop this bleeding because massive blood loss itself may deplete certain procoagulants. Only rarely are coagulation factor deficiencies responsible for this type of hemorrhage.

IDENTIFYING THE CAUSE OF THE BLEEDING

Specific factor assays will be suggested by the laboratory consultant based on the preceding screening studies. It should be noted that Table 6-5 does not include data from the defibrination syndromes, platelet abnormalities, clotting factor inhibitors, or vascular defects. These are covered in the remainder of this section. Isolated deficiencies are usually hereditary, whereas those that are acquired frequently involve multiple factors.

Hereditary Factor Deficiencies

   1. Classic hemophilia (hemophilia A) or factor VIII deficiency, a sex-linked hereditary disorder, is the deficiency most commonly diagnosed in practice. It is detected by the presence of an abnormal PTT that is corrected by barium sulfate–adsorbed normal plasma.

2. Hemophilia B (Christmas disease) or factor IX deficiency is less common. It also is a sex-linked, autosomally recessive inherited condition. The PTT is prolonged, but, in contrast to hemophilia A, the abnormality is not corrected by barium sulfate–adsorbed plasma, although normal stored plasma or serum can correct the PTT.

3. The remaining numbered factor deficiencies are rare.

4. Factor deficiencies must be confirmed by performing a specific factor assay using known factor-deficient control material.

5. Clotting factor inhibitors may be associated with some disease states, notably the connective tissue disorders. Special laboratory tests are necessary for their identification.

Vascular Defects

Vascular disorders are poorly defined and not well understood. The etiology of vascular "fragility" is not always apparent. With the exception of vascular pseudohemophilia (von Willebrand's disease), the bleeding is rarely severe.

1. Classic von Willebrand's disease exhibits autosomal dominant inheritance. It is characterized by a prolonged bleeding time and a decreased value for factor VIII. There is evidence to show that at least some patients have functional platelet deficits that contribute to the prolonged bleeding time. It is believed that there may also be some type of circulating antiaggregation factor, since platelet transfusions alone do not correct the bleeding time. Defective platelet adhesion is generally found. Sometimes aggregation abnormalities and platelet factor 3 deficiency are found, but usually the aggregation studies are normal.

2. The factor VIII deficiency differs from that found in hemophilia A. Infusion of plasma concentrates causes a prolonged elevation of factor VIII levels in von Willebrand's disease but not in classic hemophilia, in which the factor VIII activity disappears rapidly.

3. Aspirin causes an exaggerated prolongation of the bleeding time in patients with this disease.

Platelet Defects

Bleeding can occur because of too few or too many platelets. Platelets that are qualitatively defective may be unable to react normally in the clotting process even when present in adequate numbers. The normal platelet count is 150,000 to 350,000 per cubic millimeter. One-third of the platelet mass is sequestered in the spleen. It takes 5 to 7 days for platelets to mature from megakaryocytes. The platelet survival time in the circulation is about 10 days. Platelets adhere to injured vascular endothelium by contact with subendothelial collagen. The ADP released from the cytoplasmic granules of the platelets participates in the induction of aggregation and cohesion. Meanwhile, the phospholipids (platelet factor 3) and other cellular constituents that are discharged activate Hageman factor (XII), which in turn activates the intrinsic clotting pathway. Thrombin and perhaps ADP cause consolidation of the platelet plug.

Laboratory Tests

1. If bleeding is thought to be due to a platelet abnormality, the following quantitative and qualitative platelet tests are indicated. The first four tests can be done in any laboratory. The remainder may not be generally available.
   a. Direct examination of the stained smear.
   b. Platelet count.
   c. Template bleeding time.
   d. Clot retraction.
   e. Prothrombin consumption time with and without inosithin.
   f. Adhesion.
   g. Aggregation.
   h. Assay for platelet factor 3.

2. The probability of bleeding is related to the results of the quantitative and functional tests.
   a. Functionally normal platelets in numbers greater than 50,000 per cubic millimeter will ordinarily prevent hemorrhage during surgical procedures.
   b. Major hemorrhage is unusual with platelet counts in excess of 20,000 per cubic millimeter.
   c. Spontaneous hemorrhage may occur with counts of 10,000 per cubic millimeter or less, but it is not unusual for patients with such levels to go for long periods without serious complications. The major threat is intracranial hemorrhage. Patients with both anemia and thrombocytopenia are more likely to bleed than those with thrombocytopenia alone.
   d. In patients with depressed platelet counts, it is important to have some idea of the functional integrity of the platelets. Observation of clot retraction may be useful for this purpose. Studies of platelet adhesiveness and aggregation may sometimes be pertinent but are not widely available.

Quantitative Platelet Abnormalities

1. Definition. Thrombocytopenia is said to exist when the platelet count is below 70,000 per cubic millimeter. Thrombocytosis, usually a transient state, is present when the platelet count is greater than 400,000 per cubic millimeter. Thrombocythemia is a condition in which the platelet count exceeds 900,000 per cubic millimeter.

2. Etiology.
   a. Thrombocytopenia.
      (1) Diminished or defective platelet production.
         (a) Congenital.
            i) Wiskott-Aldrich syndrome.
            ii) May-Hegglin syndrome.
            iii) Chediak-Higashi anomaly.
         (b) Acquired.
            i) Aplastic anemia.
            ii) Marrow infiltration.
            iii) Radiation toxicity.
            iv) Chemotherapy.
            v) Direct toxicity to platelet production (e.g., thiazides, alcohol, estrogens).
            vi) Cyclic thrombocytopenia (premenstrual).
         (c) Nutritional.
            i) Vitamin B_{12} deficiency.
            ii) Folic acid deficiency.
            iii) Iron deficiency.
         (d) Viral infections.
         (e) Paroxysmal nocturnal hemoglobinuria.
      (2) Increased platelet destruction.
         (a) Giant cavernous hemangioma (Kasabach-Merritt syndrome).
         (b) Infection (viral, bacterial, rickettsial, fungal, mycobacterial).
         (c) Disseminated intravascular coagulation.
         (d) Thrombotic thrombocytopenic purpura.
         (e) Hemolytic-uremic syndrome.
         (f) Drug-induced.
            i) Immunologic (e.g., quinine, quinidine).
            ii) Nonimmunologic.
         (g) Posttransfusion.
         (h) Idiopathic thrombocytopenic purpura.
         (i) Connective tissue disorders.
   b. Thrombocythemia.
      (1) Myeloproliferative disorders.
      (2) Chronic inflammatory states.
      (3) Acute inflammation.
      (4) Acute hemorrhage.
      (5) Iron deficiency.
      (6) Hemolytic anemias.
      (7) Malignant diseases.

(8) Postoperative (especially splenectomy).

(9) Drug-induced.

(10) Postexercise.

c. Thrombocytopenic purpura.

  (1) Acute idiopathic thrombocytopenic purpura (ITP) is usually a disease of childhood. Onset is usually preceded by a viral infection. Spontaneous recovery within a 1- to 2-month period from onset is the general rule.

  (2) Chronic idiopathic thrombocytopenic purpura is primarily a disease of females between the ages of 20 and 50 years. Onset is usually insidious. The disease is characterized by the presence of a purpuric or petechial eruption on the distal portions of the extremities. Splenomegaly is minimal if present at all. The platelet counts may range between 10,000 and 75,000 per cubic millimeter. Bleeding is rare unless the platelet count falls below 20,000 per cubic millimeter. The number of megakaryocytes in the bone marrow is normal or increased, but the megakaryocytes are less granular and more basophilic than normal. Drug sensitivity, sepsis, disseminated intravascular coagulation, systemic lupus erythematosus, tuberculosis, sarcoidosis, and lymphoma must be excluded.

  (3) Platelet sequestration (hypersplenism). Many conditions may cause splenomegaly with hypersplenism and thrombocytopenia.

  (4) Other causes. Hemorrhage, multiple transfusions, and extracorporeal circulation may result in platelet losses and thrombocytopenia.

d. Thrombocythemia. Platelet counts above 1 million per cubic millimeter are likely to be dangerous. Bleeding from the mucous membranes may occur. Thrombotic phenomena are common. The cause of the bleeding is presumed to be mechanical interference with the normal clotting mechanisms by the presence of excessive numbers of platelets and the release of platelet procoagulant factors.

Qualitative Platelet Disorders

1. Thrombasthenia (Glanzmann's disease). This is a rare disorder with autosomal recessive transmission characterized by a prolonged bleeding time, failure of the platelets to aggregate in the presence of ADP and thrombin, abnormal clot retraction, and a prolonged Lee-White whole blood clotting time.

2. Thrombocytopathic purpura (platelet factor 3 deficiency). In this condition, the platelets lack clot-promoting activity because of defective phospholipid release. The bleeding time is prolonged, and aggregation of platelets by ADP and thrombin may be impaired, but clot retraction is normal.

3. Thrombocytopathy. This disorder is characterized by a prolonged bleeding time, impaired platelet aggregation by ADP and collagen, normal clot retraction, and normal platelet phospholipid release.

4. Aspirin inhibits platelet aggregation markedly and may prolong the bleeding time for periods of up to one week.

Acquired Disorders

Vitamin K-Dependent Factors

1. Factors II, VII, IX, and X are synthesized by the liver. All are dependent upon vitamin K for their synthesis. Deficiencies in these factors are detected by measuring the prothrombin time. However, it should be noted that different methods of PT determination exhibit different sensitivities to deficiencies in these factors.

2. Vitamin K is naturally synthesized by intestinal bacteria. It is absorbed only in the presence of bile salts because of its lipid solubility.

3. Depletion in vitamin K-dependent factors may occur in patients receiving antibiotics (especially for "bowel preps"), obstructive jaundice, malabsorption states (e.g., sprue), and hepatic parenchymal disease.

4. Parenteral vitamin K therapy can alleviate vitamin K deficiency unless hepatic cellular function is too severely compromised.

Liver Disease

1. Deficiencies may be noted in factors VII, IX, X, V, II, and I, in the order given. The degree of deficiency is related to the severity and duration of the hepatocellular disease.

2. Factor VIII paradoxically rises to extremely high levels.

3. Plasminogen and antithrombin III deficiencies may occur.

4. Fibrin split products are poorly cleared, thus predisposing to fibrinolysis.

5. Abnormal fibrinogens (dysfibrinogenemia) and antithrombin V may also be produced.

6. Marrow platelet production may be depressed. Excessive sequestration of platelets may occur in the spleen.

Renal Disease

1. Uremic thrombocytopathy may occur when the BUN exceeds 100 mg/100 ml.

2. The thrombocytopathy is manifested by an adhesive abnormality that is correctable by dialysis.

3. Urinary loss of procoagulants, especially factor IX, may occur.

4. In the connective tissue diseases with renal involvement, pathologic inhibitors of procoagulants may appear in the circulation.

Massive Transfusions

Bank blood is deficient in platelets and factor V. Factor VIII is also variably depleted. Clinical problems related to deficiencies in bank blood rarely occur unless at least 10 units of stored blood have been transfused.

Reaction to Heparin Therapy

1. Heparin is a naturally occurring substance whose greatest concentration is found in lung tissue. It interferes with clotting by a variety of actions: inhibition of factors IXa, Va, and XIII; inhibition of the proteolytic activity of thrombin (antithrombin); increased inactivation of factor Xa; and, in large doses, inhibition of platelet aggregation.

2. Heparin prolongs the Lee-White whole blood clotting time, plasma or whole blood recalcification time, PTT, and even PT. The correlation of the heparin dose with the results of these tests is imperfect.

3. No single test of heparin activity presently available is clearly superior to any other. The optimum level of anticoagulation for heparin therapy is still uncertain.

Reaction to Coumarin Compounds

1. Coumarin derivatives are drugs with similar mechanisms of action but with variable rates of absorption and duration of activity. Their principal action is inhibition of the hepatic synthesis of vitamin K-dependent factors (II, VII, IX, and X) either by interference with vitamin K transport in the liver or by direct competition with vitamin K. It is also possible that these compounds cause the liver to produce abnormal forms of factors II, VII, IX, and X, perhaps by interference with a late step in peptide chain formation.

2. Factor VII is depressed first by the action of these drugs. The PT is affected most by deficiency of this factor. Subsequently, factor IX (not measured by the PT) falls, followed by decline in factors X and II. The last two factors reach their lowest levels in about 5 to 10 days. Reversal of drug effects by intravenous vitamin K usually occurs in 6 to 12 hours, provided liver function is normal. However, factor II remains depressed for some time after the PT and PTT become normal.

3. Coumarin drugs may prolong the PTT as well as the PT.

4. The PT is the test of choice for monitoring therapy with this group of drugs. The absolute PT compared to a control is more meaningful than "percent activity."

Circulating Anticoagulants

Circulating anticoagulants are found most often in association with hemophilia A or systemic lupus erythematosus. In both instances, the substances, which may be IgG autoantibodies, are active against factor VIII. Circulating anticoagulants that are active against other factors or that are found in other diseases are rare.

Defibrination Syndromes

Classification

1. Defibrination syndromes may be divided into two major categories: disseminated intravascular coagulation and primary fibrinogenolysis.

    a. Disseminated intravascular coagulation (DIC), sometimes called secondary fibrinolysis, occurs when thromboplastin-like material enters the circulation in sufficient quantities to cause excessive deposition of fibrin in the microcirculation. The physiologic response to the fibrin deposition is extensive fibrinolysis, with the formation of soluble fibrin degradation products (fibrin split products). Some of the fibrin split products, particularly fragments X and Y, are themselves potent anticoagulants.

    b. Primary fibrinogenolysis, in contrast, occurs in the presence of excessive plasmin, which is a potent digester of fibrinogen. This disorder may also result in the production of fibrin split products.

2. Disseminated intravascular coagulation is a relatively common hemorrhagic disorder. It constitutes more than 90 percent of the defibrination syndromes. It is often associated with a treatable predisposing disease, such as bacteremia, abruptio placentae, retained dead fetus, incomplete abortion, burns, and snakebite. Other, less directly treatable causes include transfusion reactions, giant hemangiomas, surgical manipulations, and carcinoma.

3. Primary fibrinogenolysis is relatively rare. It is associated most frequently with prostatic adenocarcinoma and cirrhosis of the liver.

Diagnosis of Acute DIC and Primary Fibrinogenolysis

1. The clinical situation is generally urgent. Bleeding is extensive and characteristically occurs from multiple sites, such as the mucous membranes, incisions and wounds, needle puncture sites, the gastrointestinal tract, and the genitourinary tract.

2. In both diseases, the pathophysiologic process is essentially the conversion of plasma to serum in vivo. Thus, variable depressions of plasma fibrinogen level, the platelet count, and procoagulants are seen. The PT and PTT are usually prolonged. The fibrin split products that are produced can be measured directly or estimated from the thrombin time.

3. The tests listed below (shown with "typical" results) are recommended for the diagnosis of diffuse intravascular clotting. All of the studies can easily be completed in less than an hour by one technologist.

Test	DIC	Primary Fibrinogenolysis
Platelets	↓ ↓ ↓	Normal (↓)
Fibrinogen	↓ ↓	↓ ↓
PT	↑ ↑	Normal (↑ in cirrhosis)
PTT	↑ ↑	Normal (↑ if fibrinogen ↓)
FSP	↑ (Normal)	↑ ↑
Euglobulin lysis	Normal or shortened	Rapid

4. Comments.

    a. Fibrinogen is considerably elevated in women during the third trimester of pregnancy and in many males and females under stress. Thus, in such individuals, a "normal" fibrinogen level may actually represent a depressed one when compared to fibrinogen concentrations in the prehemorrhagic state.

    b. Not all cases show all of the features of the respective disorders; for example, the PT or PTT may be relatively normal.

    c. The euglobulin lysis time may appear abnormally short in any individual with a plasma fibrinogen level below 75 mg/100 ml.

    d. The red blood cell structure in DIC is often abnormal, with the formation of schistocytes and helmet cells. However, DIC may occur in the absence of these changes.

5. Additional studies.

    a. In both DIC and primary fibrinogenolysis, factor V is depleted. Assay for this factor may not be readily available.

    b. Factor VIII is low in both of these entities. However, factor VIII, like fibrinogen, is a stress factor and may be elevated before or concomitantly with the bleeding episode. Thus, a normal level may be misleading. Low levels may occur in liver disease.

    c. Cryofibrinogen may be detectable in DIC, but its determination is time-consuming. It is useful only retrospectively.

    d. Antithrombin III is depleted in DIC, according to some but not all methods. Since this determination is also time-consuming, it too is of retrospective value.

    e. Plasmin and plasminogen assays are not routinely available and generally are too time-consuming to perform.

    f. Plasma paracoagulation tests (ethanol gelation and protamine sulfate precipitation) have proved unreliable.

    g. Differences in clot tension are reported to exist in DIC and primary fibrinogenolysis. However, the technology required for this determination is generally unavailable and the results are as yet unverified.

Hypercoagulable State

Patients with a hypercoagulable state usually present clinically with a history of one or more thrombotic episodes. Laboratory studies to support the clinical diagnosis of hypercoagulability or to identify patients at risk from this disorder are often unrevealing. However, one or more of the following abnormalities may be found in some patients:

1. Abnormally short PTT.

2. Abnormally short antithrombin III time.

3. High platelet count.

4. Abnormal thrombin generation time.

5. Abnormalities in thromboplastin generation and thromboelastography have also been described.

7.

Renal, Electrolyte, and Blood-Gas and Acid-Base Problems

Renal and Urinary Tract Disorders

S. Robert Contiguglia
Jeffrey L. Mishell
Melvyn H. Klein

In the approach to diseases of the kidney and urinary tract, it is important to differentiate between primary renal disease and renal disease that is secondary to a systemic disorder. A strong effort should also be made to determine the anatomic localization of the lesion (e.g., the glomerulus, tubules, interstitium, vascular system, lower urinary tract). Special attention should be paid to those diseases, listed in Tables 7-1 and 7-2, that are either preventable or treatable.

Kidney and urinary tract disease may present in a number of ways.

1. In many cases, a renal abnormality is suspected because the patient's complaints are directly related to the urinary tract or urine formation. Examples of such symptoms are frequency, dysuria, burning on urination, urgency, colic, polyuria, nocturia, hematuria, oliguria, and anuria.

2. Disease of the urinary tract may also become evident because of the nonrenal manifestations of a systemic illness that involves the kidney secondarily. Examples of such conditions are as follows:

    a. Metabolic diseases (e.g., diabetes mellitus).

253

TABLE 7-1.   Possibly and Potentially Preventable Renal Diseases

1. Glomerulopathies
   a. Acute poststreptococcal glomerulonephritis
   b. Infective endocarditis
   c. Toxemia of pregnancy
2. Vascular diseases
   a. Nephrosclerosis
   b. Hypersensitivity angiitis
3. Tubular diseases
   a. Acute tubular insufficiency
   b. Hypercalcemic nephropathy
   c. Hypokalemic nephropathy
   d. Obstructive nephropathy
4. Interstitial diseases
   a. Pyelonephritis (including tuberculosis)
   b. Drugs (antibiotics, analgesics) and heavy-metal poisoning
   c. Urate nephropathy

SOURCE: Reprinted from S. Papper, *Clinical Nephrology.* Boston: Little, Brown, 1971.

TABLE 7-2.   Treatable Renal Diseases

1. Glomerulopathies
   a. Systemic lupus erythematosus
   b. Infective endocarditis
   c. Toxemia of pregnancy
   d. Disseminated intravascular coagulation
   e. "Minimal" (membranous? proliferative?) glomerulonephritis (idiopathic)
2. Vascular diseases
   a. Atherosclerosis of major artery
   b. Polyarteritis nodosa
   c. Hypersensitivity angiitis
3. Tubular diseases
   a. Hypercalcemic nephropathy
   b. Hypokalemic nephropathy
   c. Obstructive nephropathy
4. Interstitial diseases
   a. Pyelonephritis
   b. Drugs (antibiotics, analgesics) and heavy-metal poisoning

SOURCE: Reprinted from S. Papper, *Clinical Nephrology.* Boston: Little, Brown, 1971.

    b. Connective tissue diseases (e.g., systemic lupus erythematosus, polymyositis, polyarteritis nodosa, scleroderma).
    c. Infectious diseases (e.g., gram-negative sepsis, tuberculosis, malaria).
    d. Cardiovascular diseases (e.g., hypertension, congestive heart failure).
    e. Infiltrative diseases (e.g., multiple myeloma, lymphoma).

  3. Occasionally patients present with symptoms and signs of renal failure (e.g., "uremic" symptoms, anuria, hypertension, edema) without any prior knowledge of kidney disease.

4. Finally, some patients are discovered to have renal diseases because of the finding of laboratory abnormalities (e.g., proteinuria, microscopic hematuria, abnormal renal function tests, electrolyte and acid-base disturbances) during the course of a routine examination or an investigation for another purpose.

FREQUENCY, URGENCY, AND DYSURIA

General Considerations

1. This triad of symptoms is most often associated with infection of the urinary tract. However, care must be taken to evaluate each symptom, because it may represent conditions other than urinary tract infection.

2. Psychoneurotic water-drinkers and patients with polyuria from any cause may complain of frequent voiding with an increased urine flow. In contrast, bladder inflammation may cause frequency without an increase in urine flow.

3. Urgency is most often caused by bladder inflammation, although a full bladder caused by increased urine flow may also cause this symptom. The urgency of urinary tract infection is more compelling; moreover, it is paradoxical because only small amounts of urine are passed at each voiding. External compression of the bladder by masses, as in pregnancy, may also generate the feeling of urgency.

4. Dysuria is suggestive of urethral inflammation, which may be a manifestation of urinary tract or genital infection. Some patients may complain of burning during febrile states.

History

1. A history of recurrent urinary tract infections suggests underlying anatomic or physiologic abnormality of the urinary tract.

2. Other causes of this triad of symptoms, particularly genital infections, should be excluded.

3. The presence of chills and fever suggests systemic involvement. These symptoms are usually seen with upper urinary tract involvement.

4. The back pain often associated with this triad of symptoms strongly suggests upper urinary tract involvement.

Physical Examination

1. A complete physical examination is indicated.

2. The presence of costovertebral angle tenderness is compatible with renal inflammation. Suprapubic tenderness suggests cystitis. However, neither of these findings need be present to diagnose urinary tract infection.

3. Because abnormalities of the urethral meatus and along the course of the urethra may cause dysuria, specific attention should be given to these areas on examination.

4. An acutely inflamed prostate gland may cause urethral symptoms. Hence this gland should be examined carefully in all males with urinary symptoms.

Laboratory Findings

1. Pyuria and bacteriuria are consistent with the diagnosis of urinary tract infection. Leukocyte casts are pathognomonic of renal parenchymal infection.

2. Urine culture and sensitivity tests should be done. Positive cultures recovered from catheterized or suprapubic puncture specimens are significant. Bacteriuria with over 100,000 colonies per milliliter of urine (from clean-voided specimens) is considered abnormal.

3. Urethral discharge, if present, should be examined in a wet preparation and cultured appropriately.

4. Further evaluation of these symptoms may require excretory urography, voiding cystourethrography, retrograde urography, cystoscopy, and other, more specialized tests.

5. Sterile pyuria suggests renal tuberculosis.

RENAL AND URETERAL COLIC

Definition

Renal colic, which is most often unilateral, is characterized by severe crescendo-decrescendo type of pain, which usually radiates from the costovertebral angle toward the hypochondrium. The pain of ureteral colic has similar characteristics but typically radiates around the flank toward the inguinal ligament and into the scrotum or labium major.

Etiology

Renal colic is usually produced by acute inflammation of the renal capsule resulting from such diseases as acute pyelonephritis. Ureteral colic is most often associated with the passage of a renal calculus.

Associated Symptoms

The pain is commonly associated with nausea and vomiting. The presence of chills and fever suggests either a primary or secondary urinary tract infection. Gross hematuria may be seen with the passage of a stone.

Physical Examination

The physical examination is usually unremarkable except for the presence of flank tenderness.

Laboratory Findings

1. Urinalysis. Hematuria as the sole urinary abnormality supports the diagnosis of calculus. The presence of pyuria suggests infection of the urinary tract.

2. X-ray. Abdominal films may show the presence of an opaque stone. If not, an intravenous pyelogram should be performed to reveal calculi not visualized in plain films, to determine their location more precisely, and to rule out obstruction. If the affected kidney is not visualized, delayed films should be taken. When intravenous pyelography is not helpful, retrograde pyelography is necessary.

NEPHROLITHIASIS

Etiology

1. Calcium oxalate and calcium phosphate stones. Hypercalciuria is the most common cause of such stones. Hypercalciuria (>150 mg/24 hours) may occur in sarcoidosis, hypervitaminosis D, distal renal tubular acidosis, hyperparathyroidism, idiopathic hypercalciuria, prolonged immobilization, hyperadrenocorticism, and excessive milk intake. Primary and secondary oxalosis results in the formation of calcium oxalate stones.

2. Triple phosphate stones. Triple phosphate stones occur most often in patients who have had frequent urinary tract infections with urea-splitting organisms and who have undergone multiple manipulative procedures.

3. Cystine stones. Cystine stones are found exclusively in patients with congenital cystinuria.

4. Urate stones. Urate stones are usually associated with hyperuricemic states (primary gout, secondary gout, and idiopathic hyperuricemia). However, many patients with uric acid calculi do not have hyperuricemia or increased uric acid excretion.

Diagnostic Approach

History and Physical Examination

1. The history should include information concerning the following: the age at which symptoms of stones were first noted; family history of nephrolithiasis; past history of fractures or prolonged immobilization; previous urinary tract infections or manipulations; and the intake of milk, alkali, and vitamin D.

2. The physical examination should include investigation for the band keratopathy associated with hypercalcemic states.

Laboratory Procedures

1. At least two determinations of serum calcium should be performed. In addition, serum levels of phosphorus, alkaline phosphatase, total protein and albumin, uric acid, creatinine, and electrolytes should be obtained.

2. A midstream urine specimen should be collected for culture and sensitivity studies because urinary tract infections are commonly associated with nephrolithiasis.

3. The urinary pH should be determined. A persistently alkaline urine in the presence of hyperchloremic acidosis suggests renal tubular acidosis.

4. Quantitative calcium determinations should be performed on two separate 24-hour urine specimens while the patient is on a regular diet, to detect hypercalciuria.

5. The urine should be examined for the presence of cystine crystals. The diagnosis of cystinuria is based on the demonstration of such crystals in cold acidified urine, a positive nitroprusside test, increased urinary excretion of cystine (>300 mg/24 hours), and the demonstration of the specific amino-aciduria by urinary chromatography.

6. When urate stones are found, an investigation for primary or secondary causes of hyperuricemia is warranted. However, as noted previously, urate stones may occur in the absence of hyperuricemia or increased uric acid excretion.

7. Pure oxalate stones may occur with primary or secondary oxalosis.

8. Architectural and chemical analysis should be performed on all stones that are passed.

9. Plain films of the abdomen and intravenous pyelography should be obtained routinely.

POLYURIA

Definition

Polyuria is an excessive output of urine. It may occur in association with many normal or pathologic states. Polyuria per se is not hazardous, provided the lost fluid and solutes are replaced. However, polyuria may become deleterious if such losses are excessive and replacement is inadequate. Hypotension and cardiovascular collapse may then ensue.

Etiology

1. Polyuria may represent a normal physiologic response to osmolar, sodium, or fluid loads, or it may be secondary to diuretic therapy.

   a. Osmolar loads result in the excretion of isotonic urine. The following are examples of solute loads that may produce osmotic diuresis and polyuria:

      (1) Glycosuria, as in diabetes mellitus.

      (2) Administration of mannitol or urea.

      (3) Hyperalimentation therapy with amino acids, glucose, etc.

   b. Sodium loads that are accompanied by increased water intake may result in a sodium diuresis and the excretion of isotonic urine. This may occur under the following circumstances:

      (1) High dietary intake of sodium (rare).

      (2) Administration of excessive quantities of salt and water by intravenous or tube feedings.

      (3) During recovery from acute renal failure (e.g., in acute glomerulonephritis) as a result of fluid resorption.

      (4) Rapid reabsorption of edema fluid.

   c. Water loads usually produce polyuria with the excretion of hypotonic urine. Conversely, fluid restriction usually results in the excretion of hypertonic, or concentrated, urine. Increased water loading may occur in the following conditions:

      (1) Psychogenic polydipsia (compulsive water drinking).

      (2) Iatrogenic water loading (as, for example, when large quantities of fluid are administered to patients with physiologic polyuria misdiagnosed as diabetes insipidus).

      (3) Vasopressin therapy, mistakenly administered for physiologic polyuria or psychogenic polydipsia, may cause water intoxication.

   d. Diuretic therapy, especially with the more potent diuretics, may be associated with polyuria in which the urine is isosmotic with respect to serum.

2. Polyuria may represent an inappropriate response to a pathologic state.

   a. In renal disease, in spite of increased serum osmolarity, inability to concentrate the urine adequately may result in obligatory polyuria. This may occur in the following conditions:

      (1) Renal failure.

         (a) Chronic renal disease, particularly salt-losing nephropathy.

         (b) Acute tubular necrosis, during the recovery or polyuric phase.

         (c) Postobstructive uropathy.

      (2) Hypercalcemic nephropathy, in which frank renal failure may ensue.

      (3) Hypokalemic nephropathy, which rarely causes renal failure.

   b. Nephrogenic diabetes insipidus, either congenital or acquired. This
   disorder may be associated with other renal tubular defects (e.g.,
   renal tubular acidosis). The diagnosis is based on the following:
   dilute urine in the presence of hyperosmolar serum; exclusion of
   the renal disorders listed above; inability to concentrate the urine
   when fluid restriction is imposed; and failure to respond to vasopressin.

   c. True diabetes insipidus. The diagnosis is based on the same criteria
   as those listed in paragraph **b** above except that the abnormalities
   respond to vasopressin (see also the section Hypernatremia, later
   in the chapter).

   d. Adrenocortical insufficiency, in which, in rare instances, fluid replacement may cause polyuria.

Diagnostic Approach

1. Rule out administered fluid or solute loads, or both, as possible causes
of polyuria by the history and by a review of the fluid and electrolyte
balance.

2. Determine the urine and serum osmolality.

   a. If the urine osmolality is elevated above that of the serum, rule out
   glycosuria.

   b. If the urine is isosmotic with respect to serum, check for evidence
   of renal failure, and exclude glycosuria, administered diuretics, and
   solute loads as possible causes.

3. If the urine is hypotonic compared to serum osmolality, test for renal
concentrating ability by restricting the fluid intake.

   a. If the urine becomes concentrated with fluid restriction, it can be
   concluded that fluid intake was excessive and that it was either
   psychogenic or iatrogenic in origin.

   b. If the ability to concentrate urine is impaired, it can be assumed
   that the nephron is unable to conserve water adequately, indicating
   either nephrogenic or true diabetes insipidus. The patient's response
   to vasopressin should then be determined.

      (1) If the patient is responsive to vasopressin, the diagnosis is
      diabetes insipidus.

      (2) If the patient is unresponsive to vasopressin, it can be con-
      cluded that the patient has some type of renal disease (e.g.,
      postobstructive uropathy, nephrolithiasis, hypercalcemic ne-
      phropathy) causing nephrogenic diabetes insipidus.

OLIGURIA AND ANURIA

Definition

Oliguria is that amount of urine output below which the normal load of
metabolic waste products (usually 400 to 500 ml/24 hours) cannot be

excreted. Anuria is arbitrarily defined as a urinary output below 100 ml/ 24 hours.

Etiology

  1. Prerenal defects—decreased "effective" renal blood flow—hypoperfusion.
     a. In the presence of hypotension.
        (1) Extracellular fluid volume depletion.
        (2) Cardiogenic shock.
        (3) Septic shock.
     b. In the absence of hypotension.
        (1) Congestive heart failure.
        (2) Renal arterial blockade.
           (a) Thrombotic and embolic.
           (b) Vasoconstriction secondary to drugs.
        (3) Volume depletion.
        (4) "Third space" losses (e.g., peritonitis, bowel obstruction).

  2. Postrenal defects.
     a. Obstructive uropathy.
        (1) Prostatic or urethral obstruction.
        (2) Bilateral ureteral obstruction (rare).
     b. Renal vein thrombosis.

  3. Intrarenal defects.
     a. Diffuse acute glomerular disease (acute glomerulonephritis, rapidly progressing glomerulonephritis, acute vasculitis).
     b. Acute tubular necrosis.
     c. Bilateral cortical necrosis.
     d. Interstitial diseases.
        (1) Acute interstitial nephritis.
        (2) Urate nephropathy.
        (3) Hypercalcemic nephropathy.
     e. Postcontrast media (especially in patients with multiple myeloma).
     f. Chronic renal failure (oliguria occurs only at the end stage of the disease except in the presence of a prerenal component).

Diagnostic Approach

Although the history and physical examination may provide clues to the cause of oliguria, differentiation of renal from extrarenal causes is based primarily on laboratory studies. In general, glomerular lesions may be diagnosed on the basis of urinalysis. Usually the major diagnostic dilemma in the oliguric state is to differentiate acute tubular necrosis from prerenal and postrenal disease.

1. Obstructive uropathy may be diagnosed by determining the residual bladder urine volume, measurement of the urinary output during bladder catheterization, and intravenous or retrograde pyelography.

2. The BUN to creatinine ratio is usually 10 to 15:1 in renal parenchymal disease but is greater than 15 to 20:1 in prerenal disorders.

3. Determination of sodium concentration in a "spot" urine specimen may be the most reliable diagnostic aid in differentiating between renal and extrarenal causes.

   a. Prerenal disorders.   Urine sodium is less than 10 mEq per liter and is often below 5 mEq per liter. If the urine sodium concentration is more than 10 mEq per liter, it is unlikely that prerenal factors are solely responsible for the oliguria.

   b. Acute tubular necrosis.   Urine sodium is greater than 30 mEq per liter and often exceeds 40 mEq per liter. Urine sodium concentration between 10 and 30 mEq per liter is usually indicative of a combined problem, i.e., hypoperfusion superimposed on renal tubular insufficiency. One way to distinguish between prerenal disorders and acute tubular insufficiency in doubtful cases is to test the patient's capacity to excrete urine by administering 500 to 1000 ml of saline intravenously within 1 hour. An increase in urine flow suggests hypoperfusion.

   c. Postrenal disorders.   Urine sodium is variable, but may resemble that found in prerenal disease.

   d. Urine sodium concentration is of little or no diagnostic value in patients receiving diuretics.

4. Urine osmolality.

   a. Prerenal and postrenal disorders.   In these conditions, urine osmolality is usually greater than 500 mOsm per kilogram of water and may be as high as 1100 or 1200 mOsm per kilogram of water.

   b. Acute tubular necrosis.   The urine is usually isosmotic, with the urine to serum osmolality ratio between 0.9 and 1.1.

   c. Maximum concentration of urine may not occur in elderly individuals, patients on diuretics, or those with preexisting chronic renal disease.

5. Urine urea nitrogen concentration.

   a. Prerenal disorders.   The urine urea nitrogen concentration is usually greater than 500 mg/100 ml and may even be as high as 1500 to 2000 mg/100 ml, except in elderly persons or patients on diuretic therapy.

   b. Acute tubular necrosis.   The urine urea nitrogen concentration is usually less than 400 mg per milliliter.

6. Comments.

   a. In a patient with any degree of chronic renal insufficiency, the above-mentioned parameters may not be valid.

b. In patients with severe oliguria or anuria (a rare occurrence in acute tubular necrosis), consideration must be given to the diagnosis of potentially reversible obstructive uropathy and its correction. When doubt exists as to the presence of obstruction, cystoscopy and retrograde pyelography should be performed.

UREMIA

Definition

Uremia is a symptom complex found in renal failure. The gastrointestinal, cardiovascular, and central nervous systems are particularly involved. Uremic manifestations are believed to be related to the accumulation of as yet unidentified dialyzable substances in the blood. A uremic individual may also have symptoms and signs related to altered fluid and electrolyte balance. Patients sometimes present with uremic symptoms without any knowledge of antecedent renal disease.

Clinical Features

A patient with uremia may present with some or all of the following manifestations:

1. Gastrointestinal symptoms include anorexia, nausea, vomiting, diarrhea, and hiccups. The nausea and vomiting resemble the morning sickness of pregnancy. The patient may awake feeling reasonably well but have nausea and vomiting at the very sight, smell, or taste of food.

2. The spectrum of nervous system manifestations is broad. The sensorium may range from mental alertness to coma. Personality changes, irritability, delusions, and hallucinations may occur. Muscle twitching and seizures are not uncommon. Peripheral neuropathy is sometimes observed.

3. Cardiovascular manifestations include fibrinous pericarditis and sometimes cardiac tamponade. Pulmonary edema and circulatory volume overload may occur.

4. Other uremic signs include the Kussmaul breathing of metabolic acidosis, increased cutaneous pigmentation, pruritus, anemia, and a uremic breath odor.

5. The insidious onset of weakness and anemia may be the only clues to severe renal insufficiency.

6. A patient with uremia may present with some or all of the above-mentioned manifestations.

LABORATORY ABNORMALITIES IN RENAL DISEASE:

URINALYSIS

It is not unusual for a patient with renal disease to present without a history or physical findings suggestive of renal disease. Many patients are discovered to have kidney disease because of abnormal findings on routine urinalysis. Others are picked up when azotemia or electrolyte abnormalities are found on routine biochemical screening. Of course, many patients have symptoms directly referable to the urinary tract or other symptoms (e.g., edema) that bring up the possibility of a renal abnormality. The two most common urinary abnormalities that suggest renal disease are hematuria and proteinuria. These conditions are discussed separately from other aspects of the urinalysis.

1. Appearance. The appearance of the urine may give a clue to the presence of a renal or systemic abnormality. Cloudiness or turbidity on standing is usually secondary to the precipitation of urates and phosphates and, less commonly, to pyuria. Normal urine is yellow to amber in color. Bile may produce cola-colored urine. Blood, hemoglobin, and myoglobin may impart a red or reddish-brown color to the urine. Urine containing porphyrins changes to a port-wine color on standing. The urine may also be discolored by food (e.g., beets) or drugs (e.g., methylene blue, phenolphthalein). A white foam may occur when urine is shaken. Foaming is increased with proteinuria. Yellow foam suggests the presence of bile salts and bile pigments.

2. Concentration. Urine concentration is best determined by recording the osmolality. Urine concentration can be approximated by measuring the specific gravity with a refractometer (preferred method) or a urinometer. A urinometer should be calibrated before use to be sure it reads 1.000 with distilled water. A single determination of osmolality or specific gravity is of limited usefulness unless the results are related to the clinical setting (e.g., the state of hydration). Urine osmolality is of greatest value when compared to serum osmolality in a specific clinical situation (e.g., oliguria).

3. pH. Urine is almost always acid except during the alkaline tide or when there is infection with urea-splitting organism. The urine is alkaline in renal tubular acidosis. The overall clinical situation must be known for such a measurement to be useful. For example, an alkaline urine in the presence of systemic acidosis suggests a renal acidification defect, whereas an alkaline urine with systemic alkalosis is appropriate.

4. Glucose. Methods that employ glucose oxidase (e.g., dipstick) detect only glucose, whereas other methods detect not only glucose but other reducing substances as well (e.g., salicylates, dextran, urates, antibodies, pentose sugars), and thus produce false-positive results. When glycosuria is found, it should be determined whether it is secondary to hyperglycemia or renal glycosuria. This is best accomplished with an oral glucose tolerance test, which yields a normal result in renal glycosuria.

5. Other substances. Ketonemia results in a positive finding for acetone in the urine. This occurs most commonly in diabetic ketoacidosis. Ketonuria alone may be found on starvation or fasting and in methanol poisoning.

PROTEINURIA

General Principles

1. Proteinuria is often the first and occasionally the only abnormality in patients with renal disease. Proteinuria represents glomerular damage and is often associated with gross or microscopic hematuria.

2. The major protein in the urine in patients with renal disease is albumin. Globulins predominate in certain tubular disorders and plasma cell dyscrasias (e.g., multiple myeloma).

3. Qualitative tests for proteinuria should include either the heat and acetic acid method or sulfosalicylic acid.

4. The measurement of the 24-hour protein excretion is of the utmost importance in the evaluation of any patient with proteinuria.

5. Proteinuria is considered significant when urinary excretion exceeds 150 mg in 24 hours.

Etiology and Classification

1. Heavy proteinuria. Heavy proteinuria is defined as the excretion of more than 3.5 gm of protein in 24 hours. It is most often associated with the nephrotic syndrome. The causes of heavy proteinuria are: all types of glomerulonephritis; systemic illnesses such as connective tissue disease, diabetes mellitus, and multiple myeloma; allergic disorders such as bee sting and drug reactions; circulatory conditions such as pericarditis, chronic congestive heart failure, and renal vein thrombosis; and infections such as malaria, cytomegalic inclusion disease, typhus, and herpes zoster.

2. Moderate proteinuria. Moderate proteinuria is defined as a 24-hour excretion of 1.0 to 3.5 gm of protein in 24 hours. The causes of moderate proteinuria are essentially the same as those causing heavy proteinuria.

3. Minimal proteinuria. Minimal proteinuria is defined as the excretion of less than 1.0 gm of protein in 24 hours. The causes include mild glomerular disease (pyelonephritis, nephrosclerosis, hypercalcemia, obstructive uropathy, tumor, nephrocalcinosis, acute tubular necrosis, and congestive heart failure), functional proteinuria, postural proteinuria, and asymptomatic persistent proteinuria. Functional proteinuria is transient proteinuria associated with febrile illness or exercise. Postural proteinuria is proteinuria associated with the upright position. Asymp-

tomatic persistent proteinuria is almost always indicative of renal disease.

Diagnostic Approach

History
Since proteinuria may be the result of primary or secondary renal disease, evidence of systemic illness that may involve the kidney should be sought and excluded (e.g., connective tissue disease, diabetes mellitus).

Physical Examination
1. Arterial hypertension may produce minimal to moderate proteinuria. When associated with moderate to heavy proteinuria, primary glomerular disease should be considered. When hypertension and proteinuria begin simultaneously, primary renal disease should be suspected.

2. The combination of proteinuria, hypoproteinemia, and edema is suggestive of the nephrotic syndrome.

3. Arthritis, an erythematous rash, and purpura suggest connective tissue disease.

4. Retinopathy may be seen in systemic hypertension, diabetes, or vasculitis. Diabetic retinopathy is almost always associated with diabetic nephropathy.

5. Peripheral neuropathy may be observed in patients with diabetes or chronic renal failure.

Laboratory Studies
1. Urinalysis. The presence of fatty casts, oval fat bodies, and doubly refractile fat globules suggests the lipiduria of the nephrotic syndrome. Red cell casts are virtually pathognomonic for glomerulonephritis. Glycosuria suggests diabetes mellitus, although renal glycosuria may be present.

2. The 24-hour urinary protein excretion. All patients with proteinuria should have a 24-hour urine collection for total protein. Patients exhibiting minimal to moderate proteinuria should be checked routinely for postural or orthostatic proteinuria. The combined study can be performed as follows: The patient voids at 7 A.M. and discards the urine. All urine thereafter is collected in a single bottle. At 8 P.M. the patient assumes the recumbent position in bed. At 10 P.M. he voids into the same bottle without getting out of bed. At 7 A.M. the next morning, without rising, he voids into another bottle. The urine in the two bottles is the 24-hour urine collection, the second bottle representing the urine voided during recumbency. In patients with postural proteinuria, the total urinary protein excretion usually exceeds 150 mg (but is less than 1 gm), but the protein excreted during recumbency should not be greater than 75 mg.

3. Serum and urinary protein electrophoresis should be performed in every patient suspected of having a plasma cell dyscrasia. The presence of light chains in the urine may be the only manifestation of multiple myeloma.

4. Hypercholesterolemia and hypoproteinemia with a decreased albumin fraction is seen in most cases of the nephrotic syndrome.

5. Hyperproteinemia with an increased gamma globulin fraction may occur in multiple myeloma.

6. An abnormal glucose tolerance test and glycosuria may be the only other manifestations of diabetes mellitus in a patient with diabetic nephropathy. Abnormal glucose tolerance, however, may occur in renal failure from any cause.

7. Serologic tests for streptococcal antibodies, connective tissue disease, syphilis, and serum complement (C'3) should be performed.

8. Radiologic examinations.   Chest films may show the type of circulatory congestion associated with uremia or congestive heart failure. Bone films may reveal the punched-out lesions of multiple myeloma or the changes observed with chronic renal failure. Small kidneys in abdominal films denote chronic renal disease. Intravenous pyelography may reveal obstructive uropathy, polycystic disease, and other abnormalities. Asymmetric size and function on pyelography are seen in renal vein thrombosis. Renal arteriography may be useful in the diagnosis of renovascular hypertension and polyarteritis nodosa.

9. Renal biopsy is indicated when all other studies fail to reveal the etiology of renal disease, when the findings will influence the management of the disease (e.g., systemic lupus erythematosus), and as an aid in determining the prognosis. If performed, the biopsy should be examined by light and electron microscopy as well as by immunofluorescent techniques.

HEMATURIA (WITHOUT PROTEINURIA)

Hematuria may be gross or microscopic (in excess of two red cells per high-power field), painful or painless. It may occur with or without proteinuria or the presence of formed elements in the urine. Hematuria may originate anywhere in the urinary tract, i.e., the kidney, ureter, bladder, prostate gland, or urethra. At times, it may reflect a generalized disorder of the clotting mechanism.

Gross hematuria must be differentiated from myoglobinuria, hemoglobinuria, and porphyria. The finding of red cells in the urinary sediment establishes the diagnosis of hematuria. The other conditions are identified by specific laboratory tests. It should be noted that either extremely concentrated or extremely dilute urine may cause lysis of red cells with resultant hemoglobinuria.

Diffuse renal parenchymal disease usually presents with painless smoky or cloudy urine associated with proteinuria and the presence of formed elements in the urine. However, gross hematuria is not a rare occurrence in diffuse renal disease. The approach to this group of patients is discussed in the preceding section, Proteinuria.

In a patient with gross hematuria, the rate and amount of blood loss can be estimated by performing serial urinary hematocrit readings. A hematocrit value of less than 1 percent indicates that the blood loss is slight. Unless blood loss is massive, hematuria does not cause anemia. If anemia is present, other causes, such as chronic renal failure, tuberculosis, neoplasm, and blood dyscrasias, should be considered.

Etiology

1. Painless hematuria may signify primary renal disease such as tumor, polycystic kidney disease, posttraumatic damage, postexercise hematuria, infection including tuberculosis, or other disease of the urinary tract (e.g., bladder tumor).

2. Painful hematuria is usually caused by nephrolithiasis, renal infarction, or urinary tract infection.

History

1. A careful menstrual history should be obtained from any woman with a history of blood in the urine to be sure that bleeding is from the urinary tract and not vaginal in origin.

2. Hematuria associated with dysuria, frequency, urgency, and suprapubic pain usually denotes cystitis, but tuberculosis must also be considered.

3. Hematuria with ureteral or renal colic suggests nephrolithiasis or renal infarction.

4. Bleeding at the beginning of urination suggests an origin in the posterior urethra, whereas the source of terminal hematuria is usually the prostate gland or the trigonal area of the bladder.

5. Inquiry concerning the presence of a blood dyscrasia or the use of anticoagulants is warranted in any patient with hematuria. Patients on anticoagulants who develop hematuria should be investigated because they often turn out to have significant lesions of the urinary tract.

6. A history of increased sexual activity, perineal pain, dysuria, and terminal hematuria suggests prostatitis.

7. A family history of polycystic kidney disease or sickle cell anemia suggests these conditions as possible causes of hematuria.

8. An intensive search for neoplasm is always indicated if all of the foregoing conditions are excluded.

Physical Examination

1. The presence of petechiae, ecchymoses, lymphadenopathy, or splenomegaly may be indicative of a blood dyscrasia or clotting disorder.

2. A tender, boggy prostate gland suggests prostatitis.

3. Costovertebral angle tenderness and fever suggest renal inflammation.

4. Suprapubic tenderness is commonly associated with bladder inflammation.

5. Bilaterally enlarged kidneys are often found in polycystic disease.

6. A unilateral renal mass suggests neoplasm or cyst.

7. The presence of atrial fibrillation or valvular heart disease suggests renal embolism and infarction as possible causes of hematuria.

Laboratory Studies

1. Urinalysis may help to differentiate diffuse renal parenchymal disease from disease of the lower urinary tract. Dysuria and bacteriuria suggest infection of the urinary tract. Hematuria and pyuria without bacteriuria suggest the possibility of renal tuberculosis.

2. Blood count. The presence of anemia suggests renal failure or a systemic illness. Polycythemia is sometimes seen with renal cell carcinoma, polycystic disease, isolated renal cysts, uterine leiomyomata, and other conditions.

3. Intravenous pyelogram. Patients with hematuria should have intravenous pyelography before cystoscopy or other urinary tract manipulations are performed. Pyelography is important in the diagnosis of cystic disease, nephrolithiasis, and tumors. It is especially indicated in children in whom renal neoplasms are frequent causes of hematuria.

4. Cystoscopy. Cystoscopy, performed after urinalysis and intravenous pyelography, is the best procedure for evaluating the lower urinary tract.

5. Arteriography is helpful in the diagnosis of cysts, tumors, thrombosis, and infarction.

6. Ultrasound is a good method for diagnosing renal cysts and for differentiating between cystic and solid tumors.

TESTS OF RENAL FUNCTION

The best clinical guide for evaluating renal function is the creatinine clearance. This test estimates the glomerular filtration rate (GFR). The urea clearance is less reliable. Clearance procedures are particularly useful in detecting early renal function impairment and in following the course of renal disease. However, clearance tests are of little help in determining the cause of kidney disease. The blood urea nitrogen (BUN) and serum creatinine have limited usefulness as indicators of the GFR; the serum creatinine has some advantages over the BUN. In some instances, the two determinations together have some advantage over either test alone (see Serum Creatinine, paragraph **2**, below). Tests for renal concentrating ability are useful in evaluating patients with oliguria. Impaired concentrating ability is an early sign of abnormal renal function in many chronic renal disorders.

Concentration Tests

1. The normal kidney can produce urine with an osmolality that is four to five times that of plasma.

2. The most reliable test of the concentrating ability of the kidney is the determination of the osmolality of urine by freezing point depression.

3. To perform a concentration test, examine at hourly intervals freshly voided urine obtained after an overnight fast until the highest urine concentration is obtained. The fast is continued until the test is completed. A specific gravity greater than 1.020 or an osmolality greater than 800 mOsm per kilogram of water is considered normal. In patients with known or suspected azotemia, no attempt should be made to concentrate the urine by dehydrating the patient because it may be hazardous to do so.

4. Factors that affect renal medulla hypertonicity (e.g., high fluid intake prior to the test, diuretics, low-protein diet, sodium restriction) may interfere with the concentration test.

5. Concentration defects may be early findings in essential hypertension, diabetic nephropathy, hypokalemia, hypercalcemia, nephrogenic diabetes insipidus, sickle cell disease, interstitial nephritis, and polycystic kidney disease. Renal concentrating ability is also reduced with advancing age.

Blood Urea Nitrogen

The normal range for blood urea nitrogen (BUN) is 10 to 20 mg/100 ml. The BUN is not a good test for detecting early renal function impairment because the BUN may be normal with as much as a 50 percent reduction in the glomerular filtration rate. Azotemia may be produced not only by renal disease but also by extrarenal disorders, such as dehydration, hypotension, hypovolemia, gastrointestinal hemorrhage, and increased protein intake. When due consideration is given to extrarenal factors, the BUN can be used to follow the course of renal disease. It is not a satisfactory method for evaluating small changes in renal function early in the course of renal failure.

Serum Creatinine

1. The serum creatinine is a more useful guide to the glomerular filtration rate than is the BUN. However, significant changes may not always be detected. The normal serum creatinine level is 1 to 2 mg/100 ml.

2. The BUN to serum creatinine ratio is of additional clinical value. Normally, this ratio is 10 to 12:1. A high ratio suggests prerenal azotemia, and a low one, decreased protein intake, liver disease, or muscle necrosis. A proportionate rise in both the BUN and the serum creatinine concentrations, with maintenance of the 10:1 ratio, suggests renal parenchymal disease.

Endogenous Creatinine Clearance

1. Clearance is defined as the volume of blood cleared of a substance per unit of time. It is reported in milliliters per minute. The endogenous creatinine clearance is preferred over the urea clearance for estimating the GFR.

2. The creatinine clearance is measured by the formula, $C = \dfrac{U \times V}{P}$, in which C is clearance in milliliters per minute, U is the urine creatinine concentration in milligrams per 100 ml, V is urine flow in milliliters per minute, and P is the serum creatinine concentration in milligrams per 100 ml.

3. Creatinine clearances are commonly employed to estimate renal function in patients with renal disease. As a rule, the creatinine clearance tends to overestimate the true GFR, especially when the GFR is low. However, serial determinations of creatinine clearance regularly parallel the rise and fall of the actual GFR.

4. A patient in a steady state excretes a constant amount of creatinine in 24 hours. Most men excrete at least 1000 mg of this substance in 24 hours, and women, more than 700 mg in the same period. Omissions in urine collection or sudden changes in renal function are possible causes of reduced excretion of creatinine. Sometimes, a patient with frail body build has a lower than normal total urine creatinine excretion. Whenever the 24-hour urine creatinine excretion is below normal, the test should be repeated. It should also be rechecked if urine creatinine excretion is not comparable to that determined in previous studies.

5. Normal values of the creatinine clearance range from 100 to 150 ml per minute in men and 85 to 125 ml per minute in women. The GFR declines slowly above the age of 40. By the age of 70, the creatinine clearance may be 50 percent of normal even in the absence of renal disease.

Electrolyte Disorders

S. Robert Contiguglia
Jeffrey L. Mishell
Melvyn H. Klein

HYPONATREMIA

Definition

Hyponatremia is defined as an abnormally low serum sodium concentration (less than 135 mEq per liter). Since the ionic components of the serum are largely responsible for its osmolality, hyponatremia results in a lowered serum osmolality. The symptoms of hyponatremia are essentially those of reduced serum osmolality. Hyponatremia may occur in a variety of clinical disorders. Since treatment of these conditions may differ markedly, it is always important to determine the cause of hyponatremia. All hyponatremic states, with the exception of hyperlipidemia and hyperglycemia, are associated with low osmolality of the serum and extracellular fluids. In other words, total body sodium is inappropriately low with respect to total body water.

Etiology and Classification

1. Pseudohyponatremia.
    a. Hyperlipidemia.   Hyperlipemic states may be associated with spurious hyponatremia. The diagnosis is established by finding a high lipid content in the serum and normal serum osmolality.
    b. Hyperglycemia.   Hyperglycemia may induce factitious hyponatremia because every 100 mg/100 ml rise in the serum glucose concentration produces an approximate 3 mEq per liter decline in the serum sodium level. The diagnosis is based on finding hyponatremia and hyperglycemia together with a normal or elevated serum osmolality.

2. Dilutional hyponatremia is a state in which an excess of total body sodium and water results in edema or ascites, or both. Serum osmolality is low. Dilutional hyponatremia occurs in congestive heart failure, hepatic cirrhosis, and nephrosis. Increased water intake continued with marked sodium restriction or diuretic therapy, or both, may aggravate any of these conditions.

3. Hyponatremia due to sodium depletion.   Conditions associated with both sodium and water depletion are characterized by the absence of edema or ascites. Symptoms and signs of extracellular fluid volume depletion, tachycardia, decreased central venous pressure, a high hematocrit reading, and elevated serum total proteins may be noted. The history and urine sodium concentrations are important diagnostically.

    a. Decreased urine sodium concentration (<10 mEq per liter).

      (1) Gastrointestinal losses.

        (a) Vomiting or nasogastric suction, or both, commonly associated with hypokalemic alkalosis.

        (b) Diarrhea, commonly associated with hypokalemic acidosis.

      (2) Excessive perspiration with replacement of water but not sodium losses.

      (3) Volume depletion without replacement of lost fluids and electrolytes after diuretic therapy.

    b. Increased urine sodium concentration (>10 mEq per liter). Causes include adrenocortical insufficiency and salt-losing nephropathy.

  4. Hyponatremia due to other causes. The disorders included in this category are not associated with edema or sodium depletion.

    a. Iatrogenically induced hyponatremia secondary to diuretic therapy and the administration of water.

    b. Syndrome of inappropriate secretion of antidiuretic hormone (ADH). This condition may be idiopathic or may be associated with one of the following disorders: diseases of the central nervous system (e.g., strokes, mass lesions, meningitis), pulmonary disease (e.g., tuberculosis, pneumonia, bronchogenic carcinoma), chlorpropamide therapy, and exogenous vasopressin administration.

      (1) Criteria for the diagnosis.

        (a) Urine osmolality greater than 150 mOsm per kilogram of water.

        (b) Normal renal and adrenal function.

        (c) Increased urinary excretion of sodium (usually, but not always, present).

        (d) Elevated serum concentration of ADH.

        (e) Reversal of the syndrome by adequate fluid restriction.

      (2) Comment. When a steady state is reached, some of the abnormalities described may not be present.

Diagnostic Approach

Once the diagnosis of hyponatremia is made, the serum sodium level should be rechecked and the serum osmolality determined.

  1. If the serum osmolality is normal or high in the presence of confirmed hyponatremia, the possibility of hyperlipidemia or hyperglycemia, or both, should be investigated.

  2. If the serum osmolality is low, confirming the diagnosis of true hyponatremia, the status of the extracellular fluid volume should be assessed.

    a. If edema or ascites is present, the hyponatremia is dilutional.

   b. If volume depletion is present, the hyponatremia is due to sodium depletion. The diagnosis is usually revealed by the history and a determination of the urine sodium concentration.

   c. If the extracellular fluid volume appears to be normal, iatrogenic causes of hyponatremia and the syndrome of inappropriate secretion of ADH must be excluded.

HYPERNATREMIA

Definition

Hypernatremia is defined as an abnormally high serum sodium concentration (>145 mEq per liter). In hypernatremia, the total body sodium content is high with respect to total body water. Hypernatremia is usually due to excessive water loss and rarely to increased total body sodium.

Etiology

1. Hypernatremia due to increased body sodium (usually iatrogenic).

   a. Excess solute administration in proportion to water intake.

   (1) Infants inadvertently given preparations with a high sodium content.

   (2) Hyperalimentation by intravenous or nasogastric tube feeding.

   b. Volume depletion (e.g., from diuretics, gastrointestinal losses) and replacement by isotonic or hypertonic solutions.

   c. "Essential" hypernatremia.

2. Hypernatremia due to excessive water loss.   This condition is usually averted in the conscious patient because thirst causes the patient to drink until the water deficit is corrected. Fluids lost from the body are almost always hypotonic with respect to sodium. Thus, hypernatremia may ensue if the fluid losses are not adequately replaced. In the evaluation of hypernatremia due to excessive water loss, both the urine and serum osmolality should be determined.

   a. Urine maximally concentrated (hyperosmotic) in response to the hyperosmolar state.

   Non-Renal **(1)** Gastrointestinal losses.

   (2) Perspiration.

   (3) Hyperpnea.

   Note: Elderly persons and patients with renal insufficiency may not be able to concentrate the urine maximally even though the hypernatremia is due to one or more of the preceding causes.

   b. Urine not maximally concentrated (isosmotic or hyposmotic) in response to the hyperosmolar state.

   (1) Diuretic therapy.

   (2) Hypercalcemic nephropathy.

   (3) Hypokalemic nephropathy.

- **(4)** Osmotic diuresis. *hyper ? hypo?*
  - **(a)** Diabetes mellitus.
  - **(b)** Osmotic diuretics.
- **(5)** Polyuric phase of acute tubular necrosis.
- **(6)** Postobstructive uropathy.
- **(7)** Diabetes insipidus (large urine volume, dilute urine).
  - **(a)** True diabetes insipidus (secondary to hypothalamic or pituitary disease)—responsive to vasopressin.
  - **(b)** Nephrogenic diabetes insipidus—not responsive to vasopressin.

Diagnostic Approach

1. Rule out iatrogenic causes of hypernatremia. If iatrogenic causes are excluded, the hypernatremia can only be due to excessive extrarenal or renal fluid losses.

2. Measure the serum and urine osmolality.
   - **a.** If the urine is hypertonic (osmolality increased), the fluid was lost by an extrarenal route—the gastrointestinal tract, perspiration, etc.
   - **b.** If the urine is isotonic (isosmotic) or hypotonic (hyposmotic), the fluid losses were probably sustained through the kidney. The renal disorders that may be responsible for this type of abnormality are listed in paragraph **2b** above.

HYPERKALEMIA (HYPERPOTASSEMIA)

Definition

Hyperkalemia is defined as an abnormally high serum potassium concentration (>5.5 mEq per liter).

Etiology

1. Excessive intake of potassium in the presence of renal failure, particularly when associated with oliguria or anuria.

2. The crush syndrome (severe trauma) in association with massive muscle necrosis and, very often, renal failure.

3. Adrenocortical insufficiency.

4. Acidosis.

5. Rapid transfusion of large quantities of bank blood.

6. Drugs (spironolactone, triamterene).

Symptoms and Signs

1. Neuromuscular symptoms and signs predominate; they include weakness, occasionally paralysis, loss of deep tendon reflexes, irritability, and confusion.

2. The following more or less sequential changes may be seen in the electrocardiogram: progressive increase in the amplitude of the T waves; decreased amplitude of the R wave with concomitant increased depth of the S wave, ST-segment depression, and prolongation of the QRS and P-R intervals; continued widening of the QRS and T wave, and their eventual replacement by a sine curve; and finally, ventricular tachyarrhythmia or asystole.

Diagnostic Approach

The major goal is to find the cause of the hyperkalemia and to correct it if possible. When hyperkalemia is severe (7.0 mEq per liter or more), diagnostic investigations should be postponed until the life-threatening situation is controlled or corrected.

HYPOKALEMIA (HYPOPOTASSEMIA)

Definition

Hypopotassemia is defined as an abnormally low serum potassium concentration (<3.5 mEq per liter).

Etiology

1. Nonrenal causes.
   a. Decreased potassium intake.
   b. Gastrointestinal losses of potassium.
      (1) Associated with alkalosis and volume depletion.
         (a) Gastric suctioning and vomiting.
         (b) Villous adenoma.
         (c) Neoplasms of the colon.
         (d) Chronic laxative abuse.
      (2) Associated with acidosis.
         (a) Diarrheal states.
         (b) Zollinger-Ellison syndrome.
         (c) Ureterosigmoidostomy.

2. Renal causes.
   a. Potassium wasting associated with metabolic acidosis.
      (1) Renal tubular acidosis.
      (2) Postobstructive uropathy.

(3) Diuretic phase of acute tubular necrosis.

(4) Chronic pyelonephritis.

  b. Potassium wasting associated with metabolic alkalosis.

  (1) Diuretic therapy (e.g., furosemide, ethacrynic acid, thiazides). Treatment with potent diuretics may cause hypochloremic alkalosis, which is usually associated with volume depletion.

  (2) Disorders with increased aldosterone secretion and hypertension (e.g., primary aldosteronism, malignant hypertension, renovascular hypertension, and essential hypertension with vomiting and diarrhea, diuretic therapy, oral contraceptives, steroid therapy).

  (3) Disorders with increased aldosterone secretion without hypertension (e.g., salt-losing nephropathy, juxtaglomerular hyperplasia, Welt's syndrome).

  (4) Disorders with normal or decreased aldosterone and hypertension (e.g., licorice ingestion, Cushing's syndrome, certain congenital enzyme deficiency syndromes, Liddle's syndrome).

Symptoms and Signs

1. Most symptoms are nonspecific. They include anorexia, nausea, vomiting, abdominal distention, ileus, weakness, decreased deep reflexes, and a depressed sensorium.

2. The electrocardiographic findings include: lowering, flattening, notching, or inversion of the T waves; prominent U waves; depression of the ST segments; and arrhythmias.

Diagnostic Approach

1. Patients with hypokalemia require a thorough investigation to determine whether the potassium loss is the result of renal or extrarenal mechanisms. Extrarenal potassium depletion is easily recognized by the clinical picture and is correctable by appropriate treatment with potassium salts and fluids.

2. To determine whether potassium depletion is renal in origin, the 24-hour urinary excretion of potassium should be measured while the patient is on a regular salt intake. Urinary potassium excretion of less than 20 mEq/24 hours in a hypokalemic individual is excellent evidence against renal potassium wasting. On the other hand, urinary potassium excretion greater than 20 mEq/24 hours, especially if it is more than 60 mEq, is strongly suggestive of renal potassium wasting.

3. The problem of hypokalemia with hypertension is discussed in the section Arterial Hypertension, Chapter 3.

4. In patients with both metabolic alkalosis and potassium wasting, volume depletion may cause the abnormal state to persist. Every effort should be made not only to ascertain the cause of the metabolic

alkalosis but also to determine whether volume depletion is a contributing factor, and if it is, to correct it.

Blood-Gas and pH Abnormalities

N. Balfour Slonim

Abnormalities of blood O_2, CO_2, and pH are diagnostically revealing as well as clinically significant. If values are extreme or changing rapidly, such abnormal laboratory findings may be of critical importance. These three vital interrelated blood parameters should not be ignored in any diagnostic situation.

For the purpose of blood-gas and pH determination there is no substitute for *arterial* blood. When reliable information is most needed—in the care of the critically ill patient—blood samples from nonarterial sources are least reliable. Discussion of the anaerobic technique of analysis of arterial blood samples for O_2, CO_2, and pH is outside the scope of this chapter, but it should be emphasized that all techniques in present use, whether they involve physical or chemical principles, are a challenge to the precision and skill of the analyst; respiratory gas exchange occurs in the pulmonary capillaries in a fraction of a second!

PATHOPHYSIOLOGY

In the interpretation of blood-gas and pH abnormalities, physiologic principles provide the conceptual framework. Hypoxemia always precedes CO_2 retention in the course of diffuse bronchopulmonary disease for the following reasons: (1) CO_2 is about twenty times as diffusible across the pulmonary alveolocapillary membrane as O_2, and (2) the slopes of the O_2 and CO_2 dissociation curves differ so that regional hyperventilation in ventilation-perfusion mismatching can compensate for regional hypoventilation with respect to CO_2 but not with respect to O_2.

HYPOXEMIA

Definition

Hypoxemia is an arterial blood pO_2 that is less than the normal value of 100 ± 10 mm Hg for a healthy resting person at sea level. Arterial pO_2 decreases with age and is less at higher altitudes.

Symptoms and Signs

Hypoxemia is a common clinical occurrence and should be suspected when a patient exhibits tachycardia, cyanosis, dyspnea, restlessness, impaired cerebral function, and polycythemia. Unfortunately, cyanosis does not appear until arterial oxyhemoglobin saturation falls to 83 percent and the arterial pO_2 to 48 mm Hg. At least 5 gm of deoxygenated hemoglobin per 100 ml of blood must be present in the systemic capillary circulation to produce the color that characterizes cyanosis. Hence, cyanosis is seen at pO_2's higher than 48 mm Hg in polycythemia and at pO_2's lower than 48 mm Hg in anemia. Indeed, patients who have chronic severe anemia may die of hypoxemia without cyanosis. Good illumination is required to detect cyanosis, and it may be obscured by skin pigmentation. Acrocyanosis, as well as other regional cyanosis, may reflect only local conditions and not arterial hypoxemia.

Etiology

Clinical arterial hypoxemia results from any of four pathophysiologic mechanisms, which may occur singly or in combination (Table 7-3).

1. The most common mechanism is ventilation-perfusion ($\dot{V}_A/\dot{Q}_C$) abnormality, or mismatching of the distribution of inspired gas with the distribution of pulmonary capillary blood flow. This occurs in acute and chronic diffuse bronchopulmonary diseases:

    a. Chronic bronchitis.

    b. Pulmonary emphysema.

    c. Bronchial asthma.

    d. Unilateral bronchostenosis.

    e. Pulmonary atelectasis.

    f. Diffuse bronchiectasis.

    g. Extensive pulmonary tuberculosis.

    h. Extensive acute and chronic pneumonias: infectious, chemical, allergic, aspiration.

    i. Pulmonary embolism with infarction.

    j. Extensive pulmonary neoplasm.

    k. Extensive pulmonary granulomata.

    l. Adult respiratory distress syndrome.

    m. Primary pulmonary hypertension.

    n. Radiation fibrosis.

    o. Pneumoconiosis (e.g., silicosis).

    p. Acute bronchitis or bronchiolitis.

    q. Fibrothorax.

    r. Pneumothorax.

    s. Acute anterior poliomyelitis with respiratory paralysis.

    t. Mucoviscidosis or fibrocystic disease.

    u. Kyphoscoliosis.

2. The second most common mechanism is generalized alveolar hypoventilation (not to be confused with the *regional* hypoventilation that occurs in ventilation-perfusion mismatching) due to one of the following:

TABLE 7-3. The Four Pathophysiologic Mechanisms of Arterial Hypoxemia and Patterns of Response to Oxygen Breathing and Physical Exercise

Mechanism	Condition*	pO₂		pCO₂	
		Alveolar	Arterial	Alveolar	Arterial
Ventilation-perfusion mismatching	Initial	Normal to high	Low	Normal to low	Low to high
	Oxygen	Marked increase	Variable increase	Normal to high	Normal to high
	Exercise	Normal to high	Slight increase	Normal to low	Low to high
Generalized alveolar hypoventilation	Initial	Low	Low	High	High
	Oxygen	Marked increase	Marked increase	Increase	Increase
	Exercise	Varies	Varies	Varies	Varies
Pulmonary diffusing capacity decrease	Initial	High	Low	Low	Low
	Oxygen	Marked increase	Marked increase	Increase	Increase
	Exercise	Slight increase	Decrease	Decrease	Decrease
Right-to-left shunt	Initial	Normal to high	Low	Normal to low	Normal to low
	Oxygen	Marked increase	Slight increase	Increase	Increase
	Exercise	Slight increase	Decrease	Slight decrease	Slight decrease

* (1) Initial: spontaneous initial condition; physiologic measurement. (2) Oxygen: effect of breathing 100 percent O₂ for 15 minutes; oxygen breathing test. (3) Exercise: effect of physical exercise; exercise test.

    a. Skeletal abnormalities (e.g., kyphoscoliosis, trauma).

    b. Neuromuscular diseases affecting breathing.

    c. Pickwickian obesity-hypoventilation syndrome.

3. A less common mechanism of hypoxemia is decreased pulmonary diffusing capacity. There are two types:

    a. Decreased alveolocapillary membrane surface area.

    (1) Loss or destruction of lung tissue (e.g., lung resection).

    (2) Compression of lung or restriction of lung expansion (e.g., pneumothorax, "vanishing lung" syndrome).

    b. Increased length of the gas diffusion pathway—*alveolar block syndrome.* This occurs in diffuse parenchymatous bronchopulmonary diseases and certain cardiovascular conditions:

    (1) Pulmonary berylliosis.

    (2) Pulmonary sarcoidosis.

    (3) Diffuse interstitial pulmonary fibrosis or Hamman-Rich syndrome.

    (4) Pulmonary adenomatosis.

    (5) Lymphangitic carcinomatosis.

    (6) Alveolar proteinosis.

    (7) Pulmonary edema.

    (8) Mitral stenosis with chronic pulmonary vascular congestion.

4. The least common mechanism of hypoxemia is right-to-left cardiac or pulmonary circulatory shunt. Although there are innumerable small shunts that cause venous admixture in ventilation-perfusion mismatching, the term *cardiac* or *pulmonary circulatory shunt* refers to discrete gross anatomic shunts.

    a. Congenital right-to-left shunts.

    b. Acquired right-to-left shunts.

    c. Pulmonary hemangioma.

Diagnostic Approach

Unfortunately, a given bronchopulmonary disease may produce hypoxemia by more than one of these four mechanisms. Differential diagnosis of the diseases that produce hypoxemia proceeds as follows:

1. Ventilation-perfusion mismatching is established and quantified by the following tests and procedures:

    a. Single-breath nitrogen test.

    b. Closed-circuit helium equilibration mixing index.

    c. Distribution of inhaled radioactively labeled gas (e.g., xenon).

    d. Distribution of intravenously injected solution of radioactively labeled gas (e.g., xenon).

    e. Lung scan after intravenous injection of radioactively labeled particulates (e.g., radioiodinated macroaggregated serum albumin).

2. Generalized alveolar hypoventilation is established and quantified by the following tests:
    a. Spirometry.   The minute volume of breathing is less than predicted.
    b. Analysis of an alveolar gas sample reveals low pO_2 and high pCO_2.

3. Decreased pulmonary diffusing capacity is established and quantified by any of several carbon monoxide diffusing capacity tests. Tests of pulmonary diffusing capacity can measure a decrease but cannot distinguish between the conditions listed in paragraphs **3a** and **3b**, page 281. Unfortunately, the validity of these tests is decreased in patients who have ventilation-perfusion mismatching or generalized alveolar hypoventilation, or both.

4. Right-to-left shunt is established by the following tests and procedures:
    a. Chest roentgenography with special views and techniques, as indicated (e.g., tomography).
    b. O_2 breathing test with analysis of arterial blood sample. A physiologic diagnosis of right-to-left shunt.
    c. Angiocardiography.   An anatomic diagnosis of the structure and location of a right-to-left shunt.
    d. Cardiac catheterization, with calculation of right-to-left shunt flow.

5. Identification of the mechanism of arterial hypoxemia may require the O_2 breathing test and an exercise test. Table 7-3 shows the characteristic responses of each of the four pathophysiologic mechanisms of clinical arterial hypoxemia to these two tests.

ABNORMALITIES OF BLOOD pCO_2

Definition

The arterial blood pCO_2 of a healthy resting man breathing air spontaneously at sea level is 40 ± 2 mm Hg. Arterial blood pCO_2 is promptly and strongly affected by changes in alveolar ventilation rate. Although arterial pCO_2 equals alveolar pCO_2 over a wide range of clinical conditions, in moderate to severe ventilation-perfusion mismatching, arterial pCO_2 is greater than alveolar pCO_2, and hypoxemia is always already present. Although hypoxemia is the only clinically important blood pO_2 abnormality, hypocapnia and hypercapnia are both clinically important.

Hypocapnia

Pathophysiology

The clinical signs of hypocapnia are always the result of alveolar hyperventilation. Significant physiologic responses are:

1. Slightly decreased systemic arterial blood pressure.

? **2.** Systemic venoconstriction.

3. Decreased cerebral blood flow.

4. Respiratory alkalosis with decreased concentration of ionized calcium in extracellular body fluids.

5. The respiratory alkalosis of chronic hypocapnia induces the kidney to excrete HCO_3^-, producing a compensatory metabolic acidosis that corrects the pH abnormality.

Symptoms and Signs
1. Dizziness.
2. Numbness and tingling of hands and feet.
3. Psychomotor impairment.
4. Signs of tetany.
5. Carpopedal spasm.

Etiology
1. Exposure to high altitudes (physiologic).

2. Normal pregnancy (physiologic).

3. Psychogenic hyperventilation.
   a. Hysterical.
   b. Voluntary.

4. Passive hyperventilation with mechanically controlled or assisted ventilation.

✓ **5.** Compensatory alveolar hyperventilation in response to primary metabolic acidosis.

— **6.** Salicylates.

⁻**7.** Progestogens.

8. Primary central nervous system disease.

9. Severe anemia.

10. Pneumonia, asthma, or pulmonary edema.

11. Gram-negative sepsis.

12. Restrictive lung diseases, such as pulmonary fibrosis.

13. Hepatic failure.

Diagnostic Approach

The cause of hyperventilation is usually readily apparent from the following:

1. History.

2. Physical examination.

3. Mental status and neurologic examination.

4. Routine laboratory work-up.

5. The presence of primary metabolic acidosis as shown by low arterial blood pH.

6. Consideration of altitude and ambient pressure.

7. Rarely, hyperventilation and arterial hypocapnia may result from cerebrospinal fluid acidosis, stimulating the central chemoreceptors.

Hypercapnia

Pathophysiology

1. Responses to *mild hypercapnia:*
   a. Breathing frequency increases.
   b. Tidal volume increases.
   c. Body heat loss increases.
   d. Acute hypercapnia produces respiratory acidosis; chronic respiratory acidosis induces the kidney to retain HCO_3^-, producing compensatory metabolic alkalosis.

2. Responses to *moderate hypercapnia:*
   a. Cerebral blood flow increases.
   b. Intracranial and cerebrospinal fluid pressure increase.
   c. The sympatho-adrenomedullary system discharges, but catecholamines are inhibited by the concomitant respiratory acidosis.
   d. Hyperbaric O_2 convulsions are inhibited.

3. Responses to *severe hypercapnia:*
   a. Body core temperature decreases.
   b. Narcosis.
   c. Unconsciousness.
   d. Death.

Symptoms and Signs

1. Transient, throbbing headache.
2. Flushed face.
3. Nausea.
4. Sweating.
5. Tachycardia.

6. Palpitation.

7. Insomnia.

8. Somnolence.

9. Tunnel vision.

Etiology

1. Acute or chronic obstructive bronchopulmonary conditions.

    a. Pulmonary emphysema.

    b. Chronic bronchitis.

    c. Status asthmaticus.

    d. Bronchiolitis: infectious or chemical.

    e. Mechanical obstruction of trachea or bronchi by water (drowning), blood (hemorrhage), bronchial secretions, or pus.

2. Obstruction of the upper respiratory tract.

3. Generalized alveolar hypoventilation.

    a. Thoracic skeletal conditions, chest wall disease, or chest trauma affecting breathing (e.g., kyphoscoliosis, flail chest, ankylosing spondylitis).

    b. Neuromuscular conditions affecting breathing.

        (1) Muscular dystrophy.

        (2) Myasthenia gravis.

        (3) Intoxications (e.g., pesticides, curare, nerve gas).

        (4) Acute or chronic infectious diseases (e.g., poliomyelitis, Guillain-Barré syndrome, diphtheria, tetanus).

    c. Pickwickian obesity-hypoventilation syndrome.

    d. Central nervous system conditions affecting breathing.

        (1) Cerebrovascular accident.

        (2) Increased intracranial pressure (e.g., intracranial tumor, head trauma).

        (3) Meningitis or encephalitis.

        (4) Pharmacologic depression of respiratory centers (e.g., barbiturates, morphine, tranquilizers, alcohol).

    e. Hypoventilation with mechanical respirator.

    f. Extreme abdominal distention or pain, traumatic or postsurgical, interfering with diaphragmatic breathing.

    g. Other causes.

        (1) Severe hypothyroidism.

        (2) Starvation cachexia.

        (3) Severe electrolyte disturbance.

        (4) Acute intermittent porphyria.

4. Restrictive and other bronchopulmonary conditions.

    a. Pneumothorax, hemothorax, hydrothorax.

    b. Restrictive disease of the pleurae (e.g., fibrosis, calcification).

    c. Extensive infiltrative disease or fibrosis of lung parenchyma.

    d. Severe pulmonary edema.

Diagnostic Approach

The precise diagnosis of the disease or condition producing primary hypercapnia is established as follows:

1. Arterial hypoxemia is always also present, unless the patient is breathing O_2.

2. If the simultaneously determined arterial blood pH is low, then respiratory acidosis is either uncompensated or partially compensated by metabolic alkalosis. If the pH is within normal limits, then respiratory acidosis is either (a) completely corrected by compensatory metabolic alkalosis, or, rarely, (b) a primary coexisting metabolic alkalosis may be just sufficient to correct fully the low pH of hypercapnia. The combination of high pCO_2 and normal pH indicates chronicity and stability of the inciting etiologic agent.

3. If respiratory acidosis is the only primary acid-base disturbance present, differential diagnosis is then made by the following procedures:

    a. History.

    b. Physical examination.

    c. Routine laboratory studies.

    d. Chest roentgenography.

    e. Electrolyte profile.

    f. Pulmonary function tests.

    g. Neurologic examination.

    h. Special laboratory studies as indicated (e.g., porphyria, hypothyroidism).

ABNORMALITIES OF BLOOD pH

Definition

In clinical use, the term *blood pH* means "plasma pH." The normal arterial blood pH of a healthy resting man at sea level is 7.40 ± 0.05. Deviations of arterial blood pH from this range of normal values result from one or more *primary* acid-base disturbances, which induce the pH homeostatic mechanisms to respond with *secondary* pH-compensating processes. Such responses always tend to restore pH toward normal.

Etiology

Metabolic (Nonrespiratory) Acidosis

Metabolic acidosis may result from either acid excess or base deficit. It usually results from either retention of nonvolatile acids (acids other than H_2CO_3, which is excreted by the lungs) or loss of HCO_3^- from the body.

1. Hyperchloremic.
    a. Diarrhea.
    b. Acetazolamide.
    c. Interstitial renal disease.
    d. Renal tubular acidosis.
    e. Arginine hydrochloride.
    f. Ammonium chloride.
    g. Ureterosigmoidostomy.
    - h. Dehydration.

2. Increased undetermined anion.
    - a. Diabetic ketoacidosis.
    b. Renal failure with uremic acidosis.
    c. Lactic acidosis.
    d. Salicylate intoxication.
    e. Methanol intoxication.
    f. Ethylene glycol intoxication.
    g. Starvation ketoacidosis.

Metabolic (Nonrespiratory) Alkalosis
Metabolic alkalosis may result from either base excess or acid deficit.

1. Chloruretic diuretics.

2. Nasogastric suction.

3. Vomiting.

4. Alkali therapy.

5. Mineralocorticosteroid excess.   ↓K
    a. Endogenous (e.g., aldosteronism).
    b. Exogenous (e.g., deoxycorticosterone acetate, licorice intoxication).

6. Glucocorticosteroid excess.
    a. Endogenous (e.g., hyperadrenocorticism, Cushing's syndrome).
    b. Exogenous (e.g., therapy with glucocorticosteroids, ACTH).

7. Severe K+ deficit (usually depletion).

8. Cl− deficit (usually restriction).

9. Intravenous phosphate or sulfate salts in a Na+-depleted patient.

Diagnostic Approach

Precise diagnosis, and thus proper therapy, of acid-base disorders requires identification of the *primary* inciting—as opposed to *secondary* compensatory—processes. Usually one, but sometimes more than one, of the four possible primary acid-base disturbances is found; any primary disturbances and their etiologic agents must be identified and distinguished from any secondary compensatory responses. In general, respiratory compensations for metabolic pH disturbances are incomplete.

Graphic Approach

1. Review the history for potential causes of acid-base disturbance.

2. Review the physical examination for signs of acid-base disturbance.
   a. Nasogastric tube.
   b. Cyanosis.
   c. Evidence of bronchopulmonary disease.
   d. Fever.
   e. Hypotension.
   f. Jaundice.
   g. Signs of alkalemic tetany.

3. Review the laboratory values for blood CO_2 content and K^+ concentration, and calculate the undetermined anion concentration (anion gap) as follows:

$$\text{Undetermined anion concentration} = [Na^+] - [CO_2] - [Cl^-]$$

The value is normally less than 12 to 14 mEq per liter and consists of phosphates, anionic proteins, sulfates, and anions of various organic acids. Slight elevations to 15 or 16 mEq per liter sometimes occur in respiratory alkalosis. Increased undetermined anion concentration indicates metabolic acidosis. However, the converse is not true; metabolic acidosis may be hyperchloremic. Larger undetermined anion gaps are more likely due to increased organic acids. Values greater than 25 mEq per liter occur only in diabetic ketoacidosis; methanol, ethylene glycol, or salicylate intoxication; and lactic acidosis.

Acidosis is usually associated with hyperkalemia unless (a) the acidosis develops in a patient already K^+-depleted, or (b) the acidosis is due to loss of $KHCO_3$ from the body, e.g., in diarrhea, acetazolamide therapy, or renal tubular acidosis. Alkalosis is usually associated with hypokalemia, except when K^+-loading predominates due to increased K^+ intake or increased rate of tissue breakdown.

4. Review other laboratory data for acid-base clues.
   a. Polycythemia.
   b. Hyperglycemia.
   c. Elevated BUN.
   d. Elevated NH_3.
   e. Decreased pulmonary function.
   f. Positive blood culture.

5. Analyze and interpret pH, pCO_2, and HCO_3^- as follows. Plot pCO_2 and pH on any of the three available two-dimensional graphs or on the three-dimensional acid-base surface model of the Henderson-Hasselbalch buffer equation. Visual inspection of the position of this plotted acid-base point relative to both the isobar $pCO_2 = 40$ (line of pure metabolic disturbance) and the patient's CO_2 titration, or blood buffer, curve (line of pure respiratory disturbance) indicates either an apparently (but not necessarily) pure primary respiratory or metabolic disturbance or an obviously mixed disturbance consisting of one or more primary components with or without secondary compensatory responses. Using the other clinical information from paragraphs **1** through **4** above, deduce the nature, sequence, and cause of acid-base events.

Tabular Approach
See Table 7-4.

TABLE 7-4. Diagnosis of Acid-Base Disorders

	Low pH	Normal pH	High pH
High pCO$_2$	Respiratory acidosis with or without Incompletely compensating metabolic alkalosis or Coexisting metabolic acidosis	Respiratory acidosis and Compensatory metabolic alkalosis	Metabolic alkalosis with Coexisting respiratory acidosis or Incompletely compensating respiratory acidosis
Normal pCO$_2$	Metabolic acidosis	Normal	Metabolic alkalosis
Low pCO$_2$	Metabolic acidosis with Coexisting respiratory alkalosis or Incompletely compensating respiratory alkalosis	Respiratory alkalosis and Compensatory metabolic acidosis	Respiratory alkalosis with or without Incompletely compensating metabolic acidosis or Coexisting metabolic alkalosis

8.

Musculoskeletal Problems

Peripheral Joint Arthritis

Herbert Kaplan

The diagnostic challenge presented by the patient with pain or swelling in the elbows, knees, or the joints of the hands and feet will be considered in this section. Although disorders that affect the peripheral articulations may also involve the shoulders, hips, and spine, these disorders are covered separately. The following abbreviations are used in this chapter:

ANA = antinuclear antibody
ARF = acute rheumatic fever
  AS = ankylosing spondylitis
CTD = connective tissue disease
 DIP = distal interphalangeal
 ESR = erythrocyte sedimentation rate
   IP = interphalangeal
 JRA = juvenile rheumatoid arthritis
  LE = lupus erythematosus
MCP = metacarpophalangeal
MTP = metatarsophalangeal
  OA = osteoarthritis
PAN = polyarteritis nodosa
 PIP = proximal interphalangeal
  RA = rheumatoid arthritis
  RF = rheumatoid factor
 SLE = systemic lupus erythematosus

ETIOLOGY

The more common causes of peripheral joint disease diagnosed in office practice, listed in order of decreasing frequency, are as follows:

1. Osteoarthritis.

2. Bursitis, tendinitis.

3. Connective tissue diseases (rheumatoid arthritis, systemic lupus erythematosus, polymyalgia rheumatica, scleroderma, dermatomyositis, polyarteritis nodosa, acute rheumatic fever).

4. Crystalline arthropathies (gout, pseudogout).

5. Rheumatoid variants (ankylosing spondylitis, psoriatic arthritis, Reiter's syndrome, palindromic rheumatism, enteropathic arthropathy, juvenile rheumatoid arthritis).

6. Infectious arthritis (bacterial and viral).

7. Joint trauma.

8. Miscellaneous disorders (sarcoidosis, hyperparathyroidism, myxedema, hemophilia, neuropathic arthropathy, pharmacologic arthritis, Behçet's syndrome, Whipple's disease, malignancy).

DIAGNOSTIC APPROACH

History

Mode of Onset

1. The type of onset, whether abrupt or insidious, is of limited diagnostic value because cases of acute arthritis may become chronic, and chronic forms of arthritis may present during an acute exacerbation.

2. An acute, dramatic onset suggests crystalline arthropathy or infectious arthritis. However, acute rheumatic fever, rheumatoid arthritis, juvenile rheumatoid arthritis, Reiter's syndrome, and psoriatic arthritis may also begin acutely. The chronic course of osteoarthritis frequently is punctuated by acute exacerbations of painful, swollen, and occasionally warm joints.

Trauma

1. A history of trauma, recent or remote, may be significant in predisposing to osteoarthritis, tendinitis, or bursitis.

2. Acute gouty arthritis is often triggered by relatively mild trauma to the involved joint.

Antecedent Infection

1. A history of an infected skin laceration or any other bacterial focus may be the clue to infectious arthritis.

2. An antecedent streptococcal pharyngitis or scarlet fever should rouse suspicion of acute rheumatic fever.

3. Recent sexual exposure or urethritis suggests gonococcal arthritis or Reiter's syndrome.

4. Fever and a skin rash followed by polyarthritis suggests rubella, infectious mononucleosis, or arthritis associated with viral hepatitis.

Drugs
1. A history of drug ingestion should suggest the possibility of pharmacologic arthritis.

2. Penicillin, sulfonamides, and horse serum injections are common causes of foreign protein reactions (serum sickness) typified by urticaria and polyarthritis.

3. Antihypertensive drugs that produce hyperuricemia are common causes of secondary gout. Chemotherapeutic agents used in malignant disease may also cause secondary gout.

4. Anticonvulsant drugs, hydralazine, procainamide, isoniazid, and some antibiotics may cause an LE-like syndrome with polyarthritis.

5. Acute joint swelling in patients taking anticoagulants suggests hemarthrosis. However, hemarthrosis may also occur in patients with hereditary clotting disorders.

Previous Response to Therapy
1. A therapeutic response or a failure to respond to a specific drug may be of some diagnostic assistance.

2. A good result from the administration of colchicine is almost pathognomonic of gout, although a beneficial response has also been reported in both sarcoid arthritis and rheumatoid arthritis.

3. A good response to large doses of salicylates may be obtained in most acute joint inflammations. However, these drugs are less effective in Reiter's syndrome, crystalline arthropathy, and infectious arthritis.

4. Steroids may alleviate the arthritis of connective tissue disease and gout, but they are much less effective in joint infections, osteoarthritis, Reiter's syndrome, and psoriatic arthritis.

5. The response to drugs with a broad spectrum of antiinflammatory and analgesic activity, such as phenylbutazone and indomethacin, is of little or no diagnostic value in either acute or chronic arthritis.

Family History
1. A family history of "arthritis" is generally of little diagnostic significance.

2. A well-documented family history of gout, Heberden's nodes, psoriasis, ankylosing spondylitis, or hemoglobinopathy may be of value. The hereditary nature of RA and SLE is less well established.

Physical Examination

In the physical examination, extraarticular manifestations of rheumatic disorders may provide important clues to specific diagnoses. Some of the more important of these findings are listed below.

1. Mucocutaneous lesions.
    a. Alopecia may be seen in SLE and RA. The hair of the forehead is characteristically short and brittle in SLE.
    b. A combination of oral and genital ulcers with iritis suggests Behçet's syndrome. The oral lesions consist of single or multiple painful ulcers. Ulcerative lesions of the penis and scrotum, or of the vulva and vagina, are commonly observed. Pyoderma may be noted.
    c. Balanitis circinata and keratoderma blenorrhagica are features of Reiter's syndrome.
    d. Erythematous cutaneous lesions, a malar butterfly rash, and erythematous lesions of the fingertips should suggest SLE.
    e. Subcutaneous nodules in the olecranon bursa, along the extensor surface of the forearm, or along bony protuberances are almost pathognomonic of RA, although they may rarely be seen in patients with acute rheumatic fever and SLE. Subcutaneous nodules may be indistinguishable from the tophi of gout. Tophi commonly occur in the cartilage of the helix of the ear, the olecranon and patellar bursae, and tendons.
    f. Indolent ischemic ulcers on the distal portion of the leg occur in RA with Felty's syndrome or vasculitis, in SLE, and sometimes in scleroderma.
    g. Pyoderma gangrenosum is often associated with the arthropathy of ulcerative colitis.
    h. The presence of cutaneous psoriasis suggests the possibility of psoriatic arthritis. Pitted lesions of the nails are characteristic.
    i. Edematous, indurated, and atrophic changes in the skin, ulcerations, and hyperpigmentation are features of scleroderma.
    j. Erythema over the knuckles, a dusky erythematous eruption in a "shawl" distribution over the shoulders, a lilac or heliotrope discoloration of the upper eyelids, and diffuse or localized muscle induration should suggest dermatomyositis.
    k. Sweaty palms with thenar and hypothenar erythema are common in RA.

2. Ocular lesions.
    a. Keratoconjunctivitis sicca, nasopharyngeal ulceration, and parotid enlargement are manifestations of Sjögren's syndrome, which is associated with RA in about half the cases and less commonly with other connective tissue diseases.
    b. Conjunctivitis and iritis occur in Reiter's syndrome, sarcoidosis, ankylosing spondylitis, juvenile RA, and Behçet's syndrome.
    c. Episcleritis and less commonly scleritis may be seen in RA.

d. Retinal cytoid bodies are a manifestation of SLE. Retinal granulomata may be observed in sarcoidosis and tuberculosis.

3. Lymphadenopathy. Lymphadenopathy is a nonspecific abnormality noted not uncommonly in SLE, RA, juvenile RA, sarcoidosis, and the arthritis seen in lymphomas.

4. Cardiopulmonary abnormalities.

    a. Wheezing, cough, and shortness of breath may occur as a result of the pulmonary parenchymal disease sometimes found in RA, SLE, scleroderma, polymyositis, polyarteritis nodosa, and sarcoidosis.

    b. Pleural effusion is not uncommon in RA and SLE.

    c. Cardiac involvement (pericarditis, heart block) may be a feature of any of the connective tissue diseases or of Reiter's syndrome.

    d. Aortic insufficiency may occur in acute rheumatic fever, RA, ankylosing spondylitis, Reiter's syndrome, and Behçet's syndrome.

    e. Decreased chest expansion is a feature of ankylosing spondylitis.

5. Hepatosplenomegaly. Enlargement of the liver and spleen may be found in connective tissue diseases, sarcoidosis, infections, and juvenile RA. Splenomegaly is a feature of Felty's syndrome.

6. Neurologic abnormalities.

    a. Polyneuritis or mononeuritis may occur in the connective tissue diseases and neuropathic arthropathies.

    b. Long tract signs and motor weakness may result from cord compression due to C1-C2 subluxation in RA and ankylosing spondylitis.

    c. Peripheral nerve entrapment syndromes may occur in RA, myxedema, and gout.

ETIOLOGY OF PERIPHERAL JOINT DISEASE

The mode of onset, clinical course, and pattern of joint involvement provide a convenient basis for classifying the clinical patterns of peripheral joint disease. Four major categories can be identified: (1) acute polyarthritis, (2) chronic polyarthritis, (3) acute monarthritis, and (4) chronic monarthritis. It should be recognized that although this classification is useful in the diagnostic approach to joint disease, it is not all-encompassing. Moreover, it should not be implied that all cases can be grouped into these categories. The most common causes of these clinical patterns are listed below.

Acute Polyarthritis

1. Acute rheumatic fever.
2. Rheumatoid arthritis.
3. Other connective tissue diseases.
4. Rheumatoid variants.

5. Infectious arthritis (especially gonococcal).
6. Gout.
7. Pseudogout.
8. Foreign protein reaction (serum sickness).

Chronic Polyarthritis

1. Rheumatoid arthritis.
2. Other connective tissue diseases.
3. Rheumatoid variants.
4. Chronic gouty arthritis.
5. Osteoarthritis.
6. Sarcoidosis.

Acute Monarthritis

1. Gout.
2. Pseudogout.
3. Traumatic joint disease.
4. Infections arthritis (septic joint, tuberculosis).
5. Rheumatoid arthritis.
6. Osteoarthritis.
7. Palindromic rheumatism.
8. Intermittent hydrarthrosis.

Chronic Monarthritis

1. Infectious arthritis, especially tuberculosis.
2. Traumatic arthritis.
3. Osteoarthritis.
4. Gout.
5. Pseudogout.
6. Neuropathic arthropathy.

CLINICAL FEATURES OF PERIPHERAL JOINT DISEASE

The clinical manifestations and the pattern of joint involvement may provide useful clues to the diagnosis of arthritis.

Acute Polyarthritis

1. Acute migratory polyarthritis in children and young adults beginning shortly after a streptococcal infection suggests acute rheumatic fever (ARF). Typically, there is swelling, heat, redness, tenderness, pain, and limitation of motion of two or more joints, most commonly the knees, ankles, elbows, wrists, hips, and small joints of the feet. Ac-

cording to the modified Jones criteria, the presence of two major criteria, or one major and two minor criteria, of those listed below, are considered diagnostic of ARF.

a. Major manifestations.
   (1) Carditis.
      (a) Significant murmurs.
      (b) Cardiomegaly.
      (c) Pericarditis.
   (2) Polyarthritis.
   (3) Chorea.
   (4) Erythema marginatum.
   (5) Subcutaneous nodules.
b. Minor manifestations.
   (1) Clinical.
      (a) History of previous ARF or evidence of rheumatic heart disease.
      (b) Arthralgias.
      (c) Fever (>38° C).
   (2) Laboratory.
      (a) Elevated sedimentation rate and positive C-reactive protein test.
      (b) Electrocardiographic changes, chiefly prolongation of the P-R interval.
c. Supporting evidence of streptococcal infection.
   (1) Laboratory.
      (a) Positive throat culture.
      (b) Positive antibody test (ASO titer).
   (2) Recent scarlet fever.

2. Although RA usually begins insidiously, it may begin as an acute polyarthritis resembling ARF in every way and responding to salicylates in similar fashion, but the polyarthritis of ARF usually disappears within a few weeks while that of RA tends to persist. Negative findings on a battery of streptococcal antibody tests rule out ARF in the presence of arthritis, and a positive finding for rheumatoid factor supports this diagnosis. Also favoring RA are the presence of morning stiffness and symmetric involvement of the small joints of the hands and feet.

3. SLE may present as an acute polyarthritis. It differs from ARF in its tendency to occur after exposure to sunlight or after the administration of drugs. A butterfly rash, evidence of nephritis, positive findings on LE cell or ANA tests, low serum complement, and negative streptococcal antibody test results strongly support the diagnosis of SLE.

4. Rheumatoid variants, such as psoriatic arthritis, Reiter's syndrome, and enteropathic arthropathy, may begin as an acute polyarthritis. The distinguishing features are discussed below (see Chronic Polyarthritis).

5. Gonococcal arthritis is usually a febrile illness beginning 1 to 2 weeks after a gonorrheal infection with evidence of a migratory polyarthralgia or polyarthritis. Eventually, the infection localizes to one or more joints. Signs of joint inflammation and tenosynovitis may be observed. Macular, hemorrhagic, vesicular, or pustular skin lesions are present in half the cases. The diagnosis is established by culture of the synovial fluid. A good therapeutic response to penicillin but not to salicylates strongly supports the diagnosis in an appropriate clinical setting, even when bacteriologic studies are negative.

6. Infectious arthritis of other origin may present a similar picture. Joint involvement is by local extension or hematogenous spread.

7. Gout and pseudogout may present in acute polyarticular form, but this is rare. The diagnosis hinges upon the demonstration of urate or calcium pyrophosphate dihydrate crystals, respectively, in the synovial fluid.

8. Foreign protein reactions, including serum sickness, may present as an acute polyarthritis. Clues to the correct diagnosis are a history of drug or horse serum administration and the presence of urticaria.

Chronic Polyarthritis

1. A progressive, symmetric polyarthritis with fusiform swelling of the joints, muscle atrophy, and eventually deformities is characteristic of RA. There is a predilection for involvement of the proximal interphalangeal (PIP) and metacarpophalangeal (MCP) joints of the fingers, the metatarsophalangeal (MTP) joints of the feet, the toes, wrists, knees, elbows, shoulder, and hips. Stiffness after inactivity, especially in the morning upon arising, is a characteristic symptom. Subcutaneous nodules, when present, are virtually pathognomonic. The outcome of a test for rheumatoid factor is positive in 70 to 80 percent of cases.

2. A rheumatoid-like arthropathy may occur in other connective tissue diseases, especially in SLE. Clues to the diagnosis of SLE are fever, a typical eruption, evidence of polyserositis, nephritis (especially the nephrotic syndrome), retinal cytoid bodies, anemia, thrombocytopenia, leukopenia, biologically false-positive results on tests for syphilis, positive LE cells, and positive ANA tests. Recurrent or persistent small joint inflammation in the absence of deformity also suggests SLE. Ankylosis and contractures are uncommon.

3. Polyarthritis may occur in the rheumatoid variants. In these diseases, joint involvement tends to be symmetric, and progression to deformity is uncommon. Interphalangeal synovitis of the toes ("sausage toes") is a feature of Reiter's syndrome, psoriatic arthritis, and the peripheral arthritis of ankylosing spondylitis. Spondylitis and sacro-iliitis are commonly observed in this group of diseases. Findings for rheumatoid factor are usually negative.

a. Reiter's disease is characterized by a combination of urethritis, iritis and conjunctivitis, arthritis, and often diarrhea, balanitis, and keratodermia blenorrhagica. Spinal involvement similar to that of ankylosing spondylitis may occur. The disease tends to be self-limited.

b. Psoriatic arthritis may mimic RA. Involvement of the distal interphalangeal (DIP) joints, typical changes in the nails, and cutaneous psoriasis are clues to the diagnosis.

c. Ankylosing spondylitis with peripheral arthritis is not often mistaken for RA because the spinal involvement dominates the clinical picture.

d. Enteropathic arthritis (e.g., arthritis associated with regional enteritis and ulcerative colitis) may simulate the polyarthritis of RA. The association of serious gastrointestinal disease and chronic diarrhea are clues to the diagnosis.

4. Although chronic gouty arthritis may mimic RA, advanced deforming arthritic changes due to gout are uncommon nowadays. A long history of acute episodic arthritis with remissions between attacks can usually be obtained. Hyperuricemia, the demonstration of urate crystals in the synovial fluid, response to colchicine, and biopsy of a gouty tophus have confirmatory value.

5. Osteoarthritis is a polyarticular disease, but symptoms are usually related to involvement of the knees, hips, vertebral column, and hands. Heberden's nodes are bony protuberances of the DIP joints of the fingers, often associated with flexion and angulation of the distal phalanges. Local pain, tenderness, and some warmth may be present. Tender, knobby enlargement of the PIP joints (Bouchard's nodes) also is not uncommon. Degenerative changes in the knees are manifested often by pain, and occasionally by joint swelling, crepitus, and flexion contracture. Involvement of the spine and hips is discussed in the sections Painful Hip and Low Back Pain, later in the chapter.

6. The joint swelling present in cases of hypertrophic osteoarthropathy may be mistaken for a polyarthritis of other origin. The presence of clubbing and an association with chronic pulmonary disease, bronchogenic carcinoma, cyanotic congenital heart disease, cirrhosis, or enteropathic disease usually makes the diagnosis apparent. The presence of periosteal proliferation on x-ray is confirmatory.

Acute and Chronic Monarthritis

1. Acute monarticular arthritis in a male involving the MTP joint of the great toe, instep, heel, ankle, knee, wrist, hand, or elbow, with complete recovery between attacks, is virtually pathognomonic of gout. The diagnosis is established by the demonstration of urate crystals in the synovial fluid or a therapeutic response to adequate doses of colchicine. Hyperuricemia is usually present. Tophi are found in advanced cases.

2. Acute monarticular arthritis may also be due to pseudogout (chondrocalcinosis). The diagnosis depends on finding calcium pyrophosphate dihydrate crystals in aspirated synovial fluid and on the presence of calcium deposits in the menisci or the articular cartilages.

3. Trauma frequently affects only one joint. Since the trauma is usually severe, the diagnosis is generally evident from the history.

4. Pyogenic, tuberculous, or gonococcal arthritis is commonly monarticular, and evidence of antecedent or concomitant infection is not difficult to obtain. Cytologic and bacteriologic study of the synovial fluid establishes the etiologic diagnosis.

5. Although several joints are usually affected in osteoarthritis, involvement of a single weight-bearing joint, such as the knee or hip, may dominate the clinical picture. Further details may be found under the heading Chronic Polyarthritis, above, and in the section Painful Hip, later in the chapter.

6. RA and especially juvenile RA may be monarticular at the onset of the disease. Local signs of inflammation are commonly observed. The

TABLE 8-1. Examination of Joint Fluid

Measure	Normal	Group I (Noninflammatory)	Group II (Inflammatory)	Group III (Septic)
Volume (ml) (knee)	<3.5	Often >3.5	Often >3.5	Often >3.5
Clarity	Transparent	Transparent	Translucent-opaque	Opaque
Color	Clear	Yellow	Yellow to opalescent	Yellow to green
Viscosity	High	High	Low	Variable
WBC (per cu mm)	<200	200 to 2000	2000 to 100,000	>100,000*
Polymorphonuclear leukocytes (%)	<25%	<25%	50% or more	75% or more*
Culture	Negative	Negative	Negative	Often positive
Mucin clot	Firm	Firm	Friable	Friable
Glucose (mg/100 ml)	Nearly equal to blood	Nearly equal to blood	>25, lower than blood	<25, much lower than blood

* Lower with infections caused by partially treated or low-virulence organisms.
SOURCE: Reprinted from *Primer on the rheumatic diseases*, JAMA, 224:661, 1973.

diagnosis may become apparent only after a prolonged period of observation. Infectious arthritis and other causes of monarthritis must be excluded.

7. Neuropathic arthropathy (Charcot's joint) is characterized by joint hypermobility, effusion, and disproportionately little pain in association with a primary neurologic disorder such as tabes dorsalis, diabetic neuropathy, or syringomyelia.

DIAGNOSTIC PROCEDURES IN ARTHRITIS
Synovial Fluid Analysis

Synovial fluid analysis should include the following: white cell count, differential count, LE cell preparation, crystal identification, Rope's test, and when appropriate, gram and acid-fast stains, culture, and serum complement determination. The pertinent findings on examination of joint fluid are summarized in Tables 8-1 and 8-2. Table 8-3 contains information concerning commonly used laboratory tests in the diagnosis of arthritis.

TABLE 8-2. Differential Diagnosis by Joint Fluid Groups

Group I (Noninflammatory)	Group II (Inflammatory)	Group III (Septic)	Hemorrhagic
Degenerative joint disease	Rheumatoid arthritis	Bacterial infections	Hemophilia or other hemorrhagic diathesis
Trauma*	Acute crystal-induced synovitis (gout and pseudogout)		Trauma with or without fracture
Osteochondritis dissecans	Reiter's syndrome		Neuropathic arthropathy
Osteochondromatosis	Ankylosing spondylitis		Pigmented villonodular synovitis
Neuropathic arthropathy*	Psoriatic arthritis		Synovioma
Subsiding or early inflammation	Arthritis accompanying ulcerative colitis and regional enteritis		Hemangioma and other benign neoplasm
Hypertrophic osteoarthropathy†	Rheumatic fever†		
Pigmented villonodular synovitis*	Systemic lupus erythematosus†		
	Progressive systemic sclerosis (scleroderma)†		

* May be hemorrhagic.
† Groups I or II.
SOURCE: Reprinted from *Primer on the rheumatic diseases*, JAMA, 224:661, 1973.

TABLE 8-3.   Diagnostic Procedures in Arthritis

Test	Purpose	Results and Interpretation
CBC	Routine	1. Anemia common in RA, connective tissue diseases, rheumatoid variants 2. Leukocytosis in infectious arthritis, juvenile RA, crystalline arthropathy, occasionally RA 3. Leukopenia common in SLE; also occurs in Felty's syndrome and juvenile RA
ESR	Routine	1. Nonspecific sign of inflammatory disease 2. May parallel severity of RA 3. When normal, favors noninflammatory joint disease 4. Strikingly elevated in polymyalgia rheumatica 5. Normal values increase with age (20 mm up to the age of 60 years and 30 mm above this age)
Urinalysis	Routine	1. Proteinuria in nephropathy of SLE, polyarteritis nodosa, scleroderma, gout 2. Proteinuria in long-standing RA or ankylosing spondylitis suggests complicating amyloidosis 3. Pyuria in gonorrhea, Reiter's syndrome 4. Cylindruria and RBC casts in SLE nephritis
RF	Diagnosis of RA	1. Nonspecific test, not absolutely pathognomonic of RA, but strongly suggestive of the diagnosis when titer exceeds 1:80 2. May be positive in 5 to 10% of normal individuals above age of 50 years and in 20 to 30% of cases of SLE. Sometimes positive in connective tissue diseases, rheumatoid variants, and diseases associated with hypergammaglobulinemia 3. Negative RF favors osteoarthritis, infection, crystalline arthropathy
LE cell, antinuclear antibody (ANA)	Diagnosis of SLE	1. ANA more sensitive than LE cell phenomenon but less specific for the diagnosis of SLE 2. ANA rarely if ever absent in SLE but frequently positive in low titer in other connective tissue diseases and in 5% of "healthy" elderly individuals 3. LE cell factor positive in 60 to 80% of patients with SLE, 15% of cases of RA, and occasionally in patients with other connective tissue diseases 4. LE factor and ANA often positive in drug sensitivity states

TABLE 8-3.   (*Continued*)

Test	Purpose	Results and Interpretation
T₄ or equivalent	Diagnosis of hypothyroidism	Performed to rule out hypothyroidism, which may produce rheumatoid-like arthropathy
CPK, SGOT, aldolase	Diagnosis of polymyositis	1. Enzymes elevated in polymyositis 2. Enzymes often elevated in myopathy of hypothyroidism 3. Enzymes normal in polymalgia rheumatica and other connective tissue diseases
Serum calcium, phosphorus, alkaline phosphatase	Detection of arthritis associated with intrinsic bone disease	1. Hypercalcemia, hypophosphatemia, and elevated alkaline phosphatase in hyperparathyroidism 2. Hypercalcemia often present in sarcoidosis, metastatic malignancy
Serum protein electrophoresis, immunoglobulins	Detection of hyperglobulinemia and dysproteinemias	1. Hyperglobulinemia seen in sarcoidosis, enteropathic arthropathy, lymphomas, other malignancies, and advanced stages of some connective tissue diseases 2. Diffuse hypergammaglobulinemia in chronic infection, liver disease, SLE, and RA 3. Monoclonal gammopathy in myeloma, macroglobulinemia, some cases of primary amyloidosis or carcinoma, and some normal elderly persons
Serum uric acid	Detection of hyperuricemia	Causes of hyperuricemia 1. Asymptomatic, genetic 2. Gout (primary or secondary) 3. Drugs (e.g., salicylates, diuretics) 4. Hematologic disorders (e.g., polycythemia, leukemia, hemolytic anemias) 5. Renal disease 6. Hypertension 7. Hereditary disorders (e.g., Lesch-Nyhan syndrome) 8. Endocrine disorders

Suggested Work-up for Acute Polyarthritis

1. CBC.

2. Urinalysis.

3. ESR.

4. ASO titer, C-reactive protein, and sometimes a battery of antistreptococcal antibody tests; throat culture.

5. Biochemical screening (e.g., SMA-12) and serum protein electrophoresis.

6. Test for RF, including titer.

7. ANA, LE cell factor, or both.

8. Exclude infectious process clinically, and if necessary, by cytologic study and culture of synovial fluid.

9. Synovial fluid analysis to rule out crystalline arthropathy when appropriate.

10. X-rays of involved and contralateral joints.

11. Chest films.

12. Electrocardiogram.

Suggested Work-up for Chronic Polyarthritis

1. CBC.

2. Urinalysis.

3. ESR.

4. Biochemical screening (e.g., SMA-12) and serum protein electrophoresis.

5. Test for RF, including titer.

6. ANA, LE cell factor, or both.

7. Serologic test for syphilis.

8. Thyroid function tests, if appropriate.

9. X-rays of involved and contralateral joints.

10. Chest films.

11. Electrocardiogram.

12. Synovial fluid analysis.

13. Special procedures, when appropriate.
   a. Immunoglobulins.
   b. Serum complement.
   c. Creatinine clearance.
   d. Coagulation screening.
   e. Esophageal motility studies.
   f. Contrast studies of the gastrointestinal tract.
   g. Biopsy of subcutaneous nodules, tophi, or synovium.

Suggested Work-up for Monarthritis

1. CBC.

2. Urinalysis.

3. ESR.

4. Biochemical screening (e.g., SMA-12).

5. Test for RF.

6. ANA, LE cell factor, or both.

7. Serologic test for syphilis.

8. X-rays of involved and contralateral joints.

9. Synovial fluid analysis.

10. Cultures of cervix, rectum, throat, and skin lesions.

Myalgia
Herbert Kaplan

DEFINITION

Myalgia is poorly localized aching in a muscle or group of muscles. While any of the diseases that primarily affect the joints may also cause muscle pain, this discussion is limited to patients with muscle pain and minimal or no articular involvement.

ETIOLOGY

Myalgia may be secondary to rheumatic or nonrheumatic conditions. The causes are listed in order of decreasing frequency within each group.

1. Rheumatic disorders.
   a. Fibrositis and psychogenic rheumatism. Both conditions are diagnosed by exclusion. A consideration of whether they are the same condition or separate entities is beyond the scope of this discussion.
   b. Tendinitis and peritendinitis.
   c. Connective tissue diseases.
   d. Ankylosing spondylitis.
   e. Sarcoidosis.

2. Nonrheumatic disorders.
  a. Infectious diseases (viremia, bacteremia).
  b. Disease of the spinal column (intervertebral disc protrusion, spondylolisthesis, osteoporosis of the spine).
  c. Peripheral nerve entrapment syndromes (e.g., carpal tunnel syndrome).
  d. Neoplasms, including hypertrophic osteoarthropathy.
  e. Endocrine disorders (hypothyroidism, hyperparathyroidism, acromegaly).
  f. Peripheral neuritis, including diabetic neuropathy, pernicious anemia.
  g. Drug-induced myalgia.
    (1) Steroid-induced pseudorheumatism.
    (2) Hypokalemia secondary to diuretics.
    (3) LE syndrome secondary to anticonvulsants, hydralazine, procainamide, isoniazid, antibiotics, etc.
    (4) Clofibrate (Atromid-S).
    (5) Chloroquin.
  h. Reflex neurovascular dystrophy (shoulder-hand syndrome).
  i. Alcoholism, acute and chronic.
  j. Parkinson's disease.
  k. Paget's disease of bone.
  l. Postgastrectomy (subtotal).

CLINICAL FEATURES

Table 8-4 lists the clinical features of the most common causes of myalgia.

DIAGNOSTIC APPROACH
History

1. Mode of onset.
  a. An insidious onset and chronic course are typical of most of the etiologic entities. An acute onset is reported in the majority of patients with polymyalgia rheumatica and those with occult or overt infections.
  b. Acute muscle pain, often associated with muscle swelling during the course of an alcoholic bout, is seen in alcoholic myopathy.

2. Area of involvement.
  a. The more diffuse and poorly localized the myalgia, the more likely it is that the diagnosis is fibrositis.
  b. Specific localization over a tendon is helpful, as in bicipital tendinitis, de Quervain's disease, or the carpal tunnel syndrome.

c. Involvement of the muscles of neck, the pelvic and pectoral girdles, and the thighs and upper arms occurs in polymyalgia rheumatica. The muscles below the elbows and knees are not affected in this condition.

d. Concomitant arthritis in an adjacent or distant joint suggests one of the connective tissue diseases. However, one of these may present with myalgia unassociated with articular involvement.

e. Episodic or continuous aching in the low back region or shoulder girdle, in a young male with or without sciatic radiation, suggests ankylosing spondylitis.

f. Pain in the muscles of the pelvic girdle and thighs may occur in Paget's disease.

3. A history of use of any of the drugs listed above as etiologic agents (p. 306) suggests drug-induced myalgia.

4. Response or lack of response to therapy.

a. Antiinflammatory drugs (salicylates, steroids, indomethacin, phenylbutazone) may give some degree of relief in both rheumatic and nonrheumatic conditions. Hence, the response to these agents is of little diagnostic value.

b. Failure to respond to antiinflammatory analgesic treatment should suggest psychogenic rheumatism, peripheral neuritis, nerve entrapment, reflex neurovascular dystrophy, endocrinopathy, and Parkinson's disease.

System Review

In the system review, areas of inquiry specifically applicable to the evaluation of myalgia are listed below.

1. Weight loss, malaise, anorexia, and fever suggest neoplasia (with or without associated dermatomyositis), granulomatous disease (sarcoidosis, tuberculosis), or infection.

2. The well-known but nonspecific symptoms of hypothyroidism suggest the myopathy associated with this disease.

3. Recurrent and severe headaches, especially in the temporal region, a history of tender spots over the scalp, claudication of the jaw, and unilateral or bilateral blurring or loss of vision suggest temporal arteritis associated with polymyalgia rheumatica.

4. Neuropsychiatric evaluation during the history-taking process is most important in evaluating a patient with myalgia. Overemphasis by the patient of a "strong family history of arthritis," multitudinous complaints, strong denial of any emotional problems, grimacing, and autopalpation during the teary-eyed recitation of symptoms, all may be clues to psychogenic rheumatism.

TABLE 8-4. Most Common Causes of Myalgia

Cause	History	Physical Examination	Laboratory Data	Course
Fibrositis—psychogenic rheumatism	Poorly localized muscle aches; occurs predominantly in females	Negative except for hypertrophic joints	Negative	Chronic, nonprogressive
Tendinitis, peritendinitis, capsulitis	Acute or insidious onset, often associated with trauma or excessive use	Local tenderness over tendon insertion and contiguous muscle; periarticular tenderness; limited motion common	Negative	Self-limited, although it may result in joint deformity (especially with shoulder involvement)
Rheumatoid arthritis	Muscular symptoms may precede articular symptoms; often severe pain and stiffness	Usually significant synovitis in the peripheral joints; subcutaneous nodules; muscle wasting if severe	ESR elevated; RF positive; minimal inflammation on muscle biopsy	Severe muscle symptoms in RA often associated with more ominous course
Polymyalgia rheumatica	Typically, elderly female, with relatively acute onset of aching and stiffness of the proximal muscles and pelvic and shoulder girdles	Painful and tender proximal muscles without true weakness; minimal synovitis; possible temporal artery tenderness	Striking elevation of ESR; other tests negative	Dramatic response in 6 hours to steroids; may be a prodrome of RA, other connective tissue disease, or cancer

Dermatomysitis, SLE, scleroderma	Usually insidious onset except in dermatomyositis	Abnormal muscle consistency, wasting, weakness; skin induration in scleroderma; rash in SLE and dermatomyositis	Abnormal SGOT, CPK, aldolase in dermatomyositis; positive ANA in SLE; soft tissue calcification in scleroderma; abnormal esophageal motility may be present in all; muscle biopsy abnormal in dermatomyositis	Variable
Infection	Acute onset associated with overt or occult infection	Fever and signs associated with infection	Leukocytosis, elevated ESR	Improves with treatment of infection
Drug-induced	Steroids, diuretics, clofibrate, chloroquin; drug-induced SLE (anticonvulsants, procainamide)	Usually negative	Occasionally positive ANA, elevated ESR, eosinophilia	Remission occurs when offending drug is stopped

Physical Examination

General Examination

The abnormalities noted in the section Peripheral Joint Arthritis, earlier in the chapter, should also be sought in evaluating the patient who presents with myalgia. Abnormalities on the general physical examination that are specifically pertinent to the patient with myalgia are as follows:

1. Lethargy, a husky voice, dry skin and hair, edema, and delayed tendon reflex relaxation suggest hypothyroidism. The well-known facies and bone structure of acromegaly should suggest the myopathy associated with this disease.

2. The motor, sensory, and reflex changes caused by nerve root compression in the cervical or lumbar area may be observed in patients in whom myalgia is secondary to intervertebral disc protrusion. Pain or tingling in the forearm and hand, or both, while tapping over the median nerve at the wrist (Tinel's sign) suggests the carpal tunnel syndrome. A mask-like facies, a pill-rolling tremor, and rigidity suggest Parkinson's disease.

3. An erythematous, indurated rash over the "shawl" distribution of the shoulders, face, and extremities may be seen in dermatomyositis. Indurated skin is observed in scleroderma.

4. Hepatosplenomegaly, spider angiomata, and clubbed fingers, with or without other physical findings of the alcoholic, suggest alcoholic myopathy.

5. A shiny skin with swollen fingers, atrophic skin, and hyperhidrosis of palms is seen in the shoulder-hand syndrome.

6. Temporal artery thickening or tenderness and bruits over carotids or other peripheral arteries may be found in some cases of polymyalgia rheumatica.

Musculoskeletal Examination

Many of the disease entities causing myalgia may show abnormalities of the musculoskeletal system as described in the section Peripheral Joint Arthritis, earlier in the chapter. Examination of the muscles may reveal various abnormalities.

1. Moderate to exquisite tenderness in many muscle groups without anatomic localization, normal muscle tone, absence of muscle atrophy, and maintenance of a normal range of motion is characteristic of psychogenic rheumatism.

2. Striking proximal muscle stiffness without weakness, normal muscle consistency, minimal tenderness on palpation, and minimal or absent synovitis in a patient over 55 (female/male ratio 5:1) suggests polymyalgia rheumatica.

3. Proximal muscle weakness, often with induration and muscle tenderness, with or without an associated skin rash, occurs in dermatomyositis.

4. Severe low back pain, with or without percussion tenderness over one or more vertebrae, suggests osteoporosis with possible compression fracture, myeloma, or metastatic bone disease.

Laboratory Studies

The diagnostic survey outlined in the section Peripheral Joint Arthritis, earlier in the chapter, is applicable to the patient with myalgia.

1. Normal findings on a battery of tests does not rule out organic disease but strongly favors fibrositis or psychogenic rheumatism.

2. An ESR (Westergren) greater than 50 mm per hour, with or without anemia, suggests polymyalgia rheumatica.

3. Serum enzymes (SGOT, CPK, aldolase) are commonly elevated in dermatomyositis.

4. Decreased thyroid function occurs in hypothyroidism.

5. Hypokalemia is usually diuretic-induced.

6. Hypercalcemia may be associated with the myopathy of hyperparathyroidism, sarcoidosis, myeloma, and metastatic carcinoma.

7. Hyperuricemia is commonly associated with the myopathy of lymphoma, leukemia, sarcoidosis, hyperparathyroidism, and hypothyroidism.

8. The serum alkaline phosphatase is usually elevated in Paget's disease of the bone, metastatic carcinoma, sarcoidosis, and hyperparathyroidism.

9. The ANA test finding is likely to be positive in connective tissue diseases and the drug-induced LE syndrome.

10. The postprandial blood sugar or glucose tolerance level is abnormal in the occasional patient with diabetes who presents with myalgia before other abnormalities of this disease are manifested.

11. A characteristic triad of abnormalities is seen in the electromyogram in polymyositis: spontaneous fibrillations and positive, saw-toothed (spike potentials), complex polyphasic or short-duration potentials on voluntary contraction, and salvos of repetitive high-frequency action potentials.

12. Temporal artery biopsy and arteriograms may be abnormal in poly-myalgia rheumatica.

13. Muscle biopsy may show inflammatory changes in polymyositis, and although it is not yet a practical clinical tool, muscle tissue studied with histochemical techniques shows abnormalities in patients with polymyalgia rheumatica and rheumatoid arthritis.

Radiologic Findings

In a patient with myalgia, the following roentgenographic abnormalities should be sought:

1. Hilar adenopathy or parenchymal abnormalities, which suggest sarcoi-dosis.

2. Subcutaneous calcifications, which may be seen in scleroderma and dermatomyositis. Calcification about the shoulder joint is common objective evidence for tendinitis in this area.

3. Subtle changes of sclerosis of the sacro-iliac joints, squaring of the vertebrae, and spinal ligamentous calcification occur in ankylosing spondylitis. In the spine, intervertebral disc space narrowing, spondy-lolisthesis, osteoporosis, and foraminal encroachment secondary to osteo-arthritis are capable of causing muscle pain.

Painful Shoulder

Robert C. Jacobs

Shoulder pain is the symptom that causes most patients with shoulder dis-orders to seek medical attention. The pain may arise from the joint structures or the periarticular tissues, or both. It is also important to be aware that the shoulder is a common site of pain referral from cervical, intrathoracic, and diaphragmatic lesions. Contrary to popular belief, nonarticular disorders of the shoulder, not arthritis, cause the vast majority of painful shoulders. Fractures and dislocations will not be considered in this discussion.

ETIOLOGY

Omitting fractures and dislocations, approximately 80 to 90 percent of cases of shoulder disability are caused by one of the following conditions: acute and chronic tendinitis and bursitis (often calcific), bicipital tenosynovitis, adhesive capsulitis, and lesions of the musculotendinous cuff. The more common causes of shoulder pain and disability are listed in Table 8-5.

TABLE 8-5.   Common Causes of Shoulder Pain

A. Intrinsic lesions
  1. Periarticular disorders
     a. Calcific tendinitis
     b. Adhesive capsulitis
     c. Bicipital tendinitis
     d. Lesions of the musculotendinous cuff
  2. Articular disorders
     a. Inflammatory lesions
        (1) Connective tissue diseases
        (2) Rheumatoid variants
        (3) Crystalline arthropathies
     b. Osteoarthritis
     c. Neuropathic arthropathy
     d. Traumatic arthritis
     e. Infectious arthritis
     f. Neoplasms
B. Extrinsic lesions
  1. Neurologic disorders
     a. Central nervous system (e.g., cervical discs, herpes zoster)
     b. Peripheral nervous system (e.g., neuropathy)
  2. Neurovascular syndromes
     a. Thoracic outlet syndromes
        (1) Cervical and first rib syndromes, scalenus anterior syndrome
        (2) Costoclavicular syndrome
        (3) Hyperabduction syndrome
     b. Reflex neurovascular syndromes
        (1) Shoulder-hand syndrome
        (2) Sudeck's atrophy
  3. Vascular syndromes
     a. Arterial (e.g., arterial occlusion, Raynaud's phenomenon)
     b. Venous (e.g., venous occlusion, thrombophlebitis)
     c. Lymphatic (e.g., lymphangitis, lymphedema)
  4. Psychogenic disorders
  5. Viscerogenic disorders (referred pain)
  6. Idiopathic disorders (e.g., fibrositic syndromes, myalgias, arthralgias, neuralgias)

CLINICAL FEATURES

Calcific Tendinitis and Bursitis

Pain, tenderness, and limited motion of the shoulder are characteristic findings in calcareous tendinitis. The condition may be acute, subacute, or chronic. On examination, there is tenderness below the tip of the acromium, especially pronounced in acute cases. X-ray films of the shoulder show calcific deposits in the vicinity of the affected tendon.

Bicipital Tenosynovitis

Bicipital tenosynovitis is a common cause of shoulder pain. The onset is acute or insidious. The pain usually radiates along the course of the bicipital tendon, and muscle tenderness over the tendon in the bicipital groove is characteristic. Shoulder motion is generally limited, particularly in abduction and internal rotation. Yergason's sign (the production of pain on resisted supination of the forearm while the elbow is flexed at 90°) is usually positive. X-ray findings are negative. When the condition is chronic, the shoulder may become "frozen."

Adhesive Capsulitis

The onset of adhesive capsulitis is acute or insidious. It is often precipitated by trauma or strain but probably has varied causes. In some instances, it represents the end stage of other conditions. The clinical manifestations include localized pain, diffuse periarticular tenderness, and often a profound reduction in shoulder mobility that may eventually result in complete limitation of glenohumeral motion (frozen shoulder). X-ray findings are negative except for demineralization of the humerus in long-standing cases.

Lesions of the Musculotendinous Cuff

The rotator cuff is able to withstand mild to moderate injury with little effect unless the tendons are already diseased as a result of degenerative changes. The supraspinatus tendon is the one most frequently affected. Partial or complete rupture of this tendon is usually precipitated by a fall with the shoulder abducted. The injury is followed by pain, limited motion of the shoulder, and especially an inability to initiate abduction. Tenderness over the tip of the shoulder and a sulcus at the site of rupture may be noted. Assisted abduction may cause pain when the acromial process impinges on the damaged tendon. Once the arm is elevated to 90° or more, the glenohumeral joint can usually be held in abduction with little or no pain.

Neurovascular Syndromes

1. Reflex neurovascular dystrophy (the shoulder-hand syndrome). The shoulder-hand syndrome is a symptom complex characterized by painful disability of the shoulder in association with painful swelling of the hand. The latter may precede, accompany, or follow the former. Vasomotor disturbances (vasospasm or vasodilatation) are common. The condition may terminate with permanent dystrophic changes and contractures of the hand and fingers. The syndrome may be unilateral or bilateral. Provocative or associated conditions include myocardial infarction, cervical osteoarthritis, trauma, hemiplegia, and other disorders. Approximately 25 percent of cases are idiopathic. Mottled or diffuse osteoporosis of the humeral head and wrist is a characteristic x-ray finding.

2. Other neurovascular syndromes. The distinctive features of the costoclavicular, hyperabduction, and the scalenus anterior and cervical rib syndromes and their differential diagnosis from the shoulder-hand syndrome are summarized in Table 8-6 (see section The Thoracic Outlet Syndrome, chapter 10, and p. 37 for additional information).

TABLE 8-6. Neurovascular Syndromes of the Shoulder Girdle*

Syndrome	History	Pulse	Diagnostic Test
Costoclavicular syndrome	Symptoms associated with shoulders being forced downward and backward for long periods	Reduced in abnormal shoulder position	Downward and backward bracing of the shoulder reproduces symptoms and signs
Hyperabduction syndromes (costoclavicular syndrome)	Hyperabduction in sleep or at work for long periods	Reduced in hyperabduction (also blood pressure and oscillometry)	Hyperabduction: reproduction of symptoms and signs
Scalenus anterior, cervical rib, and first rib syndromes	No special postural features	Reduced in resting position or brought on by Adson maneuver	Adson maneuver may reproduce musculoskeletal, neuritic, and vascular signs; tender point at scalenus area
Shoulder-hand syndrome (reflex neurovascular dystrophy)	Trauma, intrathoracic disease, or idiopathic; no special postural features	Sometimes reduced	Stellate ganglion block produces transient or prolonged relief

* Symptoms common to some or all in each disorder: pain of shoulder, and arm or hand, or both; numbness, paresthesias of fingers; swelling of hand(s), fingers; discoloration of hand(s); Raynaud's phenomenon; weakness of hand(s); supraclavicular bruit possible in compression disorders.
Source: Modified from H. H. Friedman, T. G. Argyros, O. Steinbrocker, Neurovascular syndromes of the shoulder girdle and upper extremity—the compression disorders and the shoulder-hand syndrome, *Postgrad. Med. J.*, 35:397, 1959.

Fibromyopathies

See the section Myalgia, earlier in the chapter.

DIAGNOSTIC APPROACH

History

1. The history is of little diagnostic assistance. Inquiry should be made concerning previous involvement or the presence of systemic disease.

2. A history of minor trauma or strain is commonly elicited in musculotendinous lesions. Tendon rupture is suggested by an acute onset of pain and inability to abduct the shoulder precipitated by a fall or a sudden strain in abduction.

3. The diagnosis of a shoulder-hand syndrome should be entertained in patients who have sustained a myocardial infarct, stroke, or trauma to

the distal portion of the upper extremity (e.g., Colles' fracture). Cervical radicular syndromes, thoracotomy, and pulmonary disease (e.g., tuberculosis) are also predisposing factors.

4. Analysis of the shoulder pain may be helpful in ruling out pain referred from other localities. Diaphragmatic lesions (e.g., pleurisy) commonly cause pain in the distribution of the trapezius muscle, and disease of the biliary tract, in the right scapular area. Cardiac pain is rarely localized to the shoulder; a retrosternal component is usually present. On the other hand, pain due to intrinsic disease of the shoulder is almost always felt in the deltoid region. Vague, poorly localized pain, unassociated with limited mobility and unaffected by activity, should arouse suspicion of a fibrositic-psychogenic origin.

Physical Examination

1. Careful examination of all four articulations (glenohumeral, acromioclavicular, scapuloclavicular, and scapulohumeral) is indicated and may help to differentiate between intrinsic and extrinsic disease of the shoulder. The range of motion of the shoulder should be recorded. Localized tenderness suggests tendinitis or a fibrositic syndrome. Diffuse tenderness suggests a more extensive process. A frozen shoulder implies adhesive capsulitis.

2. Signs of joint inflammation and effusion suggest one of the following: crystalline-induced arthropathy, infectious arthritis or a connective tissue disease, tumor, or degenerative change.

3. Popping, snapping, and crepitation on movement are common abnormalities but are nonspecific. Moreover, they may occur in the absence of disease.

4. Limited or painful motion of the neck suggests disease of the cervical spine.

5. Neurovascular abnormalities—shoulder and extremity pain, numbness, paresthesias, swelling of the hand and fingers, and dystrophic changes —suggest a thoracic outlet syndrome or reflex neurovascular dystrophy. The maneuvers employed to diagnose the neurovascular compression syndromes are listed in Table 8-6.

X-ray Examination

1. All patients with shoulder disability should have roentgenograms of the shoulder taken in both internal and external rotation.

2. Cervical spine films are important in evaluating cervical radicular syndromes associated with shoulder discomfort. Chest films are indicated for the assessment of thoracic outlet and neurovascular syndromes.

Other Procedures

1. In the presence of effusion, the joint fluid should be aspirated and examined for white cell count, cytologic features, and the presence of crystals. Smears and cultures are indicated when infection is suspected.

2. Plethysmography, nerve conduction studies, and angiography may be useful in evaluating thoracic outlet syndromes.

3. Contrast arthrography is often of material assistance in the diagnosis of rotator cuff tears.

Painful Hip
Joseph C. Tyor

DEFINITION

This discussion is limited to conditions, exclusive of fractures and dislocations, that may cause hip pain in adults.

ETIOLOGY AND CLINICAL FEATURES

1. Intrinsic causes.
   a. Periarticular disorders.
      (1) Muscle rupture. A history of trauma is usual. Tenderness at the site of rupture, hematoma formation, and deformity of the muscle are usually noted. Some degree of limitation of the hip may be present.
      (2) Bursitis.
          (a) Trochanteric bursitis commonly causes pain in the thigh and along the posterolateral region of the hip. Direct manual pressure over the greater trochanter usually reproduces the pain. Pain may be noted on external rotation of the hip.
          (b) Ischiatic bursitis causes pain and tenderness over the ischial tuberosities. Straight leg raising may be painful and limited.
          (c) Iliopectineal bursitis is associated with tenderness over the superior and anterior aspect of the joint capsule, under the psoas muscle, and in Scarpa's triangle. Hip extension may be limited.
          (d) Obturator bursitis causes painful internal rotation of the hip.
   b. Articular disorders.
      (1) Connective tissue diseases. Rheumatoid arthritis, scleroderma, polymyositis, systemic lupus erythematosus, and polyarteritis

nodosa rarely cause involvement of the hip joint alone. Usually, other joints are also affected.

(2) Rheumatoid variants. Ankylosing spondylitis, Reiter's syndrome, enteropathic arthropathy, psoriasis, etc., may involve the hip joints and lead to permanent articular damage. Usually, joint involvement is not limited to the hip.

(3) Crystalline arthropathies.

(a) Gouty arthritis of the hip is quite rare.

(b) Pseudogout may cause acute arthritis of the hip. The presence of crystals of calcium pyrophosphate in the joint fluid is diagnostic.

(4) Neuropathic arthropathy. Neuropathic arthropathy due to tabes dorsalis, diabetic neuropathy, or other neurologic disorders may affect the hip. It is characterized by effusion, undue mobility and instability of the hip, and disproportionately little pain. Some authorities have suggested that neuropathic hip disease may also result from repeated intraarticular injections of steroids.

(5) Osteoarthritis of the hip. Degenerative arthritis of the hip is usually a disease of older individuals, more common in males, and more often unilateral than bilateral. It may be primary or secondary to long-standing mechanical malalignment of the hip due to congenital dislocation of the hip, Calvé-Perthes disease, slipped capital femoral epiphysis, or trauma (leg fracture, dislocation). The onset is insidious. The chief symptoms are pain, stiffness, and a limp on walking. The pain is usually located in the groin but may be felt along the medial aspect of the thigh. It is commonly referred to the buttock or knee. Initially, the pain is present on standing or walking and relieved by rest. Over a period of time, however, the pain tends to persist in the sitting position or recumbency. Backache from mechanical strain is a common accompaniment. On physical examination, the lower extremity is often found to be everted, with the hip in a flexed and adducted position. Hip motion is limited in all directions, especially on internal rotation and adduction.

(6) Tumors of the hip. Tumors of the hip, including benign cysts, giant cell tumors, osteogenic or synovial sarcomas, and metastatic carcinomas are uncommon causes of hip pain.

(7) Infectious arthritis.

(a) Septic arthritis is usually hematogenous in origin and due to staphylococci, streptococci, or, less commonly, to other organisms. Fever and other systemic symptoms are present. Pain may be located in the hip but is commonly referred to the knee. The thigh is flexed, adducted, and internally rotated. Motion is markedly limited. Local signs of inflammation and bulging of the joint capsule are noted commonly. Joint aspiration is essential for early diagnosis and proper treatment, since x-ray signs may not appear for sev-

eral days. The synovial fluid should be cultured and cytologic studies done.

(b) Tuberculosis of the hip joint is usually associated with pulmonary or visceral tuberculosis. It is more common in
adolescents than in adults. A history of preceding trauma
is often obtained. The onset is insidious. Nocturnal and
rest pain are common. Pain in the knee and thigh, a limp,
muscle spasm, fullness in the groin, tenderness over the
hip, and limited motion of the hip are usually noted. The
diagnosis should be suspected in any tuberculous individual
with chronic monarticular arthritis involving the hip. Confirmation by culture of the joint fluid or biopsy is indicated.

(8) Aseptic necrosis of the femoral head.   Aseptic or avascular necrosis of the femoral head refers to the changes that occur in
the bone after interruption of its blood supply by trauma or disease. Avascular necrosis may occur in the osteochondroses, following fracture of the neck of the femur or dislocation of the
hip, in sickle cell anemia or other hemoglobinopathies, or in
caisson disease and other conditions. The condition is painful.
The diagnosis is made radiologically.

(9) Bleeding disorders.   Hemarthrosis occurs in the vast majority
of patients with hemophilia and may lead to permanent joint
drainage and deformity.

2. Extrinsic causes.   Pain may be referred to the hip in degenerative disease of the lumbar spine, pelvic disease, and vascular insufficiency in
the lower extremities. Pain in the hip is uncommonly of psychogenic
origin.

DIAGNOSTIC APPROACH

1. In the history, the type of onset and course of the disease may be of
some help. Trauma may itself result in hip pain or may predispose to
subsequent development of osteoarthritic changes. A history of conditions such as congenital dislocation of the hip, slipped capital femoral
epiphysis, and Calvé-Perthes disease may be important in revealing the
underlying cause in osteoarthritis of the hip.

2. The location of the pain, its relationship to weight-bearing or walking,
and its constancy may provide clues to the severity of the hip joint
involvement. Pain at rest and nocturnal pain suggest inflammatory or
neoplastic disease.

3. Evidence of systemic disease suggests that hip involvement may be
secondary to the primary disorder. Infection, tuberculosis, connective
tissue disease, and the rheumatoid variants should be ruled out. Usually
this can be accomplished on clinical grounds alone.

4. Examination of the hip joint should include observation for the presence of an abnormal gait, limp, or deformity. Palpation of the joint and periarticular structures may help to localize the source of difficulty. The range of motion of the hip and the length of the extremity should be measured.

5. Routine laboratory studies should include CBC, urinalysis, and sedimentation rate. In the presence of effusion, the synovial fluid should be aspirated. When an infectious etiologic agent is under consideration, appropriate cultures and cytologic studies are indicated. Examination for urate and calcium pyrophosphate crystals should be done if crystalline arthropathy is suspected.

6. X-ray examination is essential for the proper evaluation of hip pain. An AP roentgenogram of the pelvis, including both hips, and a lateral view of the hip should be taken. Salient features of the more common abnormalities causing hip pain are listed below.

   a. Rheumatoid arthritis and the rheumatoid variants.   Early, there is juxtaarticular demineralization of the bone, which is followed by narrowing of the joint space, the appearance of marginal erosions, pseudocyst formation, and eventually bony ankylosis. Protrusio acetabuli may occur occasionally in rheumatoid arthritis.

   b. Osteoarthritis.   Reduction of the joint space without osteoporosis is an early finding. Later, spur formation is found at the acetabular margins and around the head of the femur. Sclerosis of the subchondral bone and cyst formation eventually appear. The head of the femur tends to drift laterally and becomes flattened.

   c. Pseudogout.   Roentgenograms show calcification of the articular cartilage and acetabular labra. The calcification is indistinguishable from that produced by degenerative joint disease.

   d. Neuropathic arthropathy.   The radiologic picture is that of degenerative arthritis "gone wild," with acetabular erosions, irregularity of the joint space, marked osteophyte formation, bone destruction, the presence of fragmented bone in the joint space, and ossification of the soft tissues.

   e. Infectious arthritis.   In septic arthritis, the earliest finding is narrowing of the joint space. Later, destruction of the articular margin and adjacent bone occurs. Eventually, hypertrophic changes and bony ankylosis may occur. Tuberculous arthritis may show little change early in the course of the disease. Later, demineralization without narrowing of the joint space appears. This is followed by destructive changes at the joint margins and contiguous bone. Joint destruction may eventually become quite extensive. Sinus tract formation is often present in advanced cases.

   f. Avascular necrosis of the femoral head.   Initially there is separation of the subchondral bone from the articular margin and apparent condensation of the separated fragment within the femoral head, leaving a crescentic lucent area between the two. Over a period of time there are formed intermingled areas of increased and decreased bone density.

Low Back Pain

Charley J. Smyth

Low back pain is one of the most common complaints and causes of disability in persons seen in office practice. Despite the frequency with which low back complaints occur, the etiologic diagnosis is often elusive and imprecise. Sometimes it is impossible to determine whether the cause is primarily musculoskeletal, neurologic, or visceral. In this discussion, primary consideration will be given to musculoskeletal causes of low back pain.

ETIOLOGY

The most common causes of pain in the low back region, in order of decreasing frequency, are as follows:

1. **Low back strain.** Low back strain may be acute, subacute, or chronic. Conditions that predispose to strain include postural defects, disc degeneration, osteoarthritis, spondylolisthesis, and repeated trauma.

    a. Acute low back strain usually follows injury, the severity of which may be variable. The clinical picture is one of trauma followed by diffuse low back pain accompanied by muscle spasm, tenderness, and limited painful motion of the back. The course is usually of relatively short duration.

    b. Subacute or chronic low back strain is probably the most common disorder causing low back pain. A history of antecedent injury is often lacking. The course is chronic, but it may be punctuated by repeated acute exacerbations. Usually there is stiffness and some degree of painful motion of the back. Limitation of motion may or may not be present. Tenderness to palpation or percussion is common. Neurologic findings are negative, although pain may be referred in dermatomal distribution.

    c. Herniated intervertebral disc is a common cause of low back pain. The L4-L5 and L5-S1 discs are most frequently affected. The L3-L4 disc is involved less frequently, and the other lumbar discs, rarely. More than one disc may herniate in the same patient. Herniation of the L5-S1 disc causes compression of the S1 nerve root; L4-L5 herniation causes L5 compression; and L3-L4 herniation, L4 compression. Degenerative changes in the discs predispose to herniation. Disc trouble often begins with a popping or snapping sensation in the back followed by low back pain. Although the initial episode may subside, there is a tendency for recurrence. During the attack, the pain is likely to be severe and incapacitating. After a period of time, the pain usually begins to radiate in sciatic distribution. On examination, one observes difficulty in standing and walking. A list to the side opposite the pain is common. Tenderness of the musculature on the affected side is often marked. The straight leg raising, sitting knee extension, and popliteal compression findings are usually positive. Neurologic changes are variable. Compression of S1 is suggested by a decreased or absent ankle jerk, hypoesthesia of the lateral foot and sole, and weakness of the calf muscles. Compression of L5 is commonly manifested by sensory loss in the lateral leg and in the dorsomesial aspects of the foot, and by weakness of the toe extensors. Compression of L4 usually results in a decreased or absent knee jerk, hypoesthesia of the medial aspect of the leg, and weakness of the knee extensors.

2. Osteoarthritis.   Osteoarthritic changes are the result of degenerative changes in the discs, vertebral bodies, and apophyseal joints. The clinical picture is similar to that of chronic low back strain. However, degenerative changes in the discs may occasionally lead to herniation with attendant nerve root compression and radicular pain. In some instances, however, radicular pain may be simulated by pain referred along dermatomes related to specific areas of spinal involvement. The radiologic features are discussed later in the section (p. 325). Although osteoarthritis is usually a primary disorder, its occurrence may be secondary to trauma, neuropathic disorders, steroid therapy, epiphyseal dysplasia, Wilson's disease, ochronosis, infections, vertebral osteochondritis, or chondrocalcinosis.

3. Other causes.
   a. Ankylosing spondylitis.   Ankylosing spondylitis is a common cause of low back pain, especially in young men. The disease usually begins in the sacro-iliac joints and spreads cephalad. Typically, there is continuous low back pain, often with radiation to the buttocks and thighs, accompanied by stiffness, muscle spasm, limitation of motion, and tenderness to palpation. With thoracic involvement and attendant inflammation of the costovertebral joints, root pains and decreased chest expansion become manifest. Spread to the cervical spine produces limitation of motion of the neck. When the disease is advanced, there is loss of the lumbar lordotic curve, dorsal kyphosis, and protrusion of the head and neck. The shoulders and hips are commonly diseased, and arthritis of the peripheral joints is not unusual. Iritis and spondylitic heart disease occur in some patients. The radiologic abnormalities, described later in the section (p. 326), are characteristic.
   b. Other rheumatoid variants.   Diseases such as Reiter's syndrome, ulcerative colitis, regional enteritis, Whipple's disease, psoriasis, and juvenile rheumatoid arthritis may affect the spine and produce sacroiliac arthritis. The radiographic changes in the sacro-iliac joints in these conditions are indistinguishable from those seen in ankylosing spondylitis. The differential diagnosis of these disorders is based on the more characteristic extraarticular and systemic manifestations of each disease.
   c. Osteoporosis.   Osteoporosis of any origin is another cause of back pain, especially in the elderly, in whom senile or postmenopausal osteoporosis is common. Osteoporotic vertebrae are susceptible to pathologic fracture. The diagnosis is made by x-ray study, but additional laboratory studies are needed to differentiate between the various causes.

d. Fractures.   The relationship between trauma and fracture is usually obvious. The diagnosis is established by physical examination and roentgenographic findings. In pathologic fractures, the relationship of trauma is less evident. Aside from osteoporosis, pathologic fractures are most frequently caused by metastatic carcinoma (usually arising in the breast, kidney, lung, or thyroid gland), multiple myeloma, tuberculosis, eosinophilic granuloma, and other conditions.

e. Infections.   Back pain may occur as a symptom of such systemic infections as viral diseases. Meningitis may, of course, cause backache, but it is usually easily distinguished by the presence of nuchal rigidity, a positive Kernig's sign, and spinal fluid abnormalities. Nontuberculous as well as tuberculous infections may cause backache by direct involvement of the spine and its associated structures. Herpes zoster involving the lumbar nerve roots may present a diagnostic problem until the characteristic rash appears.

f. Psychogenic rheumatism.   Back pain is a common feature of psychogenic rheumatism. The diagnosis should be suspected in neurotic individuals with multitudinous complaints in whom the symptoms fail to fit any anatomic pattern of disease and in whom there is a discrepancy between the multiplicity of symptoms and the paucity of objective findings. Laboratory findings are normal. The diagnosis should be approached with caution because the neurotic individual may have organic disease.

g. Fibrositis.   Fibrositis may cause backache. This is the "lumbago" of a generation ago. The characteristic symptoms are pain and muscle stiffness aggravated by tension, fatigue, immobilization, and chilling, and relieved by heat and physical activity. Although the pain is diffuse, one or more "trigger" points may be found on palpation. Laboratory findings are normal. Patients with the fibrositis syndrome should be reexamined frequently to rule out underlying disease.

DIAGNOSTIC APPROACH

Initial Evaluation

The preliminary investigation of every patient with low back pain should include a complete history and physical examination with special attention to the back, CBC, sedimentation rate, urinalysis, and x-rays of the lumbosacral spine (AP and lateral views usually suffice, but oblique and special views may be needed to delineate specific pathologic processes more clearly).

History

1. A history of back pain initiated by injury or strain suggests low back strain, herniated disc, or fracture. Absence of trauma does not exclude these diagnostic possibilities.

2. Occupational and recreational activities that may be related to back pain should be investigated. An effort should be made, when trauma is involved, to learn whether compensation insurance or legal questions are pending.

324 Ch. 8 Musculoskeletal Problems

3. Diagnostic clues to rheumatoid disorders and other systemic disease may be obtained from the general history and system review (see the section Peripheral Joint Arthritis, earlier in the chapter).

4. The pain should be analyzed with respect to its chronology, its character, and the response to previous treatment. The severity of the pain, its localization, radiation, and duration, and the effects of aggravating (cough, sneezing, straining) and alleviating (rest, exercise, activity, drugs) factors should be determined.

   a. Low back pain with sciatica is caused most commonly by herniation of a nucleus pulposus. The pain is characteristically aggravated by cough, sneezing, straining, bending, or lifting.

   b. In the elderly, lumbar nerve root irritation may be caused not only by osteoarthritis but by collapse of a vertebral body due to osteoporosis, metastatic carcinoma, or infection.

   c. Continuous, severe back pain that is worse at night and is not relieved by ordinary analgesics should arouse suspicion of metastatic carcinoma, multiple myeloma, lymphomas, and abdominal or retroperitoneal malignancy.

   d. In young men, continuous, aching low back pain with radiation to the buttocks and thighs or low back pain in sciatic distribution should suggest ankylosing spondylitis.

   e. Retroperitoneal or abdominal malignancy should always be considered in individuals with intractable low back pain associated with constitutional symptoms of fatigue, anorexia, and weight loss.

   f. A history of back or leg pain, lower extremity weakness, and unsteady gait should suggest disease of the cervical rather than the lumbar spine. Such a history is suggestive of spinal cord compression either by osteoarthritic changes or by posterior dislocation of the odontoid process caused by rheumatoid arthritis.

Physical Examination

1. The examination of every patient with backache should include abdominal, pelvic, and rectal examinations, to exclude visceral causes of low back pain. Examination of the hip is also warranted to exclude hip joint involvement (e.g., in ankylosing spondylitis) or hip joint disease causing backache (e.g., osteoarthritis of the hip).

2. The physical examination of the back involves inspection, palpation, determination of the range of motion of the spine, and observation of the gait. The presence or absence of pain during movement should also be noted.

   a. A mechanical cause of low back pain is suggested by poor posture, scoliosis, kyphosis, and obesity. A sharp, angular deformity in the dorsal or lumbar area may suggest tuberculosis. The appearance of the patient with ankylosing spondylitis is characteristic.

   b. Reduction of chest expansion suggests ankylosing spondylitis.

   c. Loss of lumbar lordosis, with muscle spasm and tenderness, is a sign pointing to ankylosing spondylitis, spondylolisthesis, or other congenital lesions with secondary degenerative changes.

    d. Tenderness over the sacro-iliac joints is, when supported by a positive iliac compression test, a sensitive indicator of the sacro-iliitis found in ankylosing spondylitis and other rheumatoid variants.

    e. Restricted motion of the spine and muscle spasm are nonspecific abnormalities found in many low back disorders.

    f. Localized lumbar spine pain associated with tenderness and muscle spasm suggests involvement of a vertebra or its processes by fracture, tumor, or infection.

    g. The presence of tender or "trigger" points without other abnormalities is suggestive of fibrositis. Disappearance of this pain following local injection of procaine or lidocaine into the tender spot is both diagnostic and therapeutic. However, underlying disease or psychogenic rheumatism is not ruled out by this maneuver. Psychogenic pain is suggested by the presence of cutaneous hyperoesthesia at the tender point. It is demonstrable when pain is elicited by lifting and gently pinching a fold of skin over the affected site. Further presumptive confirmation is secured when relief of pain is obtained by the intracutaneous, rather than the intramuscular, injection of the local anesthetic.

3. Special tests are useful in assessing specific problems. Straight leg raising, allowing for tightness of the hamstrings, is a valuable but not infallible indicator of nerve root compression. The sitting knee extension and popliteal compression tests confirm nerve root compression when results are positive. The Patrick's test yields a positive result in hip joint disease. A positive jugular compression test (Naffziger) result is indicative of spinal cord or nerve root.

4. A neurologic examination including tests for reflex, sensory, and motor functions should be done routinely. It is essential for the diagnosis of nerve root compression or lesions of the spinal cord. The findings in L4, L5, and S1 nerve root compression by herniated discs are listed earlier in the section (pp. 321 and 322).

Radiologic Examination

Although different pathologic conditions may cause similar clinical pictures, the radiologic findings are often specific or sufficiently characteristic to establish a diagnosis. Reference will be made to the more common diseases whose skeletal lesions have distinctive roentgenographic appearances.

1. Generalized osteoporosis of the spine is a common but nonspecific radiologic abnormality. Partial or complete collapse of one or more vertebral bodies may be an associated finding. Osteoporosis may be due to many causes.

2. Osteoarthritis of the lumbar spine is manifested radiologically primarily by disc narrowing and spurring, which is most often located anteriorly. Anterior spurs rarely have clinical significance. Changes in the apophyseal joints consist of narrowing of the joint spaces, spur formation, and bony sclerosis. It should be emphasized that the presence of x-ray findings of osteoarthritis do not necessarily imply that symptomatology is related to these changes.

3. Sacro-iliac arthritis is a characteristic feature of ankylosing spondylitis and the other rheumatoid variants. The sacro-iliitis is manifested early by irregularity and blurring of the joint margins; later, by sclerosis of the adjacent bone; and eventually, in some cases, by bony ankylosis. The sacro-iliac changes in these diseases are radiologically indistinguishable. Osteitis condensans ilii may mimic sacro-iliitis by the presence of sclerosis of the iliac bone adjacent to the sacro-iliac joints. The joints themselves, however, are uninvolved. Osteoarthritic sacro-iliac disease is differentiated by the absence of destructive changes and the presence of sclerosis of subchondral bone with marginal spur formation.

4. Spinal ankylosis may be seen in several disorders:
   a. In ankylosing spondylitis, the vertebrae have a "squared" appearance in lateral views. Other typical radiologic findings include: paravertebral ossifications leading eventually to a "bamboo spine"; apophyseal narrowing, sclerosis, and fusion; loss of lumbar lordosis; and occasional destruction of a disc and its adjacent vertebra with pseudoarthrosis formation.
   b. Senile ankylosing hyperostosis is a condition seen in elderly patients, characterized by irregular ossification of the anterior longitudinal ligament. The hyperostosis produces typical "candle-flame" shadows along the anterior aspect of the vertebral bodies.
   c. Paravertebral ossifications bridging adjacent vertebral bodies, limited to one or a few areas, may be seen following trauma or infection, and in psoriatic arthropathy and Reiter's syndrome.

5. Destruction of vertebral bodies may be seen with infection (e.g., tuberculosis, pyogenic organism), neoplasm, and neuropathic disorders.

6. Paget's disease (osteitis deformans) is characterized by a mottled increase in bone density, coarse trabeculation, and at times fractures.

7. Spondylolysis is a unilateral or bilateral congenital vertebral arch that can be detected only by radiologic studies. Spondylolisthesis is the anterior displacement of a vertebra on the one below, found in some cases of bilateral spondylolysis.

8. Disc rupture may show disc narrowing or no abnormality. When the condition is of long standing, secondary osteoarthritic changes occur. Conclusive x-ray diagnosis depends on myelography or discography.

Subsequent Evaluation

1. Usually the diagnosis of broad categories of disease can be established on the basis of the initial examination. Thus, a history of trauma followed by backache with characteristic symptomatology is diagnostic of low back strain. No further work-up is indicated, and therapy should

be instituted. Failure to respond to conservative management may or may not suggest the need for further investigation. The diagnosis of chronic low back strain is really nonspecific because the clinical picture may be caused by recurrent minitrauma, osteoarthritis, or fibrositis. Again, no further work-up is necessary unless there is poor response to treatment or unusual features develop that suggest the original diagnosis was in error.

2. Pantopaque myelography may be indicated for the precise diagnosis of disc herniations. It may also be helpful in differentiating disc herniations from tumors or other obstructive lesions. Myelography is customarily performed only when conservative therapy fails, when the diagnosis is uncertain, or preoperatively to confirm the presence and site of disc herniations. Electromyography and discography have more limited applications in the diagnosis of herniated discs.

3. A radiologic survey of other bones and joints may be indicated when osteoporosis, metabolic bone disease, malignancy, connective tissue diseases, or rheumatoid variants are suspected.

4. Additional laboratory tests may be advisable under certain circumstances.
   a. Serum calcium, phosphorus, and alkaline phosphatase, in suspected hyperparathyroidism, malignancy, osteoporosis, and Paget's disease.
   b. Serum uric acid, which is elevated in gout, lymphomas, leukemia, etc.
   c. Serum protein electrophoresis and immunoglobulins may be useful in the diagnosis of multiple myeloma, lymphomas, and connective tissue diseases.
   d. Spinal fluid examination, for the diagnosis of disease of the central nervous system and spinal cord.

5. Systemic or visceral disorders with low back pain (e.g., enteropathic arthropathy) may require barium studies of the gastrointestinal tract or other diagnostic measures (e.g., lymph node biopsy), as suggested by the symptoms and physical findings.

6. In patients with persistent, intractable low back pain of unknown cause, bone marrow biopsy and radioisotope scanning of the skeleton may reveal the presence of malignancy or other conditions undetectable by conventional examinations.

9. Endocrine and Metabolic Problems

Hyperglycemia

Walter A. Huttner

DEFINITION

Hyperglycemia is the presence of elevated blood glucose levels in fasting or postprandial specimens.

BLOOD GLUCOSE DETERMINATIONS

1. Blood glucose determinations performed on plasma or serum are preferable to those performed on whole blood. Plasma or serum methods are not dependent on the hematocrit value and are more suitable for use in autoanalyzers. Plasma and serum glucose levels, which are about equal, are approximately 15 percent higher than those obtained from whole blood.

2. Venous blood is customarily used for glucose determinations except in children, in whom capillary blood may be more convenient. In the fasting state, venous and capillary glucose levels are comparable, but the values tend to be higher in capillary than in venous blood for at least 2 hours after eating.

3. Glucose determinations by true glucose methods (e.g., glucose oxidase) are preferred because their use avoids the spuriously elevated values produced by hemolysis, uremia, or other sugars such as fructose or galactose.

CRITERIA FOR THE DIAGNOSIS OF HYPERGLYCEMIA

The diagnosis of hyperglycemia should be considered if the following glucose values are obtained on whole blood:

1. Fasting blood glucose exceeding 110 mg/100 ml.

2. Random blood glucose greater than 160 mg/100 ml.

3. Blood glucose 1 hour after a carbohydrate meal or after a 75- to 100-gm glucose load, above 160 mg/100 ml.

4. Blood glucose 2 hours after a carbohydrate meal or after a 75- to 100-gm glucose load, more than 120 mg/100 ml.

An oral glucose tolerance test should be performed when hyperglycemia is discovered unless the diagnosis of diabetes is unequivocal (see below).

CRITERIA FOR THE DIAGNOSIS OF DIABETES MELLITUS

1. Fasting whole blood glucose values above 150 mg/100 ml and random or postprandial values above 200 mg/100 ml are considered diagnostic of diabetes mellitus, provided the results are trustworthy and confirmed by a second determination to rule out laboratory error.

2. The standard oral glucose tolerance test is abnormal.

3. No other cause can be found for the abnormal tests listed in paragraphs **1** and **2** above.

THE ORAL GLUCOSE TOLERANCE TEST

1. When hyperglycemia is found but the concentration of glucose in the blood is not diagnostic of diabetes mellitus, an oral glucose tolerance test (GTT) should be performed.

2. Prior to the test, the patient should be on a diet containing at least 150 gm of carbohydrate per day for 3 days. Standardized conditions should prevail so that they can be reproduced if that is desired. The patient should be ambulatory and free from any complicating acute or chronic illness that might impair carbohydrate tolerance.

3. The standard oral GTT is a 3-hour procedure. If reactive hypoglycemia is suspected, the test should be extended to a 5-hour period. Urinary sugar determinations are no longer considered significant, but a qualitative glucose determination on the total urine collection during the test period may be worthwhile.

Criteria for the Oral Glucose Tolerance Test

The GTT is considered abnormal by the Fajans-Conn criteria when the following values for whole blood and plasma (given in parentheses) are equaled or exceeded: 1-hour or peak value, 160 mg (185 mg)/100 ml; 1½-hour, 140 mg (160 mg)/100 ml; and 2-hour, 120 mg (140 mg)/100 ml. According to the United States Public Health Service criteria for whole blood and plasma (given in parentheses), the GTT is abnormal if at least three values are equal to or higher than the following: fasting, 110 mg (125 mg)/100 ml; 1-hour, 170 (195 mg)/100 ml; 2-hour, 120 mg (140 mg)/100 ml; and 3-hour, 110 mg (125 mg)/100 ml. The test is also considered abnormal if both the fasting and the 3-hour values are 110 mg (125 mg)/100 ml or higher. Most workers in the field employ the Fajans-Conn criteria.

The Effects of Age on the Oral Glucose Tolerance Test

It is generally agreed that glucose tolerance decreases with age. For this reason, some authorities add 10 mg/100 ml to each of the maximum normal values (whole blood glucose) for each decade above the age of 50 years. Other authorities feel that with adequate dietary preparation, the effect of age on the GTT is insignificant. Still other investigators feel that a 3-hour whole blood value of 110 mg/100 ml or greater is the most reliable criterion for the diagnosis of diabetes in the elderly.

Effect of Pregnancy on the Oral Glucose Tolerance Test

The normal GTT during pregnancy is characterized by a lower fasting level, a lower peak value, and a slower decline to the baseline. The oral GTT finding is diagnostic of gestational diabetes if two or more whole blood values equal or exceed 90 mg/100 ml fasting, 165 mg/100 ml at 1 hour, 145 mg/100 ml at 2 hours, and 125 mg/100 ml at 3 hours. The corresponding values for plasma glucose are 105 mg/100 ml, 190 mg/100 ml, 165 mg/100 ml, and 145 mg/100 ml.

Nondiabetic Causes of an Abnormal Glucose Tolerance Test

1. Fasting hyperglycemia, otherwise unexplained, is virtually diagnostic of diabetes mellitus, especially in a patient with a family history of diabetes. The same holds true for a GTT that is clearly abnormal. However, the final decision depends on the exclusion of nondiabetic causes of impaired glucose tolerance.

2. The major nondiabetic causes of an abnormal GTT are as follows:
   a. Inadequate dietary preparation.
   b. Hepatocellular disease.
   c. Chronic disease and prolonged physical inactivity (bed rest).
   d. Malnutrition and starvation.
   e. Potassium depletion due to diuretics, primary aldosteronism, renal disease, alcoholism, etc.

f. Stress secondary to strokes, myocardial infarction, surgery, and febrile illnesses.

g. Endocrinopathies, such as acromegaly, Cushing's syndrome or disease, adrenocortical hyperfunction, prolonged steroid therapy, islet cell tumors (insulinomas, glucagonomas), pheochromocytoma, and thyrotoxicosis.

h. Chronic renal disease and uremia.

? i. Alimentary hyperglycemia following gastric surgery.

j. Drugs (e.g., steroids, diuretics, oral contraceptives, nicotinic acid).

3. An abnormal GTT found in any of the above-mentioned conditions should be considered nondiabetic until proved otherwise, provided the fasting blood sugar is normal. Patients with these disorders should be retested with an oral GTT after recovery has taken place and normal physical activity has been resumed. Adequate dietary preparation prior to the test is most important. The intravenous GTT is helpful in differentiating between alimentary hyperglycemia and diabetes mellitus.

Effect of Drugs on the Oral Glucose Tolerance Test

Drugs may raise or lower blood sugar values. Drugs that can impair glucose tolerance include steroids, some oral contraceptives, diuretics, and nicotinic acid. Drugs that may produce falsely normal GTT are salicylates administered in large doses, alcohol, propranolol, and monamine oxidase inhibitors. As a general rule, a normal GTT found in patients on any of these medications can be considered valid.

DIAGNOSIS OF DIABETES IN THE PRESENCE OF CONDITIONS THAT THEMSELVES MAY IMPAIR GLUCOSE TOLERANCE

There are six conditions, listed below, in which, although the fasting blood sugar is normal, the oral GTT is abnormal. It is often difficult and sometimes impossible to determine whether the glucose intolerance is a reflection of the underlying disorder or is the result of coexisting diabetes mellitus.

1. Obesity. An abnormal GTT in an obese individual should be considered prima facie evidence of diabetes and treated accordingly.

2. Pregnancy. The criteria for the diagnosis of gestational diabetes are listed above (see p. 331).

3. Hyperlipoproteinemia. Familial hyperlipoproteinemia, including types III, IV, and V in the Frederickson classification, is often associated with abnormal glucose tolerance. Until more is known, one should treat patients with hyperlipoproteinemia and glucose intolerance as he would other diabetics by standard regimens including weight reduction and carbohydrate restriction.

4. Degenerative vascular disease.   Strokes, intracerebral hemorrhages, and heart attacks are commonly associated with transitory hyperglycemia. Unless the diagnosis of diabetes is unequivocal, a final decision as to whether or not such patients are diabetic should be postponed until complete recovery has taken place and normal physical activity has been resumed.

5. Chronic liver disease.   Hepatocellular disease may produce an abnormal GTT, but fasting hyperglycemia is a rare occurrence. Usually, the glucose intolerance disappears when the liver function returns to normal. There is no available test that distinguishes between hepatic and diabetic glucose tolerance curves.

6. Gout and hyperuricemia.   A much higher incidence of glucose tolerance abnormality is found in gouty and hyperuricemic individuals than in the general population. The usual criteria for the diagnosis of diabetes are applicable.

INTRAVENOUS GLUCOSE TOLERANCE TEST

The intravenous GTT is primarily a research tool. It has no demonstrable clinical advantage over the oral test. Its major usefulness is in differentiating between diabetes and alimentary hyperglycemia secondary to gastric surgery.

Hypoglycemia
Walter A. Huttner

DEFINITION

Hypoglycemia is a symptom complex associated with abnormally low blood glucose levels. Plasma glucose values below 50 mg/100 ml are usually diagnostic of hypoglycemia. For blood glucose determinations and the preparation and precautions in performing the oral glucose tolerance test, see the preceding section, Hyperglycemia. For the diagnosis of hypoglycemic states, the standard 3-hour oral GTT is extended to a 5-hour period.

SYMPTOMS

The occurrence of hypoglycemic symptoms is related to both the rapidity and the severity of the decline in the blood glucose level. Symptoms that accompany a rapid fall in the concentration of blood glucose include a sensation of "not feeling well," shakiness, sweating, palpitation, restlessness, anxiety, hunger, nausea, and vomiting. Loss of consciousness and even coma may occur. These symptoms, which are largely due to epinephrine release, are alleviated promptly by correction of the hypoglycemia. The symptoms are usually different when the fall in glucose levels is slow and prolonged or severe. Neuroglycopenic symptoms, such as headache, restlessness, reduction in spontaneous conversation and activity, mental confusion, prolonged sleep, stupor, coma, and hypothermia or fever, may occur. Sensory and motor disturbances and bizarre behavior may also be noted.

ETIOLOGY

The causes of hypoglycemia can be divided into three major groups: reactive, fasting, and factitious hypoglycemia. The two types of hypoglycemia found most commonly in practice are reactive functional hypoglycemia and reactive hypoglycemia secondary to diabetes mellitus. The distinction between fasting and reactive hypoglycemia is important clinically because fasting hypoglycemia is not a feature of either reactive functional hypoglycemia or reactive hypoglycemia secondary to diabetes mellitus.

1. Reactive hypoglycemia.
   a. Reactive functional hypoglycemia. Reactive functional hypoglycemia is the most common cause of hypoglycemia in adults. This disorder, which seems to have a predilection for individuals with emotional problems, is characterized by transient postprandial hypoglycemia that occurs 2 to 4 hours after the ingestion of food containing carbohydrate. The symptoms are predominantly those of hyperepinephrinemia, brought about by the rapid decline in the blood sugar concentration. The symptoms usually subside spontaneously within half an hour after their onset. Reactive functional hypoglycemia does not predispose to the subsequent development of diabetes.
   b. Reactive hypoglycemia secondary to diabetes mellitus. Reactive hypoglycemia secondary to mild diabetes mellitus is the second most common type of hypoglycemia found in adults. Low blood sugar values accompanied by symptoms of hyperepinephrinemia typically occur 3 to 5 hours after meals. A family history of diabetes is commonly obtained.
   c. Alimentary hypoglycemia. Alimentary hypoglycemia is found in approximately 5 to 10 percent of patients who have had partial to complete gastrectomies or gastroenterostomies. However, it sometimes occurs in individuals who have not had gastric surgery. The rapid gastric emptying time leads sequentially, to accelerated absorption of glucose, hyperglycemia, and hypoglycemia. Symptoms usually occur 1½ to 3 hours after meals, corresponding to the time when blood glucose levels are low.
   d. Hereditary fructose intolerance. Patients with familial fructose intolerance may have postprandial reactive hypoglycemia following the ingestion of fructose-containing foods. Since the disease occurs primarily in children and is seldom found in adults, it is not dis-

cussed here. The diagnosis is established by the use of an oral fructose tolerance test.

2. Fasting hypoglycemia.

   a. Pancreatic islet cell disease. The symptoms of hypoglycemia due to islet cell tumors (insulinomas) are produced by the excessive secretion of insulin. Approximately 85 percent of these tumors are benign and 15 percent malignant. They occur most frequently between the ages of 35 and 55 years. Insulinomas may be solitary or multiple and may be either macroscopic or microscopic in size. Multiple islet cell tumors are sometimes associated with multiple endocrine adenomatosis and peptic ulceration (Zollinger-Ellison syndrome). Hypoglycemic symptoms usually develop insidiously, but with the passage of time hypoglycemic episodes tend to increase in frequency and severity. Most attacks occur in the early morning or late afternoon hours. They are often precipitated by fasting and physical activity. Neuroglycopenic symptoms predominate over those caused by epinephrine release. Whipple's triad, consisting of symptoms of hypoglycemia, low blood sugar levels, and relief with administration of glucose, is suggestive of organic hypoglycemia but is not specific for hyperinsulinism due to islet cell disease.

   b. Glucagon deficiency. Glucagon deficiency is an extremely rare cause of hypoglycemia. The failure of plasma glucose and glucagon to rise following an arginine infusion is diagnostic of this condition.

   c. Extrapancreatic tumors. Severe fasting hypoglycemia may occur in the presence of such tumors as mesotheliomas, fibromas, fibrosarcomas, leiomyosarcomas, etc., particularly when they are large. The neoplasms are usually found in the pelvis, retroperitoneum, or thorax. The diagnosis is usually based on the association of hypoglycemia with easily identified abdominal or thoracic masses.

   d. Liver disease. Glycogen storage disease and galactosemia are examples of congenital anomalies that may be associated with hypoglycemia. Hypoglycemia may also occur in severe, diffuse liver disease (e.g., fulminating hepatitis, hepatic necrosis due to toxic agents, cholangitis, cirrhosis) and in some patients with hepatomas.

   e. Leucine sensitivity. Leucine-induced hypoglycemia is an extremely rare disorder in adults but is a not uncommon cause of fasting hypoglycemia in children below the age of 4 years. The administration of leucine may produce hypoglycemia in patients with islet cell tumors or in those on sulfonylureas.

   f. Alcohol-induced hypoglycemia. Ethanol-induced hypoglycemia occurs most frequently in alcoholics who are eating little or no food. Occasionally, following a 2- to 3-day fast, the ingestion of alcohol may produce hypoglycemia in a young, healthy person. Patients with hypopituitarism or adrenocortical insufficiency exhibit increased sensitivity to the hypoglycemic effects of alcohol. Ethanol-induced hypoglycemia is promptly corrected by the administration of glucose.

   g. Malnutrition. Hypoglycemia is relatively common in children with kwashiorkor, but in adults, even severe protein depletion and malnutrition rarely lead to hypoglycemia.

h. Endocrine disorders. Fasting hypoglycemia may occur in patients with hypopituitarism or Addison's disease, but it is a relatively uncommon finding in these disorders. The endocrine cause of the hypoglycemia is usually apparent from the clinical picture.

3. Factitious hypoglycemia. Hypoglycemia may be induced by ingestion of salicylates in large amounts, monamine oxidase inhibitors, barbiturates, and other drugs. It may be precipitated in diabetics receiving insulin, when the dose of insulin is too high, when physical activity is excessive, or when food intake is inadequate or delayed. Sulfonylureas may induce hypoglycemia, especially in the presence of renal failure or the use of alcoholic beverages. Insulin has sometimes been used by medical personnel, diabetics, and the relatives of patients with malingering or with suicidal or homicidal intent. However, insulin overdosage is most commonly accidental.

DIAGNOSTIC APPROACH TO REACTIVE HYPOGLYCEMIA

1. A 5-hour oral GTT is the mainstay of the diagnostic approach to suspected reactive hypoglycemia.

a. In reactive functional hypoglycemia, the fasting blood sugar level is normal. The curve is not remarkable except for the occurrence of abnormally low plasma glucose values (50 mg/100 ml or less) between the second and fourth hours of the test.

b. In reactive hypoglycemia secondary to mild diabetes mellitus, the glucose tolerance curve generally shows a normal or slightly elevated fasting blood sugar level, hyperglycemia at the peak value and at 2 hours, and low plasma glucose levels (50 mg/100 ml or less) during the third to fifth hours.

c. In alimentary hypoglycemia, the oral GTT reveals a normal fasting glucose level, peak hyperglycemia at ½ to 1 hour, normal glucose concentration at 2 hours, and hypoglycemia shortly thereafter.

2. Since the intravenous GTT is normal in alimentary hypoglycemia but abnormal in diabetes mellitus, it is useful in differentiating between the two.

3. Once an oral GTT has been performed, when fasting hypoglycemia has to be ruled out, the procedures outlined below (Diagnostic Approach to Fasting Hypoglycemia) should be followed.

DIAGNOSTIC APPROACH TO FASTING HYPOGLYCEMIA

In addition to the oral 5-hour GTT, the following procedures are recommended in the evaluation of patients with suspected fasting hypoglycemia:

1. Determine, on at least two or three occasions, the plasma glucose and insulin levels after an overnight fast. Plasma glucose values of 50 mg/

100 ml or less together with plasma insulin levels exceeding 40 μU per milliliter occurring in association with hypoglycemia symptoms are considered virtually diagnostic of insulinoma.

2. If the plasma glucose and insulin levels are not diagnostic, the overnight fast should be prolonged for 4 hours and the plasma glucose and insulin determinations repeated. If the results still prove to be inconclusive, the fast should be extended for an additional 48 to 72 hours, with only black coffee permitted. During this time, multiple plasma glucose determinations should be obtained. These are usually done at 6-hour intervals or whenever symptoms appear. As soon as low glucose levels and symptoms of hypoglycemia are induced, the test is terminated. Otherwise, at the conclusion of the 3-day period, the patient is exercised and a blood sample is drawn thereafter.

3. In patients with islet cell tumors, the plasma glucose concentration normally falls below 50 mg/100 ml at some time during the fast. Hypoglycemia of this severity is uncommon in patients who do not have disease of the islet cells. Exercise is a valuable adjunct in the evaluation of hypoglycemia since it produces a further drop in plasma glucose concentration in patients with insulinomas or other conditions associated with fasting hypoglycemia and a rise in plasma glucose levels in patients with reactive hypoglycemia.

4. The measurement of plasma insulin levels in conjunction with plasma glucose concentrations is extremely valuable in the diagnosis of islet cell disease. Elevated plasma levels in connection with low fasting plasma glucose levels confirm the diagnosis of insulinoma. However, not all patients with islet cell tumors show fasting hyperinsulinemia. Moreover, normal fasting plasma insulin levels not only do not exclude the diagnosis but may actually support it if they occur in association with low plasma glucose concentrations. During the fast, a fall of plasma glucose to hypoglycemic levels while the plasma insulin remains unchanged or rises is also a significant finding. High fasting plasma insulin levels are not always pathognomonic of insulinoma because they may sometimes occur in obese persons without fasting hyperglycemia, in children with idiopathic hypoglycemia, and, rarely, in patients with nonpancreatic neoplasms. It has also been reported that assay of fasting plasma proinsulin levels may be helpful in the diagnosis of islet cell disease, particularly when fasting plasma insulin levels are not elevated.

5. Tests that induce the secretion of insulin are useful in confirming the diagnosis of islet cell tumors and in the differential diagnosis of hypoglycemia. The procedures used most commonly are the intravenous tolbutamide, leucine, and glucagon tests, in which serial determinations of plasma glucose and insulin are performed following the administration of the test substance. Details of the test procedures and information concerning their interpretation can be found in standard textbooks. These provocative tests for insulin secretion are abnormal in a high percentage of patients with insulinomas. However, false-

positive and false-negative results may occur with any of them. All three tests should be employed in suspected islet cell disease because an abnormal response may be obtained with one test but not with another. False-positive results may occur with the tolbutamide test in patients with nonpancreatic causes of hypoglycemia, uremia, or malnutrition, but not in patients with reactive hypoglycemia. With the leucine test, false-positive results may occur in individuals on the sulfonylureas. In children, the leucine test does not differentiate between insulinoma and the so-called idiopathic hypoglycemia of children. It is the writer's opinion that the glucagon test may prove to be the most reliable of the provocative tests for insulin secretion.

6. Once the diagnosis of islet cell tumor is made on the basis of the foregoing tests, arteriography should be performed to help localize the tumor. Skull films and serum calcium and phosphorus determinations are indicated to rule out multiple endocrine adenomatosis. If carcinoma is suspected, a liver scan should be done to rule out metastatic disease.

7. Extrapancreatic neoplasms merit consideration as possible causes of hypoglycemia after islet cell tumor has been ruled out, particularly in elderly individuals. Radiologic examinations such as chest and abdominal films, intravenous pyelography, and contrast studies of the gastrointestinal tract are useful diagnostic studies for this purpose.

8. If glucagon deficiency is suspected, an arginine test should be performed. The failure of plasma glucagon and glucose to rise following the administration of arginine by infusion is diagnostic of glucagon deficiency.

9. If pituitary and adrenal hypofunction are suspected causes of hypoglycemia, appropriate laboratory studies to confirm the diagnosis are indicated.

10. The relationship of diffuse liver disease to hypoglycemia is usually apparent from the clinical picture. Liver function tests show abnormalities. Hepatic hypoglycemia is easily corrected by the administration of glucose. Glucagon should be avoided because it may fail to cause hyperglycemia in the presence of severely impaired glyconeogenic reserve.

11. The diagnosis of alcohol hypoglycemia is supported by a fall in plasma glucose levels following an infusion of ethanol.

12. When factitious hypoglycemia due to malingering is suspected, the following procedures merit consideration:
   a. Serum insulin antibody levels. The presence of such antibodies is proof of the administration of insulin.
   b. Sulfonylurea blood levels.
   c. Examination of the urine for tolbutamide excretion products.

d. Leucine sensitivity test, which produces elevated insulin levels in patients with hypoglycemia due to sulfonylurea compounds.

13. Many investigators rely heavily on encephalographic changes for the diagnosis of questionable cases of hypoglycemia. The disappearance of alpha waves when blood sugar values are low and their reappearance after correction of the hypoglycemia are regarded as specific evidence, provided hyperventilation and severe anoxia are ruled out. The test is considered to be especially valuable in the diagnosis of organic hypoglycemia.

Failure to Mature

Janet E. Schemmel

DEFINITION AND ETIOLOGY

Failure to mature or the failure to develop secondary sex characteristics is a relatively common disorder. It is frequently, but not always, associated with delayed growth. The condition has many causes. This discussion will be limited to males; the problem as related to females is considered in the following section, Amenorrhea. The age of presentation varies, often depending on the family history and the patient's identification with his peers. Usually, the patient is seen between the ages of 12 and 17 years; within the last decade, at a slightly younger age. The various abnormalities that can occur are listed below.

1. Failure to mature, with growth retardation or failure.
   a. Delayed puberty (constitutional retardation)—most common; commonly familial; cause unknown.
   b. Pituitary-hypothalamic disease.
      (1) Idiopathic hypopituitarism (with isolated or multiple tropic hormone losses).
      (2) Pituitary tumor, nonsecreting, with multiple tropic hormone losses.
      (3) Pituitary tumor, secreting, as in Cushing's disease.
      (4) Suprasellar or parasellar tumor.
      (5) Infiltrative disease of the hypothalamus (e.g., sarcoidosis).
      (6) Vascular abnormalities (e.g., internal carotid aneurysm).
   c. Hypothyroidism, juvenile, with or without goiter.
   d. Chronic systemic disease (e.g., congenital heart disease, pulmonary disease, steroid treatment for asthmatic and dermatologic patients, chronic renal disease).
   e. Cushing's syndrome.
   f. Cryptorchidism.

    g. Testicular failure.

        (1) Infection.

        (2) Trauma.

    h. Anorchism and testicular dysgenesis.

2. Failure to mature, without growth retardation.

    a. Hypogonadotropic hypogonadism.

    b. Klinefelter's syndrome and associated syndromes.

3. Delayed puberty secondary to other disease states (e.g., myotonia dystrophica, and the obesity, mental retardation, and polydactylism or syndactylism seen in the Laurence-Moon-Biedl syndrome).

SYMPTOMS

Multiple symptoms may occur. They are usually related to the underlying cause and to the state of growth of the patient.

1. Failure to mature with growth retardation.

    a. Immature genitalia.

    b. No beard.

    c. Delay in growth.

    d. Considered younger than chronological age by peers and adults.

    e. Immature voice.

    f. In patients with pituitary or hypothalamic disorders (or both), additional symptoms may be present: (1) headaches, (2) visual complaints, (3) polydipsia and polyuria, (4) easy fatigability or episodic weakness, or both, and (5) failure to tan.

    g. In addition to the general symptoms, patients with hypothyroidism may have (1) somnolence, (2) poor concentration, (3) cold intolerance, (4) constipation and obstipation, (5) mass in neck, (6) hearing defects, and (7) joint pain, especially hip pain.

    h. Patients with systemic disease frequently have symptoms of their underlying disease. Cushing's disease or syndrome, uncommon at this age, is discussed in the sections Amenorrhea and Obesity, later in the chapter.

2. Failure to mature without growth retardation. Patients without growth retardation may have few complaints except those of delayed maturity. Patients with hypogonadotropic hypogonadism may complain of inability to smell. Enlarged breasts are common symptoms in patients with Klinefelter's syndrome.

SIGNS

Failure to Mature with Growth Retardation

1. Below height and weight for chronological age.

2. Immature facies for chronological age.

3. Immature voice and larynx for chronological age.

4. Paucity or absence of axillary or pubic hair.

5. Absence of any pubertal breast tenderness or tissue.

6. Span and upper and lower segment heights that are compatible with normal prepubertal dimensions, although occasionally a eunuchoidal habitus may be seen.

7. Tanning may be absent, or the skin may be pale, yellowish, or dry.

8. Blood pressure may be variable, depending on the underlying disease.

9. Genitalia are prepubertal, compatible with the patient's somatic age; the testes may be inguinal or impalpable.

10. In patients with pituitary disorders, additional findings may be noted:
    a. Changing visual acuity and visual field defects.
    b. Cranial bruit.
    c. Pale or yellowish, dry skin when multiple tropic hormones are lost.

11. Patients with chronic disease frequently demonstrate findings of the underlying disease (e.g., hepatosplenomegaly). The findings in Cushing's disease and syndrome are discussed in the sections Amenorrhea and Obesity, later in the chapter.

Failure to Mature without Growth Retardation

1. Normal height or taller than predicted on the basis of the family height history.

2. Commonly, increased span, with the lower segment height greater than the upper segment height.

3. Absent or small scrotal testes and a small phallus.

4. Gynecomastia.

5. Sparsity or absence of the beard and axillary and pubic hair.

6. Obesity (not uncommon).

DIAGNOSTIC APPROACH

Initial Evaluation

Initial studies should be carried out to help clarify the diagnosis, to determine the need for further investigation, and to determine proper treatment. These studies should include the following tests:

1. Hemoglobin and hematocrit values.

2. WBC and differential counts.

3. Platelet count.

4. Sedimentation rate.

5. PBI or T_4 and T_3 resin uptake.

6. Electrolytes.

7. BUN, creatinine.

8. Serum calcium, phosphorus, and alkaline phosphatase.

9. Urinary gonadotropins, plasma FSH and LH, or both.

10. Buccal smear for chromatin pattern.

11. X-rays: chest, skull, and AP, hands and wrists, for bone age.

12. 24-hour urine collection for 17-ketogenic steroids or 17-hydroxycorticoids and creatinine.

Patients with idiopathic delayed puberty (constitutional retardation) usually have normal findings except for a delayed bone age that correlates with height, facial maturity, and genital development. Urinary gonadotropins may be low or absent. The span is usually prepubertal, occasionally eunuchoidal. A family history of delayed puberty with good response to therapy supports this diagnosis.

In contrast, patients with pituitary disease may demonstrate the following findings: absent growth hormone; normal or low-normal thyroid function; reduced 17-ketogenic steroids or 17-hydroxycorticoids, and 17-ketosteroids; and absent gonadotropins. Skull x-rays are abnormal if a pituitary tumor is present. Enlargement of the sella turcica, with or without intracranial calcification, is a common finding. In idiopathic hypopituitarism, the sella turcica is usually normal. The BUN is frequently low. The serum phosphorus and alkaline phosphatase are reduced. Slight anemia may be present. Bone development is delayed. The body proportions and span are prepubertal.

Subsequent Evaluation

Further evaluation should include the following tests to determine tropic hormone losses:

1. Measurement of 17-ketogenic steroids or 17-hydroxycorticoids before and after metyrapone administration.

2. Plasma TSH or RAI uptake studies before and after exogenous TSH administration, or both.

3. Growth hormone response to insulin-induced hypoglycemia.

4. Further radiologic investigation, including sellar tomography and arteriography, as indicated.

If the diagnosis of primary hypothyroidism is established, tests for thyroid antibodies are indicated; a positive result suggests Hashimoto's struma. If a goiter is present or hearing is abnormal, other members of the family should be examined for familial goiter. A perchlorate test may be indicated in the presence of a goiter when the RAI uptake is elevated (see section, Thyroid Enlargement, later in the chapter). Other tests to determine thyroxin-synthesizing defects are not yet available. It should be remembered that patients with juvenile hypothyroidism frequently have normal to accelerated puberty in the presence of delayed growth.

Ordinarily, the history, physical findings, and initial laboratory tests suggest the presence of an underlying chronic disease as the cause of the patient's failure to mature. Electrocardiogram, pulmonary function tests, liver function tests, long bone x-rays, skin tests, urinary electrolyte excretion, and other tests should be carried out when applicable.

Hypogonadotropic hypogonadism may occur as an isolated abnormality or in association with other conditions, such as palatal abnormalities and anosmia. The initial work-up usually discloses a eunuchoidal or normal habitus, prepubertal scrotal testes, negative urinary and plasma gonadotropins, and delayed bone age. Further investigation for tropic hormone losses should be undertaken to ensure that the defect is isolated. These should include:

1. Metyrapone test (see p. 357), with measurement of 17-ketogenic steroids or 17-hydroxycorticoids before and after administration of the drug.

2. Growth hormone measurements before and after insulin-induced hypoglycemia.

3. Plasma TSH or RAI uptake before and after exogenous TSH administration, or both.

Testicular biopsy is not necessary. Follow-up study may be indicated in selected patients because tropic hormone losses theoretically may occur at a later date.

More common than hypogonadotropic hypogonadism is Klinefelter's syndrome (and its variants). These patients frequently are eunuchoidal and have small testes. Gynecomastia may be present. The buccal smear is positive, bone age is delayed, and urinary and plasma gonadotropins are elevated. A karyotype determination may be indicated.

Amenorrhea

Janet E. Schemmel

DEFINITION

Amenorrhea is the failure of menstruation to occur in a female of menstrual age. It is considered primary if menstruation has never occurred, and secondary if menses have ceased in a woman who has menstruated previously. The normal menarche is variable, but generally occurs between 12 and 15 years of age in this country. A somewhat wider age range, 11 to 17 years, has been reported for other countries. In recent years, the age of onset of menstruation appears to be younger than formerly.

PRIMARY AMENORRHEA

Etiology

The causes of primary amenorrhea are many and varied. Occasionally, the past or family history provides clues to the diagnosis, particularly in the presence of chronic disease or a familial disorder. Primary amenorrhea is commonly associated with delayed growth. The most frequent causes are listed below.

1. Delayed puberty of unknown cause.

2. Ovarian dysgenesis (agenesis, dysplasia).

3. Secondary hypogonadism: pituitary-hypothalamic disease, associated with idiopathic onset, tumors, infiltrative disease, vascular anomalies.

4. Testicular feminization syndrome.

5. Cushing's syndrome or disease occurring at puberty.

6. Juvenile hypothyroidism.

7. Systemic disease (e.g., chronic renal disease, cystic fibrosis, congenital heart disease).

8. Cervical or uterine abnormalities.

9. Other endocrine disorders, including congenital or acquired adrenal hyperplasia, pseudohermaphroditism, true hermaphroditism, and ambiguous sexual differentiation.

Symptoms

1. Delayed puberty of unknown cause and ovarian dysgenesis are probably the two most common causes of primary amenorrhea. Delayed growth usually accompanies these conditions. Patients with systemic disease and Cushing's syndrome or disease may also have retardation in growth.

2. The usual symptoms encountered in patients with primary amenorrhea are (a) amenorrhea, in association with absent or delayed development of breast tissue and absence or paucity of pubic and axillary hair, (b) retardation in growth, and (c) a younger appearance than expected for the patient's chronological age.

3. When primary amenorrhea is due to pituitary-hypothalamic disorders, additional symptoms related to its underlying cause or to the loss of specific tropic hormones may occur, such as (a) headaches, (b) visual disturbances, (c) polydipsia, (d) polyuria, (e) easy fatigability or episodic weakness, or both, and (f) failure of the skin to tan.

4. Patients with hypogonadotropic hypogonadism and testicular feminization may complain only of amenorrhea.

5. The symptoms found in young patients with Cushing's syndrome or disease are similar to those encountered in adults. The usual symptoms are (a) obesity that is not due to excessive food intake and that is chiefly truncal in distribution, (b) easy fatigability and weakness, (c) irritability and difficulty in concentrating, (d) skin problems such as acne and easy bruisability, and (e) growth retardation.

6. Patients with underlying chronic disease frequently have symptoms related to the basic disorder. Delayed growth often coexists.

7. Patients with congenital adrenal hyperplasia due to a 21-hydroxylase defect are usually diagnosed shortly after birth because of the presence of pseudohermaphroditism or adrenal insufficiency, or both. However, when acquired, this rare anomaly may present primarily with amenorrhea and, sometimes, with mild hirsutism but without any abnormality in growth. Other rare causes of congenital adrenal hyperplasia are the 11-hydroxylase and 17-hydroxylase deficiencies, both of which may be associated with systemic hypertension. However, significant growth problems are not encountered in these disorders.

8. Patients with ambiguous sexual differentiation may have few symptoms other than amenorrhea and delayed growth.

Physical Findings

Primary Amenorrhea with Associated Growth Retardation

1. Delayed height and weight for the chronological age.

2. Immature facies for the chronological age.

3. Immature voice and larynx for the chronological age.

4. Paucity or absence of axillary and pubic hair.

5. Minimal or absent breast development.

6. An arm span and upper and lower segment heights that are more compatible with normal prepubertal than with postpubertal dimensions.

7. Normotension, but occasionally systolic hypertension.

8. Skin changes, consisting of absence of tanning or a dry skin that is pale and yellowish.

9. Abnormalities that are suggestive of ovarian dysgenesis: strabismus, webbing of the neck, increased carrying angle of the arms, pedal edema, pes cavus, and shortened metacarpals.

10. External genitalia that are normal but prepubertal in appearance.

11. Findings suggestive of chronic underlying disease, such as chest deformities, heart murmurs, and hepatomegaly.

12. Diminished visual acuity, visual field defects, cranial bruits, and a pale yellow or dry skin in some patients with pituitary disorders.

Primary Amenorrhea without Associated Growth Retardation

This group of patients includes those with sexual ambiguity, some cases of ovarian dysgenesis, the testicular feminization syndrome, hypogonadotropic hypogonadism, some patients with congenital (11-hydroxylase or 17-hydroxylase deficiency) or acquired (21-hydroxylase deficiency) adrenal hyperplasia, and some patients with chronic systemic illness. Cases with these disorders may show the following features:

1. Immature but otherwise normal facies for the chronological age.

2. Immature voice and larynx for the chronological age, although the larynx is sometimes enlarged and the voice low-pitched.

3. Paucity or absence of axillary and pubic hair except in patients with acquired adrenal hyperplasia, who may show hirsutism.

4. Variable breast development—minimal to absent, or normal.

5. Arm span and upper and lower segment heights may be normal, or the arm span and lower segment height may be greater than normal.

6. External genitalia which may show normal prepubertal development, clitoral hypertrophy, ambiguity, a vaginal dimple, or urethral abnormalities.

DIAGNOSTIC APPROACH

Initial Work-up

1. Careful measurement of the arm span, total height, and upper and lower segment heights.

2. Skull films to determine the size of the sella turcica and to search for other abnormalities (e.g., intracranial calcification).

3. AP x-rays of the wrists and hands to evaluate bone age.

4. Chest films to detect bony abnormalities and to determine the heart size.

5. A buccal smear for the chromatin pattern.

6. Thyroid function tests (PBI or T_4 and T_3 resin uptake).

7. A 24-hour urine collection for 17-ketogenic steroids or 17-hydroxycorticoids, 17-ketosteroids, and creatinine.

8. Serum electrolytes, BUN, creatinine, calcium, phosphorus, and alkaline phosphatase.

9. Plasma FSH and LH determinations, urinary gonadotropins, or both.

10. Fasting serum growth hormone determination.

11. Pelvic examination.

Patients with primary amenorrhea due to delayed puberty, ovarian dysgenesis, pituitary-hypothalamic disease, or hypothyroidism show evidence of delayed bone maturation. The arm span and the upper and lower segment heights are prepubertal in character. Normal skull films virtually exclude pituitary tumors. Buccal smears are negative in many cases of ovarian dysgenesis. Thyroid function studies may be normal in each of these conditions. However, they may be borderline or low in pituitary disorders and, occasionally, in ovarian dysgenesis. They are almost always abnormal in hypothyroidism. Urinary gonadotropins and plasma FSH and LH are absent or low in hypopituitarism and delayed puberty, but are elevated in patients with ovarian dysgenesis. The serum electrolyte, BUN, and creatinine levels are normal unless a systemic disease or hypothyroidism is present. The BUN may be less than 10 mg/100 ml in patients with pituitary disease. It may be slightly elevated in some patients with hypothyroidism. The serum calcium is usually normal unless chronic disease is present. Elevated serum phosphorus and alkaline phosphatase values suggest that body growth is occurring. Such a finding is helpful because the results of growth hormone assays often are not reported until several weeks after specimens were collected and submitted for analysis. On pelvic examination, the genitalia are usually prepubertal in size, but the uterus may be absent or impalpable in ovarian dysgenesis.

Subsequent Work-up in Primary Amenorrhea with Delayed Growth

The diagnosis of delayed puberty is suggested when the serum electrolytes, BUN and creatinine, growth hormone assay, thyroid function tests, and excretion of 17-ketogenic steroids and 17-ketosteroids are normal, the buccal smear is positive, urinary gonadotropins and plasma FSH and LH are low or absent, bone maturation is retarded, and serum phosphorus and alkaline phosphatase are elevated.

Ovarian dysgenesis should be suspected if the skull films are negative, the fasting growth hormone level is normal, buccal smears are negative, bone age is delayed, and urinary gonadotropins exceed 105 MUU or plasma FSH is elevated, or both. The karyotype should be determined; usually it is XO, but a mosaic pattern may occur with or without other obvious extragenital abnormalities. Because diabetes mellitus is common in ovarian dysgenesis, a glucose tolerance test should be performed on all patients with this disorder. Thyroid antibodies are commonly present in patients with this anomaly.

A pituitary tumor should be suspected when skull films reveal an abnormality of the sella turcica or show suprasellar calcification. Confirmatory findings of hypopituitarism include delayed bone growth, absent urinary gonadotropins, low or absent plasma FSH and LH, absent growth hormone, low or normal thyroid function tests, positive buccal smears, normal or low BUN, and a normal or reduced serum alkaline phosphatase and phosphorus. To establish the diagnosis of pituitary hypofunction, additional studies are indicated:

1. Plasma TSH or RAI uptake before and after TSH stimulation, or both. (Measurement of TSH before and after the administration of TRH is not yet available.)

2. Metyrapone test (see p. 357). Dexamethasone should be administered along with the metyrapone when adrenal insufficiency is suspected.

3. Insulin tolerance test to measure the release of growth hormone and plasma cortisol with insulin-induced hypoglycemia. Prior to the test a fasting blood sample is drawn for glucose determination, growth hormone assay, and plasma cortisol. Regular insulin is then injected intravenously in a dose of 0.05 to 0.10 units per kilogram of body weight. Blood samples are collected at 15, 30, 45, and 60 minutes after the injection for glucose determinations. Samples at 30 and 60 minutes are also used for growth hormone assay and plasma cortisol.

Normally, insulin-induced hypoglycemia causes a rise in growth hormone levels to at least 20 ng at 60 minutes and a threefold rise in plasma cortisol.

4. Plasma FSH and LH.

5. Visual acuity and visual field tests.

6. Radiologic studies, such as sellar tomography, pneumoencephalography, and arteriography, depending on the circumstances.

7. Patients with suspected hypothyroidism should have a TSH assay and thyroid antibody determinations.

8. Patients with Cushing's syndrome or disease generally show elevated 17-ketogenic steroids or 17-hydroxycorticoids on initial work-up unless a pituitary tumor is present. Further investigation should include urinary steroid excretions before and after the administration of dexamethasone, metyrapone, or ACTH (see the section Obesity, later in the chapter).

9. Patients with chronic systemic disease may show abnormalities in the initial work-up that are primarily related to the underlying disorder. Usually, bone maturation is delayed and the urinary gonadotropin levels are lower than expected for the chronological age. Additional studies to elucidate the diagnosis are advisable.

Subsequent Work-up in Primary Amenorrhea without Delayed Growth

1. Patients with suspected hypogonadotropic hypogonadism should have work-ups similar to those performed on patients with hypopituitarism. Even though hypogonadotropic hypogonadism occurs as a separate entity without other tropic hormone losses, some patients with hypogonadotropic hypogonadism due to hypopituitarism may develop them eventually. Therefore, determination of all tropic hormone functions should be done not only at the time of the initial examination but also at appropriate intervals thereafter.

2. Patients with the testicular feminization syndrome have normal breast development together with abnormalities of the external genitalia, negative buccal smears, and usually normal excretion of testosterone, 17-ketogenic steroids, and 17-ketosteroids. A karyotype should be obtained in patients with this syndrome. Also, because the mode of inheritance is consistent with either an X-linked recessive or a sex-limited autosomal dominant trait, other members of the family should be studied.

3. The diagnosis of ambiguous sexual differentiation is suggested by abnormality of the external genitalia and pelvic examination findings. In such cases, even if the buccal smear is positive, a karyotype preparation should be made. Intravenous pyelography, cystography, vaginog-

raphy, and urethroscopy are indicated to further elucidate the renal and uterovaginal abnormalities commonly seen in true hermaphroditism or pseudohermaphroditism.

4. Patients with the common type of congenital adrenal hyperplasia (21-hydroxylase deficiency) rarely present with amenorrhea because they are usually diagnosed at a much earlier age. The acquired form of the disease may occur without any associated abnormality of growth. The urinary excretion of pregnanetriol should be determined in cases demonstrating increased excretion of 17-ketogenic steroids.

5. Congenital adrenal hyperplasia due to 11-hydroxylase deficiency is a rare cause of amenorrhea. This syndrome is associated with excessive production of 11-desoxycorticosterone and ultimately with the development of hypertension. The external genitalia are abnormal. The urinary excretion of aldosterone and 17-hydroxycorticoids is reduced.

6. Another variant of congenital adrenal hyperplasia, the 17-hydroxylase deficiency syndrome, is also associated with amenorrhea and hypertension. The external genitalia are underdeveloped. The urinary excretion of corticosterone and desoxycorticosterone is elevated, and that of aldosterone and 17-hydroxycorticoids is reduced.

7. Diagnostic pelvic exploration is usually indicated in ambiguous sexual differentiation once congenital or acquired adrenal hyperplasia has been ruled out by appropriate testing.

SECONDARY AMENORRHEA

Patients with secondary amenorrhea may have an abrupt cessation of menses, or the amenorrhea may be preceded by a period of oligomenorrhea. Investigation is usually warranted after four to six menstrual periods have been missed. Pregnancy is an obvious cause and should be excluded before proceeding with further investigations.

Etiology

1. Polycystic ovary syndrome—probably the most common cause in patients in their teens or early twenties.

2. Pituitary-hypothalamic disease.
   a. Tumors.
      (1) Pituitary, nonsecretory.
      (2) Pituitary, secretory.
         (a) Acromegaly.
         (b) Prolactin-secreting.
         (c) Cushing's disease.
      (3) Suprasellar, parasellar and, rarely, intrasellar tumors.

b. Hypopituitarism.
    (1) Idiopathic (Simmond's disease).
    (2) Infarction (Sheehan's syndrome).
c. Infiltrative disease (e.g., sarcoidosis).
d. Internal carotid aneurysm and other vascular anomalies.
e. Prolactin secretion in the absence of tumor (idiopathic and drug-induced).
f. Postpubertal hypogonadotropic hypogonadism.
g. Cushing's disease.
h. Empty sella syndrome.

3. Adrenal disease.
  a. Cushing's syndrome.
    (1) Tumor.
    (2) Carcinoma.
  b. Adrenal tumors with virilization.
  c. Addison's disease.

4. Ovarian disease.
  a. Ovarian failure.
    (1) Premature menopause (before the age of 40 years), usually idiopathic.
    (2) Acquired anatomic lesions, including tumors, carcinoma, and infection.
    (3) Normal menopause.
  b. Ovarian tumors.

5. Chronic systemic disease (e.g., kidney, liver, lung).

6. Anorexia nervosa.

7. Drug-induced: contraceptives, spironolactone.

8. Idiopathic.

Symptoms

The symptoms in secondary amenorrhea are quite variable. The more common ones are listed below:

1. Amenorrhea, either abrupt in onset or preceded by a period of oligomenorrhea.

2. Changes in body weight.
  a. Weight loss, which may be marked, occurs in anorexia nervosa, panhypopituitarism, Addison's disease, some tumors and carcinomas, and idiopathic amenorrhea.

    b. Weight gain may be noted in patients with polycystic ovaries, Cushing's syndrome or disease, adrenal and ovarian tumors, acromegaly, prolactin-secreting tumors, and idiopathic amenorrhea.

3. Weakness and fatigability, which are most prominent in Cushing's disease, panhypopituitarism, Addison's disease, ovarian and adrenal malignancies, and chronic systemic illness.

4. A variety of specific or nonspecific symptoms related to the cause of the amenorrhea may be present. Thus, symptoms of hypopituitarism, hyperadrenocorticism, adrenal insufficiency, hypothyroidism, etc., may be reported by the patient.

Physical Findings

There are no physical signs that are specifically related to secondary amenorrhea. The findings, if any, are those of the primary disorder.

Diagnostic Approach

Clinical Features

1. Weight loss without skin changes suggests anorexia nervosa, acquired anatomic lesions, systemic disease, infiltrative hypothalamic lesions, etc.

2. Weight loss in a patient with a pale, thin, sallow, yellowish skin suggests possible hypopituitarism.

3. Weight loss with hyperpigmentation and increased numbers of freckles and moles is commonly seen in Addison's disease.

4. Weight gain, with or without skin changes, may be observed in acromegalic patients, many of whom have increased numbers of papillomata and moles as well as a slight increase in body hair.

5. Weight gain, in association with plethora, acne, and striae, is common in Cushing's syndrome or disease.

6. Weight gain, in association with lactation, suggests a prolactin-secreting tumor.

7. The association of obesity with mild hirsutism is often noted in patients with the polycystic ovary syndrome.

8. Hirsutism of mild to severe degree may accompany ovarian or adrenal disease.

9. Patients with postpubertal hypogonadism and premature ovarian failure rarely demonstrate any significant change in body weight.

Initial Work-up

The following preliminary studies are recommended in the work-up of patients with secondary amenorrhea:

1. CBC and platelet count.

2. Sedimentation rate.

3. Chest and skull films.

4. Urinary gonadotropins or plasma FSH and LH, or both.

5. Urinary 17-ketogenic steroids or 17-hydroxycorticoids, 17-ketosteroids, and creatinine.

6. Thyroid function tests (PBI or T_4 and T_3 resin uptake).

7. Careful pelvic examination to establish the size of the uterus and ovaries and to detect the presence of infection or masses. (A single index of maturation is usually not helpful.)

Subsequent Work-up

1. If the skull films are abnormal, additional studies, such as sellar tomography, pneumoencephalography, and arteriography, may be indicated.

2. If acromegaly is suspected, appropriate bone x-rays should be done. A glucose tolerance test, including simultaneous determinations of the glucose and growth hormone levels, should also be performed.

3. Pituitary function studies are indicated in the presence of lactation. Prolactin determination should be performed if available.

4. Appropriate diagnostic studies are warranted whenever systemic disease is suspected.

5. High urinary gonadotropic levels (>100 MUU) and elevated plasma FSH determinations are indicative of primary ovarian failure.

6. Urinary gonadotropins and plasma FSH may be absent or low in prolactin-secreting tumors, hypopituitarism, massive obesity, and anorexia nervosa. Urinary gonadotropin levels and plasma FSH are usually normal in Cushing's disease or syndrome, polycystic ovary disease, and in adrenal and ovarian tumors. Urinary gonadotropin values and plasma FSH may be quite variable in acromegaly.

7. Further evaluation of pituitary function is indicated in all patients with absent urinary gonadotropins or plasma FSH and LH, to determine whether other tropic hormone deficiencies exist.

8. Additional studies for the diagnosis of Cushing's disease or syndrome, polycystic ovaries, and suspected ovarian or adrenal tumors are discussed in the section Obesity, later in the chapter.

9. Psychiatric evaluation is indicated in patients presenting with massive obesity or anorexia nervosa.

10. The response to progestational agents is often of some help diagnostically. The occurrence of withdrawal bleeding following the administration of medroxyprogesterone acetate (10 mg per day for 4 days) is indicative of previous endometrial stimulation by endogenous estrogen. Failure of such bleeding to occur suggests either estrogen deficiency or a lack of endometrial responsiveness.

Adrenocortical Insufficiency

Janet E. Schemmel

DEFINITION AND ETIOLOGY

Adrenocortical insufficiency is a symptom complex that results from deficiency of adrenocortical hormones. It may be primary, as in Addison's disease, or secondary, as in hypopituitarism. The onset may be acute or insidious.

1. Primary adrenocortical insufficiency. The term *Addison's disease* refers to primary adrenocortical insufficiency. The course of the disease may be chronic or acute, or an acute phase may be superimposed on a chronic state. Primary atrophy, tuberculosis, and fungal infections are common causes. Adrenal hemorrhage (due to anticoagulants or idiopathic in origin), surgical removal of the adrenal glands, drugs (e.g., OP-DDD, aminoglutethemide), congenital adrenal hypoplasia, congenital adrenal hyperplasia, and metastatic carcinoma may also produce primary adrenocortical insufficiency. In present-day medical practice, adrenal suppression from prolonged steroid therapy is probably the most commonly diagnosed cause.

2. Secondary adrenocortical insufficiency. Adrenocortical insufficiency may also be secondary to hypopituitarism from pituitary or hypothalamic disease. Destruction of pituitary or hypothalamic tissue may be caused by infarction, granulomatous disease (e.g., sarcoidosis, tuberculosis), chromophobe adenoma, suprasellar meningioma, craniopharyngioma, aneurysm, etc.

SYMPTOMS

The onset of adrenocortical insufficiency is usually insidious but it can be acute. The spectrum of symptoms in both primary and secondary adrenocortical insufficiency is variable. The following symptoms may be described by the patient: (1) asthenia, weakness, and lethargy, (2) weight loss, (3) easy fatigability, especially in the afternoon, (4) dizziness and syncope, (5) anorexia, nausea, vomiting, and diarrhea, (6) nervousness, irritability, apathy, and (7) nonspecific complaints such as myalgias, loss of libido, or heat and cold intolerance.

Primary Adrenocortical Insufficiency

Any of the aforementioned symptoms can occur in primary adrenal disease, but chronic weakness, fatigue, weight loss, and gastrointestinal symptoms are the most frequent complaints. Changes in the color of the skin or increased numbers of moles and freckles are sometimes noted by the patient or his friends. Salt craving and increased salt intake are also common symptoms.

Secondary Adrenocortical Insufficiency

In addition to the symptoms noted above, patients with hypopituitarism may have local symptoms related to its underlying cause and systemic symptoms resulting from specific tropic hormone deficiencies, as follows: (1) impairment of vision or visual field defects, (2) headaches (frontal, vertical, temporoparietal, or varying combinations of these locations), (3) failure to tan after exposure to sunlight, (4) mental confusion and somnolence, (5) loss of libido, amenorrhea, or impotence, (6) loss of body hair and decreased beard growth, (7) growth failure in children, and (8) polydipsia and polyuria. Salt craving does not occur.

Acute Adrenocortical Insufficiency

Adrenal crisis is characterized by headaches, malaise, restlessness, vomiting, abdominal pain, hyperpyrexia, and shock, which may progress to coma and death. Acute adrenal insufficiency may occur under the following circumstances: (1) failure of the patient with adrenocortical insufficiency to take the prescribed replacement therapy; (2) following acute illness, stress, anesthesia, or surgery in patients with decreased adrenocortical reserve; (3) failure to increase the dosage of steroids in patients with Addison's disease complicated by acute disease or other stressful situations; (4) abrupt withdrawal of adrenocortical hormones in steroid-treated individuals; (5) following injury to the adrenals by trauma, thrombosis, or hemorrhage; (6) after bilateral adrenalectomy; and (7) overwhelming sepsis, with or without hemorrhagic phenomena.

PHYSICAL FINDINGS

Primary Adrenocortical Insufficiency

The physical findings may be normal, but patients with symptoms of weakness, lethargy, and weight loss usually exhibit changes in the pigmentation of the skin. Sometimes this is the only abnormality detectable on examination. The skin changes observed include hyperpigmentation or tanning of both the exposed and unexposed parts of the body (especially prominent over pressure areas), increased numbers of freckles, and sometimes vitiligo.

Brownish-blue discoloration of the lips and gums and other mucous membranes may be present. The blood pressure may be normal, although postural hypotension is more common. The heart size is often reduced. ✓

Secondary Adrenocortical Insufficiency

The physical findings may be normal, although the examination may provide evidence suggestive not only of adrenocortical insufficiency but also of hypothyroidism and hypogonadism. Changes in visual acuity or visual field defects may be demonstrable. In the preadolescent age group, growth failure and delayed puberty are almost universal findings. The skin of the exposed portions of the body may be pale.

DIAGNOSTIC APPROACH

Primary Adrenocortical Insufficiency

1. A simple procedure called the Cortrosyn (tetracosactrin) test is useful for initial screening. The plasma cortisol level is determined from a blood sample drawn between 7 and 9 A.M. Cortrosyn (0.25 mg) is then injected intramuscularly. Plasma cortisol levels are then obtained 30 and 45 minutes after the injection. In normal subjects, plasma cortisol levels rise by at least 7 μg/100 ml in 30 minutes or the total value exceeds 18 μg/100 ml. Usually there is at least a twofold rise above the control value. The plasma cortisol value at 45 minutes should approximate that in the 30-minute sample. A normal response excludes primary adrenocortical failure. A subnormal response suggests the need for further testing.

2. If the Cortrosyn test elicits an abnormal response, additional tests should be performed.
   a. CBC and urinalysis.
   b. Serum electrolytes.
   c. BUN.
   d. Skin tests for tuberculosis and fungal diseases.
   e. Chest films, which may show a small heart.
   f. A KUB film to demonstrate adrenal calcification, which suggests tuberculosis or fungal disease.
   g. Skull films to exclude pituitary lesions.
   h. Serum calcium and phosphorus.
   i. Liver profile.
   j. Antithyroglobulin antibodies, which if present suggest an autoimmune basis for the adrenal disease.
   k. Thyroid function tests (PBI or T_4 and T_3 resin uptake).
   l. Urinary 17-ketogenic steroids or 17-hydroxycorticoids and creatinine excretion.

3. The most specific and sensitive test for adrenocortical insufficiency is the intravenous ACTH test. On the day before the test, a 24-hour

urine collection is made, and the quantities of 17-ketogenic steroids or 17-hydroxycorticoids and creatinine excreted are determined. Subsequently, on three consecutive days, 25 units of ACTH in 1000 ml of 5% dextrose in normal or 0.45 normal saline is infused intravenously over a period of exactly 8 hours. Daily 24-hour urine specimens are collected for 17-ketogenic steroids or 17-hydroxycorticoids and creatinine. A rise in steroid excretion of less than 100 percent of the control value is diagnostic of adrenocortical insufficiency. Normally, a threefold or greater excretion occurs on the first day of the test, with a further increase on the second day and maximum excretion on the third day. The urinary creatinine determinations are made to check on the reliability of the urine collections.

Secondary Adrenocortical Insufficiency

1. Patients with secondary adrenocortical insufficiency generally require a more extensive work-up than those with primary disease, not only for the purpose of determining the cause but also to ascertain which tropic hormones are deficient.

2. The tests listed below are recommended for this type of comprehensive survey.
   a. CBC and urinalysis.
   b. Serum electrolytes.
   c. BUN.
   d. Skull films.
   e. Chest films.
   f. Visual acuity, including visual fields, if appropriate.
   g. PBI or T_4 and T_3 resin uptake.
   h. Plasma TSH or RAI uptake before and after exogenous TSH administration, or both.
   i. Fasting serum growth hormone determination.
   j. Insulin tolerance test with growth hormone determinations in selected cases.
   k. Urinary gonadotropins or plasma FSH and LH, or both.
   l. Metyrapone test. This test is carried out by collecting 24-hour urine specimens for 17-ketogenic steroids or 17-hydroxycorticoids and creatinine on the day before and the day following the administration of metyrapone. The drug is given orally in a dosage of 750 mg every 4 hours for six doses. A normal response is characterized by an increase of 2.8 times or greater in steroid excretion on the day after the test compared to the control value. The metyrapone test can also be performed by measuring the plasma cortisol and deoxycortisol levels before and after the oral or intravenous administration of metyrapone. However, deoxycortisol determinations are expensive and not widely available. The responses with this type of metyrapone test are more difficult to evaluate.
   m. Plasma ACTH and vasopressin assays are currently not readily available commercially.

3. If skull x-rays show a pituitary tumor or abnormality of the sella turcica, then pneumoencephalography, arteriography, ultrasound testing, and brain scans may be indicated.

4. If surgical intervention is necessary before the appropriate laboratory studies can be completed, blood samples should be drawn for the following tests: CBC, urinalysis, electrolytes, BUN, creatinine, PBI or T_4 and T_3 resin uptake, plasma TSH, plasma cortisol, fasting growth hormone, and plasma FSH and LH.

Obesity

Janet E. Schemmel

DEFINITION

Obesity may be defined as an excess quantity of body fat. The diagnosis of obesity is usually based on statistics given in life insurance tables. A patient is considered overweight if his weight is 20 pounds greater than the norm established for his age, sex, height, and body build. However, the tables should be considered only as an approximate clinical guide. Skin fold measurements and determinations of total body composition using deuterium oxide or radioactive potassium are more helpful but are not readily available. Fat normally constitutes 15 to 20 percent of the total body weight. The degree and interpretation of obesity relates to cultural values.

ETIOLOGY

Obesity is most commonly due to overeating, but it may be associated with the conditions listed below. Although this list is not all-inclusive, it encompasses the more common and some of the unusual syndromes usually reported.

1. Diabetes.

2. Pregnancy.

3. Use of contraceptives.

4. Genetic influences (probably more environmental than genetic).

5. Hypothalamic injuries or abnormalities.

6. Hyperlipemic states.

7. Miscellaneous diseases.

   a. Cushing's syndrome or disease.

   b. Acromegaly.

   c. Islet cell tumor.

   d. Hypothyroidism.

   e. Polycystic ovary syndrome.

   f. Laurence-Moon-Biedl syndrome—obesity, hypogonadism, polydactylism.

   g. Pseudohypoparathyroidism—hypocalcemia, obesity, bone abnormalities.

   h. Babinski-Fröhlich syndrome—hyperphagia and hypogonadism due to hypothalamic lesions.

SYMPTOMS

Most obese patients are otherwise asymptomatic. When obesity is marked, easy fatigability, exertional dyspnea, depression, anxiety, and somnolence are likely to occur. Many of the symptoms attributed to obesity actually result from an underlying or associated disorder rather than from the obesity itself. The more common symptoms encountered in obese individuals are listed below.

1. Easy fatigability.

2. Depression with anxiety.

3. Malaise.

4. Weakness, hunger, fatigue, and dyspepsia—common in pregnancy.

5. Symptoms of reactive hypoglycemia—weakness, hunger, palpitation, and sweating—often seen in obese adult-onset diabetics about 3 to 5 hours after meals.

6. Excessive hunger—not uncommon in patients with adult-onset diabetes mellitus, islet cell tumors, or the Babinski-Fröhlich syndrome, pregnant women, or women taking oral contraceptives.

7. Excessive weight gain in spite of a normal or reduced caloric intake, frequent in Cushing's disease or syndrome.

8. Weight gain not due to overeating, often in association with loss of libido, headaches, increased hair growth, and enlargement of the hands and feet—common in acromegaly.

9. Muscle cramps, numbness of the hands, feet, and face, seizures, and obesity—suggestive of pseudohypoparathyroidism.

SIGNS

Some physical findings are produced by obesity per se, but most of the signs encountered in obese individuals are primarily related to the underlying disease.

1. Obesity that is generalized in distribution is typical of exogenous obesity. However, truncal accentuation (presumably genetic) is frequently observed.

2. Pink striae are commonly distributed over the axillae, breasts, abdomen, flanks, thighs, and buttocks, particularly in young women if the weight gain has been rapid. Usually, the pink color tends to fade and eventually disappear, leaving the striae shiny and white.

3. The blood pressure is usually normal, unless systemic hypertension due to another cause coexists.

4. Intertrigo is quite common in the folds below the breasts and in the inguinal regions.

5. Ankle edema is occasionally noted.

6. Plethora involving the cheeks and neck is not unusual.

7. When obesity is massive, tachypnea may be evident.

8. The presence of a thyroidectomy scar, typical changes in the skin, and a delayed return of deep tendon reflexes suggest hypothyroidism.

9. Purpura, moon facies, trunkal obesity, plethora, and weakness are common in Cushing's syndrome or disease.

10. Xanthomata, xanthelasma, and arcus senilis suggest hyperlipoproteinemic abnormalities.

11. Brachydactylia, a round facies, a stocky build, and tetany are found in patients with pseudohypoparathyroidism.

12. Excessive growth of the hands, feet, and jaw are typical of acromegaly.

13. Hypogonadism may occur in the hypothalamic obesity syndromes.

14. Hirsutism may occur in the polycystic ovary syndrome.

DIAGNOSTIC APPROACH

Initial Evaluation

1. CBC and platelet count.

2. Urinalysis.

3. Glucose tolerance test.

   a. A 3-hour glucose tolerance test is adequate for screening in most cases.

   b. A 5-hour test may be indicated in patients with symptoms of reactive hypoglycemia.

4. Total lipids and lipid fractions.

5. Thyroid function tests (PBI or T_4 and T_3 resin uptake).

6. BUN and serum electrolytes.

7. Serum uric acid, primarily to obtain a baseline value, because hyperuricemia often occurs with restricted caloric intake and after weight loss.

8. Chest films.

9. Electrocardiogram.

10. Psychiatric consultation is especially valuable in planning treatment and estimating prognosis in patients with serious weight problems.

As a rule, the aforementioned laboratory tests are normal in patients with exogenous obesity who have not been on diuretic therapy or on a dietary regimen. However, serum triglyceride levels frequently are elevated, particularly when obesity is marked.

Subsequent Evaluation

In patients in whom the symptoms, signs, or initial laboratory studies suggest the possibility of an associated disorder or systemic disease, additional work-up, as follows, is indicated.

1. Lipoprotein electrophoresis, when the serum triglycerides or cholesterol levels are markedly elevated, or if the glucose tolerance test is abnormal.

2. Pulmonary function studies and arterial blood gases, if somnolence or exertional dyspnea is present.

3. TSH determination, RAI uptake, and thyroid antibodies, when thyroid dysfunction is suspected.

4. Growth hormone measurement in association with a glucose tolerance test, if acromegaly is being considered. Growth hormone levels are measured while fasting, and at 1- and 2-hour intervals after glucose administration.

5. Skull films (and, if indicated, pneumoencephalography and arteriography), when acromegaly, Cushing's disease, or infiltrative pituitary-hypothalamic disease is suspected.

6. Fasting insulin and fasting blood sugar determinations. Both of these parameters should be measured serially during a 72-hour fast if hyper-

insulinism is suspected. Insulin levels may also be helpful in the evaluation of patients who exhibit symptoms of reactive hypoglycemia during glucose tolerance tests. A tolbutamide test with measurement of insulin levels may be useful if islet cell tumor is suspected.

7. If truncal adiposity, weakness, plethora, and other symptoms or signs suggest concomitant Cushing's disease or syndrome, an overnight dexamethasone suppression test should be performed in the following manner: A plasma cortisol level is obtained in a blood sample drawn at 8 A.M. on the day of the test. Dexamethasone (1.0 mg) is given at midnight. The plasma cortisol level is determined on a sample drawn at 8 A.M. the next morning. Normally, the administration of dexamethasone causes a reduction in the plasma cortisol level to 5 to 7 μg/ 100 ml or less. If the plasma cortisol level is not suppressed by this maneuver or if Cushing's disease or syndrome is suspected, further evaluation of adrenal function is necessary. The following procedure is recommended: Daily 24-hour urine specimens for 17-ketogenic steroids, 17-ketosteroids, and creatinine are collected before and during the test period. After an adequate collection of baseline urine (two specimens) has been obtained, dexamethasone is given orally (0.5 mg every 6 hours for a 2- to 3-day period, followed by 2.0 mg every 6 hours for an additional 2- to 3-day period). Normally, steroid excretion is reduced to at least 50 percent of the control values by the second day of dexamethasone administration. In patients with adrenocortical hyperplasia, suppression of steroid excretion is ordinarily apparent by the fourth to sixth day of dexamethasone therapy. Steroid excretion is usually not suppressed in patients with neoplasms of the adrenal cortex. When the test results are equivocal, the study can be repeated. The metyrapone and ACTH stimulation tests are important adjuncts that are helpful in differentiating between adrenal hyperplasia, tumor, and carcinoma.

8. Measurement of plasma testosterone, urinary testosterone, plasma or urinary gonadotropins or both, and determination of urinary 17-ketosteroids and testosterone excretion following dexamethasone and chorionic gonadotropin administration may be helpful in those cases in which the polycystic ovary syndrome, hyperthecosis ovarii, ovarian neoplasm, etc., is suspected. Occasionally, laparoscopy may also be useful.

Thyroid Enlargement
Janet E. Schemmel

DEFINITION

Enlargement of the thyroid gland is referred to as goiter. A goiter may be congenital or acquired, endemic or sporadic. Throughout the world, regions exist in which goiter is endemic. In such areas, the incidence of thyrotoxicosis, thyroiditis, and thyroid malignancy is increased.

ETIOLOGY

Enlargement of the thyroid gland may be due to many causes. Various classifications of goiter, based on the palpatory findings, the histologic examination, the state of thyroid function, or the results of laboratory tests, have been proposed. The more common causes of goiter are as follows:

1. Diffuse goiter.
    a. Euthyroid.
        (1) Endemic or sporadic diffuse goiter.
        (2) Drug-induced goiter.
        (3) Abnormality of hormone synthesis.
        (4) Thyroiditis.
            (a) Acute.
            (b) Subacute.
            (c) Chronic.
            (d) Hashimoto's struma.
    b. Hypothyroid.
        (1) Cretinism.
        (2) Juvenile hypothyroidism.
        (3) Thyroiditis and Hashimoto's struma.
        (4) Drug-induced goiter.
        (5) Abnormality of hormone synthesis.
    c. Hyperthyroid.
        (1) Graves' disease.
        (2) Subacute thyroiditis.

2. Multinodular goiter: endemic or sporadic.
    a. Nontoxic.
    b. Toxic.

3. Solitary nodular goiter.
    a. Nontoxic.
        (1) Benign.
        (2) Malignant.
    b. Toxic.

SYMPTOMS

1. Many patients with goiters are asymptomatic. The mass in the neck may be the presenting complaint, having been discovered by the

patient or brought to his attention by a relative or friend. At other times, the goiter is found by a physician during the course of a routine physical examination.

2. Absence of symptoms is common in patients with endemic or sporadic goiter, drug-induced goiter, multinodular goiter, solitary nodular goiter, early thyrotoxicosis, and Hashimoto's struma.

3. The presence or absence of systemic symptoms may provide a clue to the state of thyroid function or the presence of coexisting disease.

4. Fatigue, lethargy, a 10- to 20-pound weight gain, intolerance to cold, dry skin, and arthralgia suggest hypothyroidism. This may be the result of inadequate or abnormal thyroid hormone synthesis, thyroiditis, multinodular goiter, or drug-induced goiter.

5. Weakness, weight loss, heat intolerance, palpitation, and exophthalmos suggest thyrotoxicosis.

6. Pain in the thyroid during deglutition, or its radiation to the ear or jaw, may be indicative of subacute thyroiditis, cancer, or hemorrhage or other degenerative changes in an adenoma or cyst.

7. Dyspnea may occur when large thyroids encroach on the trachea.

8. Dysphagia suggests esophageal obstruction due to chronic thyroiditis or carcinoma but may occur whenever the gland is massively enlarged.

9. Symptoms of systemic illness, such as rheumatoid arthritis or nontuberculous Addison's disease, should raise the possibility of associated Hashimoto's struma.

10. Growth retardation in infants and children is common in hypothyroidism. Precocious puberty may also occur infrequently.

SIGNS

1. The findings on general examination depend largely on the status of thyroid function. Every patient with a goiter should be examined for clinical evidence of thyrotoxicosis or hypothyroidism. If the patient is euthyroid, the findings are usually limited to the neck area.

2. A diffusely and symmetrically enlarged thyroid that is smooth or lobulated is found in neonatal and childhood goiters, endemic or sporadic goiters, thyroiditis, and Graves' disease. The gland is usually soft in colloid goiter and classic hyperthyroidism. In Hashimoto's thyroiditis, the gland tends to be firmer than normal. Stony hard glands are usually indicative of malignancy or Riedel's struma. The presence of a vascular thrill or bruit over the thyroid gland suggests hyperthyroidism.

3. Multinodular enlargement of the thyroid gland may be observed in toxic or nontoxic endemic or sporadic goiters and, occasionally, in carcinoma or chronic thyroiditis.

4. The occurrence of a solitary nodular goiter suggests toxic or nontoxic adenoma or carcinoma.

5. The presence of cervical lymphadenopathy suggests carcinoma but may occur in Hashimoto's thyroiditis.

6. Evidence of tracheal or esophageal obstruction, or both, may occur in carcinoma, retrosternal goiter, Hashimoto's struma, or whenever the gland is massively enlarged.

7. Fixation of the gland is typical of carcinoma but occurs occasionally in thyroiditis.

8. Hoarseness due to compression of the recurrent laryngeal nerve suggests a malignant neoplasm of the thyroid.

DIAGNOSTIC APPROACH

Clinical Features

1. The duration of a goiter, the age, sex, and geographic origin of the patient, the family history, and evidence of previous exposure to goitrogenic agents may provide important clues to the cause of thyroid enlargement.

2. The nodularity of the thyroid gland is of diagnostic significance. Multinodular goiters are most often nontoxic and are rarely malignant. Solitary nodular goiters occur much more frequently in women than in men, but the incidence of carcinoma is higher in men than in women and is greatest below the age of 40 years. Functioning nodules are more likely to be benign than are nonfunctioning nodules. Solitary nodules may be toxic or nontoxic.

3. When signs of thyrotoxicosis are present, the thyroid gland is usually diffusely enlarged, although it is sometimes nodular or lobulated. Thyrotoxicosis rarely coexists with malignancy.

Initial Laboratory Studies

1. CBC and platelet count. Leukopenia and a relative lymphocytosis are common in thyrotoxicosis.

2. PBI or T_4 and T_3 uptake. These values are usually normal unless hyperthyroidism or hypothyroidism is present. Abnormal values sometimes occur in thyroiditis or when thyroid hormone synthesis is faulty. The many factors that may affect the results of these tests are beyond the scope of this discussion.

3. Thyroglobulin antibodies. Increased serum levels of antithyroglobulin antibodies may occur in Hashimoto's thyroiditis, simple goiter, thyrotoxicosis, and malignancy. Usually the incidence of positive tests and the antibody titer are higher in Hashimoto's struma than in the other conditions. The test should not be considered specific for Hashimoto's struma.

4. RAI uptake. This test is usually carried out at 6 and 24 hours after the administration of [131]I. An abnormally low level may occur in hypothyroidism, iodine contamination, and acute and subacute thyroiditis. An elevated value may be seen in iodine deficiency, certain types of thyroid hormone synthesis abnormalities, thyrotoxicosis (both diffuse and nodular types), and Hashimoto's struma. It may be normal in thyroiditis, multinodular goiter, toxic nodular goiter, and T_3 thyrotoxicosis.

5. Radiologic examination. X-ray examination may be useful in revealing the presence of retrosternal goiter, compression of the trachea, and, during a barium swallow, extrinsic pressure on the esophagus. Calcification within the thyroid gland may be demonstrable. The nature of the calcification may help to differentiate between benign and malignant lesions. Thus, the occurrence of concentrically layered calcium deposits within the gland is strongly suggestive of the presence of a follicular or medullary carcinoma, whereas spotty calcium deposits may suggest a degenerating cyst or adenoma.

6. Cytomel suppression test. When the RAI uptake is elevated, it is sometimes difficult to determine whether or not thyrotoxicosis or Hashimoto's struma is the underlying cause. A Cytomel (liothyronine) suppression test may be helpful. The drug is administered in a daily dosage of 100 μg for a 3- to 7-day period. The RAI uptake study is then repeated. Normal subjects respond with a reduction of the RAI uptake to less than 10 percent or a reduction that is greater than 50 percent of the control value. The RAI uptake of thyrotoxic glands is not affected by this procedure, whereas the uptake of the gland with Hashimoto's disease is usually, but not always, suppressed by the administration of Cytomel.

7. TSH stimulation test. This procedure can be used to differentiate between primary and secondary hypothyroidism and to determine the responsiveness of suppressed thyroid tissue surrounding a toxic nodule.

8. TSH assay. This determination is of value in distinguishing between primary and secondary hypothyroidism: TSH values are increased in the former condition but are low or immeasurable in the latter.

9. Perchlorate study. This test is indicated if an organification defect is suspected. A tracer dose of RAI is given. After a suitable interval, 500 mg of potassium perchlorate is administered by mouth. Normally, because of the rapid organic binding of the iodide, no thyroid loss of ^{131}I occurs. However, when organification is impaired, the potassium

perchlorate causes a partial or complete discharge of ^{131}I from the thyroid gland within a 30-minute period. This test is also useful in the occasional case of Hashimoto's struma in which the RAI uptake is elevated.

Further Investigations

1. Thyroid scan is usually not necessary in the thyrotoxic patient with diffuse thyroid enlargement and exophthalmos. However, a scan may be helpful in differentiating between toxic and nontoxic nodular goiter. It is particularly valuable when the iodine uptake is within the normal range. Under such circumstances, the demonstration of a single area of intense uptake is significant. In the case of nontoxic solitary nodules, radioisotope scanning may be helpful in management of the patient.

2. Indirect laryngoscopy is indicated in dysphonic patients to exclude intrinsic lesions of the larynx.

3. Thyroxin-binding globulin determination may be indicated when thyroid function tests (PBI or T_4 and T_3 resin uptake) do not correlate with the clinical picture, when hepatitis or nephrosis is present, when there is an uncertain history of previous drug therapy (e.g., diphenylhydantoin, estrogens), or if the diagnosis of primary thyroxin-binding globulin deficiency is suspected. T_4 and free T_3 tests should accompany this determination.

4. T_3 by radioimmunoassay. When the T_3 uptake is elevated in the presence of a normal T_4, the diagnosis of T_3 thyrotoxicosis is suggested. Determination of T_3 by radioimmunoassay should clarify the diagnosis.

5. Thyroid biopsy is employed chiefly to obtain tissue for enzyme studies. The diagnostic accuracy of this procedure is low.

6. Serum calcium and phosphorus levels are occasionally abnormal in both hyperthyroidism and hypothyroidism.

7. Liver function tests. A liver profile should be obtained in the presence or suspected presence of systemic disease.

8. Investigation of other family members is indicated when familial disease is suspected.

9. Ultrasonography is useful in differentiating between thyroid cysts and solid nodules.

10. Hearing and taste tests should be carried out in children with thyroid enlargement in whom either multinodular goiter or Pendred's syndrome (familial goiter with deafness) is suspected.

11. Other tests of thyroid function, the determination of iodinated products in serum, and chromatography of thyroid hormone percursors are either research procedures or are as yet not readily available clinically.

12. Therapeutic trials and surgery.   Despite the number of available tests, the cause of a goiter is not always easily determined. In such cases, thyroid hormone suppression treatment over a 6-month period may be indicated. If at the end of this period no reduction in thyroid size has occurred, surgical exploration may be advisable. Surgical exploration for both diagnostic and therapeutic purposes is indicated whenever malignancy is a reasonable possibility.

Hypocalcemia

Janet E. Schemmel

DEFINITION

Hypocalcemia exists when the serum calcium is less than 8.5 mg/100 ml as determined by the autoanalyzer using the Gitelman modification of the Kessler and Wolfman colorimetric method. This value may vary depending upon the normal values of the method as established by the individual laboratory.

ETIOLOGY

The most common cause of hypocalcemia is surgically induced hypoparathyroidism. Hence, if a thyroidectomy scar is present, the diagnosis is usually obvious. A history of antecedent illness, past gastrointestinal surgery or known underlying renal disease may elucidate the cause in other cases. The various causes of hypocalcemia include the following conditions:

1. Hypoparathyroidism.
   a. Surgically induced, partial or complete—most common.
   b. Idiopathic.
   c. Transient hypoparathyroidism of infancy (newborn)—usually partial.

2. Reduction in serum albumin.
   a. Malabsorption states.
   b. Short bowel syndrome.
   c. Chronic liver disease and liver failure.
   d. Nephrotic syndrome.
   e. Malnutrition.

3. Pancreatitis.

4. Renal disease.
   a. Renal tubular dysfunction.
   b. Acute tubular necrosis.
   c. Chronic renal failure.

5. Rickets and osteomalacia.

6. Pseudohypoparathyroidism.

7. Hypoparathyroidism in association with other disease states.
   a. Addison's disease.
   b. Pernicious anemia.
   c. Candidiasis.

8. Medullary carcinoma of the thyroid with or without associated endo-crinopathies.

SYMPTOMS

Symptoms of hypocalcemia usually occur when the serum calcium is below 7.5 mg/100 ml, but sometimes occur at higher levels when there has been a rapid decrease in the serum calcium concentration. The symptoms are generally those of neuromuscular irritability. Patients with chronic renal disease have such symptoms infrequently because of coexisting metabolic acidosis. Patients with primary gastrointestinal disease may have remarkably few symptoms, complaining chiefly of weakness, weight loss, diarrhea, increased number of stools, and abdominal cramping. Children and adults with pseudohypoparathyroidism often complain of weight problems. Patients with rickets or osteomalacia may have bone pain or problems related to the growth of bone. Hypocalcemic individuals may be asymptomatic or exhibit one or more of the following symptoms:

1. Numbness and tingling of the face, hands, and feet.

2. Muscle cramps in the arms, hands, abdomen, legs, and feet.

3. Increased number of stools or diarrhea.

4. Headaches, usually frontal; irritability; anxiety.

5. Difficulty in breathing, particularly noisy breathing during exercise or sleep.

6. Seizures, which are common; in infants this may be the only complaint.

7. Decreased vision.

8. Nail growth abnormalities and infections.

9. Dry skin, often infected.

10. Weight problems.
    a. Weight loss in association with chronic systemic disease.
    b. Difficulty in losing weight in pseudohypoparathyroidism.

11. Bone growth abnormalities or pain (in rickets and osteomalacia).

SIGNS

Physical signs may help to clarify the underlying disease. Signs of neuro-muscular irritability occur most often. It should be remembered that even when a patient has previously undergone thyroidectomy, other signs may suggest a coexisting disease. The following findings may be noted on physical examination:

1. None.

2. Thyroidectomy scar.

3. Dry skin.

4. Abnormal or infected nails.

5. Cataracts.

6. Chvostek's sign.

7. Trousseau's sign.

8. Crowing noises during sleep.

9. Seizure disorder—may be the only finding in infants.

10. Hypotension—infrequently seen.

11. Coma—rare, but does occur.

12. Bone pain or bone abnormalities, including abnormal growth, bowing, and brachydactylia—findings which suggest rickets, osteomalacia, or pseudohypoparathyroidism.

13. Goiter, if present, may suggest medullary carcinoma of the thyroid.

14. Other findings suggestive of underlying chronic disease (e.g., hepatomegaly, edema, surgical abdominal scars).

DIAGNOSTIC APPROACH

Initial Investigation

As mentioned previously, the most common cause of hypocalcemia is surgically induced hypoparathyroidism. The demonstration of hypocalcemia, hyperphosphatemia, and normal serum alkaline phosphatase, BUN, and serum albumin in a patient with a thyroidectomy scar is virtually diagnostic of hypoparathyroidism. The initial work-up should include the following tests:

1. Several determinations of serum calcium and phosphorus.
2. BUN, creatinine.
3. Serum albumin and globulin.
4. Hemoglobin and hematocrit determinations.
5. WBC and differential counts.
6. Platelet count.
7. Urinalysis.
8. Electrolytes.
9. Thyroid function tests, if the patient is not on replacement therapy.

Subsequent Investigation

1. If surgically induced hypoparathyroidism has been documented by the initial investigation, the following studies should be carried out:
   a. Slit lamp examination of the eye for cataracts.
   b. Skull films for evaluation of calcification.
   c. EEG to evaluate seizure activity.
   d. Routine chest x-rays.
   e. Routine ECG (may show Q-T interval increase).

2. Since many patients with hypocalcemia due to hypoparathyroidism may have an increased number of stools, it may be difficult to know whether primary gastrointestinal disease coexists. In these patients, the following tests may be helpful:
   a. Serum carotene—usually within normal limits.
   b. D-Xylose absorption test—usually within normal limits, but may be reduced.
   c. Seventy-two-hour stool fat—usually abnormal, with a high fat content, resembling that seen in steatorrhea of gastrointestinal origin.
   d. Serum magnesium.

3. Following therapy and restitution of the serum calcium level to normal, a 72-hour stool fat determination can be repeated. It should be normal if the hypocalcemia is secondary to surgically induced hypoparathyroidism.

4. Further investigation is indicated if the patient is thought to have another underlying disease or if no previous thyroid surgery has been performed. In addition to the aforementioned tests, the following tests may be warranted if symptoms and signs suggest other disease states:

   a. Liver function tests.

   b. Creatinine clearance, urine electrolyte excretion, urine amino acid chromatography, and ammonium chloride loading in patients with renal dysfunction from varying causes.

   c. Throat, urine, and blood fungus cultures in patients suspected of candidial infections.

   d. Long bone and hand films in patients with obesity, round face, and brachydactylia, as may be seen in patients with pseudohypoparathyroidism.

   e. Glucose tolerance test—frequently abnormal in pseudohypoparathyroidism.

   f. Barium enema, upper GI series, small bowel study, serum iron, and vitamin B_{12} and folic acid levels in patient with malabsorption or short bowel syndrome.

   g. Long bone, skull, and rib films in rickets (osteomalacia in adults).

   h. If idiopathic hypoparathyroidism is proved, the patient should be followed and studied, as indicated, for Addison's disease and pernicious anemia, which are sometimes associated with hypoparathyroidism.

   i. If a goiter is present, RAI uptake and scan should be carried out. If medullary carcinoma is suspected, neck x-rays, urinary catecholamines and VMA, and thyrocalcitonin assay, if available, should be determined.

   j. Finally, parathyroid hormone assay may be helpful in determining the cause of hypocalcemia. It is immeasurable or very low in idiopathic and surgically induced hypoparathyroidism in the few cases in which it has been determined.

Hypercalcemia

Janet E. Schemmel

DEFINITION

Hypercalcemia is said to exist when the serum calcium is 10.5 mg/100 ml or greater, as determined by the autoanalyzer, using the Gitelman modification of the Kessler and Wolfman colorimetric method. This figure may vary slightly depending upon the normal values of the method as established by the individual laboratory. Hypercalcemia is emerging as an even more complex diagnostic problem than it was in the past. With automation of laboratory procedures, biochemical screenings or profiles are often done routinely, both in the physician's office and in the hospital. The serum calcium is generally included in these screenings, and elevations are often seen in otherwise asymptomatic patients.

ETIOLOGY

Multiple causes for hypercalcemia have been elucidated, hence the diagnosis may be difficult. Sometimes the diagnosis can be established only by observation of the patient over a period of time. The various known causes of hypercalcemia include the following conditions:

1. Malignancy—most common.
   a. Carcinoma.
   b. Multiple myeloma.
   c. Leukemia; lymphoma.
   d. Nonendocrine, parathyroid hormone secreting carcinoma (e.g., lung, kidney, ovary, colon, cervix, pancreas), ectopic hyperparathyroidism.
2. Primary hyperparathyroidism.
   a. Tumor.
   b. Hyperplasia.
3. Drug-induced hypercalcemia, including the thiazides and spironolactone —increasingly common.
4. Vitamin D intoxication.
5. Milk-alkali syndrome.
6. Multiple endocrine adenomatosis; Zollinger-Ellison syndrome.
7. Others.
   a. Hypothyroidism and hyperthyroidism.
   b. Adrenal insufficiency.
   c. Sarcoidosis.
   d. Acromegaly.
   e. Immobilization.

SYMPTOMS

It is obvious from the many possible causes of hypercalcemia that a variety of symptoms may occur. Frequently, an asymptomatic patient is found to have an elevated serum calcium on routine biochemical screening. As a general rule, patients with slightly elevated serum calciums usually have fewer symptoms than those with higher values. Usually, most patients with serum calciums below 11 mg/100 ml are relatively asymptomatic, whereas most patients with serum calciums above 12 mg/100 ml are symptomatic. The following symptoms may occur:

1. None—particularly common at this time.

2. Nocturia—perhaps the earliest symptom.

3. Polydipsia, polyuria—both early symptoms.

4. Easy fatigability.

5. Irritability, difficulty in concentrating, depression, confusion.

6. Constipation, obstipation.

7. Urinary tract stones and urinary tract infections—may antedate other modes of presentation by a number of years.

8. High blood pressure—may antedate other symptoms by a number of years.

9. Muscle weakness, generalized or involving the shoulders and hips.

10. Anorexia, nausea, vomiting, abdominal pain.

11. Weight loss.

12. Joint pain.

13. Deep pain (e.g., arms, legs, back).

14. Instability when walking.

15. Headache.

16. Difficulty in focusing the eyes.

SIGNS

The physical examination may yield no abnormalities, particularly if hypercalcemia has been of short duration or if the serum calcium is 11 mg/100 ml or less. In patients with malignancy, marked weight loss may occur. Physical findings in hypercalcemia may include the following:

1. Elevated systolic blood pressure with or without elevated diastolic pressure. This is a common finding.

2. Band keratopathy on slit lamp examination of the eyes. This is an uncommon finding.

3. Rarely, a parathyroid tumor may be palpable and then usually is more than 4 gm in weight. (Most palpable anterior neck masses are of thyroid origin.)

4. Bone or muscle tenderness on pressure.

5. Proximal or generalized muscle weakness.

6. Dysequilibration.

7. Emotional lability, mental confusion.

8. Coma.

9. Weight loss, varying from 10 to 30 pounds, although none may be noted.

10. Reflexes may be normal or reduced; hypotonia may be present.

11. Skin lesions, such as purpura, ecchymosis, and petechiae may be present.

12. An enlarged liver or spleen may be palpable; lymphadenopathy may be present.

DIAGNOSTIC APPROACH

Initial Work-up

In view of the paucity of signs that may be present, the work-up may be particularly difficult. The purpose of the initial study is to establish a diagnosis, or failing that, to reduce the number of diagnostic possibilities. Patients with marked hypercalcemia should be treated immediately and diagnostic studies performed at a later, more appropriate time. The following initial studies are recommended:

1. Serial determinations of serum calcium and phosphorus to establish that hypercalcemia is present. These should be obtained while the patient is not on excessive intake of phosphate because this ion may reduce the serum calcium levels.

2. A careful review of all of the patient's medications and diet. All drugs that are not essential or that are known to influence serum calcium levels (e.g., calcium, vitamin D, thiazides, and spironolactone) should be withheld.

3. Hemoglobin and hematocrit determinations.

4. WBC and differential counts.

5. Platelet count.

6. Serum electrolytes.

7. BUN and serum creatinine.

8. Serum alkaline phosphatase.

9. Serum protein electrophoresis.

10. Urine protein electrophoresis.

11. Serum immunoglobulins.

12. Sedimentation rate.

13. X-rays—chest (PA and lateral), lumbar spine (AP and lateral), skull, and PA views of both hands.

If continuous hypercalcemia and associated hypophosphatemia are documented, the most likely diagnosis is primary or ectopic hyperparathyroidism, myeloma, or sarcoidosis. However, if normal phosphate levels are found, the diagnosis remains uncertain. If the drug history indicates the use of medications known to influence serum calcium, the drugs should be withdrawn and the patient reevaluated for hypercalcemia after approximately 4 to 6 weeks.

Patients with hypercalcemia may demonstrate slight anemia. Profound anemia is usually seen only in patients with leukemia, myeloma, malignancy, and secondary renal disease. The white blood cell, differential, and platelet counts may not be helpful except in leukemia and occasionally in myeloma. The erythrocyte sedimentation rate is frequently normal in primary hyperparathyroidism but may be elevated in malignancy, leukemia, and myeloma. It may also be elevated in patients with vitamin D intoxication and, presumably, in patients with parathyroid hormone secreting nonendocrine tumors. The serum sodium and potassium levels may be normal or reduced in primary hyperparathyroidism. The serum chloride is frequently, but not always, elevated in this disease. In patients with adrenal crisis, the serum sodium and chloride may be normal or reduced in association with elevated calcium and phosphorus levels. Elevation of the BUN and serum creatinine can be expected if hypercalcemia has been present for a long period of time or if the serum calcium is over 12 mg/100 ml. Obtaining the BUN and creatinine is helpful in determining the duration of the disease, the selection of additional tests, the appropriate treatment, and the prognosis of the renal disease that may be present.

The serum alkaline phosphatase may be normal in the presence of hypercalcemia. Elevation of this enzyme suggests the bone disease of hyperparathyroidism. However, patients with malignancy of any type may have high alkaline phosphatase levels. Measurement of the serum enzyme, gamma glutamyl transpeptidase (GGPT), may help to clarify whether an elevated alkaline phosphatase level is hepatic or bony in origin.

Routine protein electrophoresis is useful in excluding sarcoidosis and multiple myeloma. Urine protein electrophoresis should also be performed to identify the rare patient who may have an abnormal protein in the urine that is not detectable by serum protein electrophoresis. Immunoglobulins are determined for the same reason, but their usefulness in all cases is not yet known.

X-ray studies may provide the following information:

1. Chest films may disclose the presence of a hilar or peripheral lung lesion. The distal portions of the clavicles should be examined for subperiosteal reabsorption.

2. Lumbar spine films may reveal the lytic lesions of multiple myeloma. In addition, nephrolithiasis and urinary tract stones may be visualized.

3. Hand films may be normal, may demonstrate subperiosteal reabsorption, or may reveal osteoporosis. Subperiosteal reabsorption of bone is pathognomonic of hyperparathyroidism. Its absence, however, is not helpful in clarifying the diagnosis. At present, osteoporosis is perhaps the most common radiologic finding in hyperparathyroidism.

4. Skull films may demonstrate osteoporosis or the presence of a pituitary tumor, or both. Occasionally, intracranial calcification suggestive of sarcoidosis can be identified.

Subsequent Work-up

Further evaluation of the patient with hypercalcemia is dependent upon the results of the initial studies and their correlation with the symptoms and signs. If the patient has lost a considerable amount of weight, has anemia, has an elevated sedimentation rate, and has normal serum alkaline phosphatase and phosphorus levels, malignancy should be strongly suspected. If the chest x-rays are normal, further radiologic investigation should be made. A barium enema, an upper GI series, and an intravenous pyelogram are indicated. The IVP should be delayed until the results of the protein electrophoresis and immunoglobulins are known and the diagnosis of multiple myeloma has been virtually excluded. The latter is important because acute renal failure may be precipitated by pyelography in myeloma patients. In addition, sigmoidoscopy should be carried out. A bone marrow biopsy is usually indicated, especially in the presence of anemia, abnormal white cell, differential, or platelet counts, or if multiple myeloma, leukemia, or lymphoma is suspected.

A 24-hour urine collection (with the patient on a normal phosphate intake) for calcium, phosphorus, and creatinine determination may be useful. Hypercalciuria and hyperphosphaturia are commonly seen in primary or ectopic hyperparathyroidism. However, they may also occur in vitamin D overdose, myeloma, and sarcoidosis. The creatinine clearance and phosphate clearance can be calculated from the 24-hour urine collection. Phosphate clearance is almost always elevated unless creatinine clearance is markedly reduced. The tubular reabsorption of phosphorus (TRP) can be calculated (on either a random or a timed urine specimen) if the serum creatinine is 1.4 mg/100 ml or less. The formula is $TRP = 1 - \dfrac{(UP \times SC)}{(UC \times SP)}$, in which UP is urine phosphorus, SC is serum creatinine, UC is urine creatinine, and SP is serum phosphorus, in milligrams per 100 milliliters. TRP values may be subnormal or normal in hyperparathyroidism. However, it should be recalled that with prolonged oral phosphate deprivation, urinary phosphate excretion may be reduced and the tubular reabsorption of phosphorus may, therefore, appear to be normal or even elevated.

Measurement of the serum level of ionized calcium, if available, may be helpful. Although this value is high in hyperparathyroidism, it is sometimes elevated in other conditions associated with hypercalcemia.

A steroid test can be carried out to determine whether calcium suppression can be induced in patients suspected of having sarcoidosis, subclinical hyper-thyroidism, or malignancy. Dexamethasone (1 mg three times a day for 7 days) is administered. The serum calcium is determined before and after the test periods. Suppression of the calcium level occurs in myeloma, sarcoi-dosis, vitamin D intoxication, hyperthyroidism, and occasionally with im-mobilization. Unfortunately, suppression also occurs occasionally in both primary and ectopic hyperparathyroidism and in approximately 50 percent of the malignancies thus far tested. It is theoretically possible and it has been postulated that the steroid suppression test can be utilized to differenti-ate hypercalcemic, nonendocrine, parathyroid hormone secreting tumors from other malignancies associated with hypercalcemia.

If hyperparathyroidism seems likely, a barium swallow may show extrinsic pressure at the site of the tumor. Calcium infusions with measurements of the urinary calcium and phosphorus concentrations before and after infusion have not been particularly successful in elucidating the cause of hypercal-cemia. Parathyroid hormone assay, which has recently become available clin-ically, may eventually clarify the diagnostic problem. To date, the results with various assays are very promising. Certain radiologic techniques, in-cluding selenomethionine scans, esophograms, toluidine blue, and arteriog-raphy, have been used to localize parathyroid tumors. At this time, arteriog-raphy and scanning techniques can localize only parathyroid tumors that are relatively large. Measurements of parathyroid hormone in blood samples obtained by catheterization of the thyroid venous plexus have also been used to localize parathyroid tumors. More experience is needed to determine the value of all these procedures in the diagnosis of hyperparathyroidism.

At present, there is no practical or widely available method for differenti-ating hyperparathyroidism due to an adenoma from that caused by hy-perplasia or parathyroid carcinoma. The latter condition, however, is rare.

If hyperparathyroidism is considered the most likely cause of hypercal-cemia, other associated endocrine abnormalities should be considered. These include pituitary tumor, islet cell tumors, pheochromocytoma, and medullary carcinoma of the thyroid. Acromegaly is sometimes associated with hyper-calcemia and may occur in the setting of multiple endocrine adenomatosis. Even if other endocrine syndromes are not found in hypercalcemic patients with hyperparathyroidism, repeated examinations for this purpose over a period of years are advisable because of the frequency with which this association occurs. Also, since hyperparathyroidism may be familial, other members of the family should be evaluated.

Occasionally, a diagnosis cannot be made with any of the aforementioned procedures. Under such circumstances, the patient should be followed and laboratory studies repeated at appropriate intervals.

10.

Neurologic Problems

Headaches and Facial Pain

Sidney Duman
Stanley Ginsburg

HEADACHE

Headache is a symptom, not a disease.

Diagnostic Approach

History
1. Age, sex, occupation.
   a. Migraine headaches are more frequent in teenagers and young adults, with a slight predilection for females. Migraine may occur in later years coincident with the development of systemic hypertension.
   b. Cluster headaches occur almost exclusively in males.
   c. Cranial arteritis occurs more frequently in late middle age and in the elderly.
   d. Exposure to occupational toxins (e.g., carbon monoxide, lead, nitrates) may predispose to headache.

2. Duration.
   a. Tension headaches often present with symptoms of long duration.
   b. Headaches due to expanding intracranial disease are usually of short duration. It should be mentioned that patients with chronic subdural hematoma may give no history of head trauma (often the injury is forgotten).

   c. Headaches due to meningeal causes (e.g., spontaneous subarachnoid hemorrhage, acute meningitis) are usually acute in onset.
   d. Posttrauma headache, although of variable duration, tends to be self-limiting. Undue prolongation of symptoms suggests nonorganic factors.
   e. Vascular and migraine headaches are usually recurrent over a long period of time with symptom-free intervals between attacks.

3. Location of headache.
   a. As a general rule, localized headache is of greater significance than diffuse headache.
   b. Tension headaches are typically generalized, band-like, or bioccipital.
   c. Classic migraine is often unilateral and frequently more prominent anteriorly. Although the side of involvement may alternate, one side tends to be affected more frequently.
   d. Common or simple migraine is frequently bilateral.
   e. The cluster variety of migraine is invariably limited to the same side of the head in any given attack. It is usually periorbital.
   f. Headache early in the course of expanding intracranial lesions is often appreciated at the site of the expanding mass. When there is a progressive increase in intracranial pressure, the headache may become generalized.
   g. The headache of acute subarachnoid hemorrhage not only is sudden in onset but usually is generalized with predominant occipital localization.
   h. Headache due to meningitis is often predominantly occipital.
   i. Cranial arteritis is initially manifested by localized temporal headache.

4. Quality of the pain.
   a. Tension headaches are pressing, squeezing, tight, or heavy.
   b. Vascular or migraine headaches are usually throbbing or pounding.
   c. The headache associated with an expanding intracranial lesion is usually relatively mild.
   d. In acute subarachnoid hemorrhage, the pain tends to be explosive and intense. Unruptured intracranial aneurysms are usually not associated with pain. Cerebral infarction is commonly painless.

5. Prodromal symptoms.
   a. Migraine headaches are commonly preceded by such systemic complaints as euphoria, anorexia, or nausea.
   b. Migraine headaches are often preceded by such neurologic symptoms as scintillating scotomata, transient hemianopias, hemimotor or hemisensory disturbances, and dysphasia.

6. Associated symptoms.
   a. Tension headaches are usually associated with other psychophysiologic disturbances.

b. Migraine headaches may be accompanied by all of the prodromal symptoms listed above. On occasion, transitory blindness or paresis of eye movements may occur.

c. Cluster headaches are typically associated with ipsilateral lacrimation, conjunctival injection, rhinorrhea, and facial flushing. Focal cerebral symptoms or signs are absent.

d. In the case of intracranial mass lesions, the associated symptomatology is often more prominent than the headache. The symptoms that occur depend on the anatomic location of the lesion. Some intracerebral lesions (e.g., tumors, arteriovenous malformations) may exhibit seizures whereas extracerebral masses (e.g., chronic subdural hematoma) are less likely to be accompanied by seizures.

e. Cranial arteritis is often associated with systemic symptoms, including fever, anorexia, and rheumatic symptoms (polymyalgia rheumatica). Focal cerebral symptoms may be related to intracranial arterial occlusion. Ocular involvement is frequent.

7. Precipitating and aggravating factors.

a. Tension headaches and vascular headaches are commonly induced or aggravated by emotional factors.

b. Factors such as alcohol, hypoxia, systemic hypertension, and hormonal changes (e.g., menses, oral contraceptives, pregnancy) may affect the frequency of vascular headaches.

c. The headache of intraventricular and posterior fossa tumors may be accentuated by changes in head position, coughing, and the Valsalva maneuver.

8. Frequency, duration, and diurnal variation of headaches.

a. Tension headaches are often relentlessly persistent and may worsen as the day progresses.

b. The frequency of migraine headaches is variable and unpredictable. Although the usual duration is from 6 to 36 hours, they may persist for days. Migraine headaches frequently begin in sleep but may occur at any time of the day.

c. Cluster headaches usually occur repetitively over a period of weeks or months. Often there are one or two attacks daily. The headaches are typically nocturnal and of brief duration (30 minutes to a few hours). The peak incidence is in the spring and fall.

d. Expanding intracranial lesions exhibit no specific pattern.

e. The headache of acute spontaneous subarachnoid hemorrhage is persistent.

9. Family history.

a. There is usually a strong family history of migraine in patients with this type of headache. Cluster headaches are not familial.

b. Some brain tumors, especially the phakomatoses, may be reported in the family history.

Physical Examination

1. General physical examination.

   a. A flushed face, lacrimation, and unilateral rhinorrhea may be noted in cluster headaches.

   b. Facial hemangiomas and neurofibromatosis may be observed in the phakomatoses.

   c. Systemic signs of disease, such as fever, weight loss, and anemia, may be seen in the following conditions:

      (1) Infectious disease.

      (2) Specific infections of the central nervous system.

      (3) Metastatic disease to the brain or meninges, or both.

      (4) Cranial arteritis.

2. Neurologic examination.

   a. No neurologic abnormalities are noted in patients with tension headaches.

   b. A small percentage of patients with migraine may exhibit permanent residual neurologic evidence of cerebral ischemia. Most patients, however, show no neurologic abnormalities.

   c. Horner's syndrome is sometimes seen during a migraine headache, but it is rarely permanent.

   d. With any expanding intracranial lesion, localizing signs are the rule. The findings depend upon the location of the lesion.

      (1) Chronic subdural hematomas may not present with localizing or lateralizing physical signs.

      (2) Midline neoplasms may have no localizing neurologic signs.

      (3) Confusion and obtundation may be the only positive findings in chronic subdural hematomas and in midline intracranial lesions.

   e. Papilledema is observed in intracranial lesions producing increased intracranial pressure.

   f. Bruits may be audible over the eyes or cranium in vascular malformations of the brain.

   g. Signs of meningeal irritation are noted in lesions affecting the meninges.

Diagnostic Studies

1. If the history does not suggest significant neurologic disease and the clinical examination reveals nothing remarkable, no further investigation is warranted.

2. If either the history or the examination suggests organic disease, additional studies are indicated. These should include an electroencephalogram, skull x-rays, a brain scan, mapping of the visual fields, and an echoencephalogram (if available).

3. If such preliminary studies confirm the presence of a structural lesion of the brain, further studies, such as angiography, pneumoencephalography, and ventriculography, may be required.

4. Lumbar puncture is indicated in suspected subarachnoid hemorrhage, encephalitis, or meningitis. It may also be of value in the investigation of other neurologic diseases producing headache. A spinal tap is contraindicated in the presence of increased intracranial pressure, with an occasional specific exception (e.g., bacterial meningitis with associated papilledema).

5. The need for other studies is ordinarily suggested by the history and physical examination (e.g., sedimentation rate and biopsy in suspected cranial arteritis, various diagnostic x-ray studies to rule out primary neoplasm metastatic to the brain).

FACIAL PAIN

Neuralgia

Neuralgia may be defined as recurrent, usually brief, paroxysmal, intense, lancinating pain of unknown cause, localized to the distribution of a specific nerve, and not associated with objective evidence of nerve dysfunction.

1. Trigeminal neuralgia (tic douloureux).
  a. Trigeminal neuralgia may involve one or more of the sensory divisions of the trigeminal nerve.
  b. The condition usually occurs in older people. Its occurrence in patients under 35 years of age is rare and should suggest the possibility of multiple sclerosis.
  c. The frequency of episodes of pain is variable. Pain may occur many times each day or may occur infrequently. Various stimuli, such as talking, eating, exposure to cold, and local pressure, may trigger paroxysms of pain.
  d. The presence of signs of dysfunction of the fifth cranial nerve in association with neuralgia should suggest the possibility of such entities as multiple sclerosis or tumors of the nerve.
  e. The diagnosis is entirely based on the history and the absence of neurologic, radiologic, and laboratory abnormalities.

2. Glossopharyngeal neuralgia.
  a. This condition is found much less frequently than trigeminal neuralgia.
  b. The pain is generally referred to the throat or ear.
  c. The frequency of attacks is variable.
  d. The pain is often triggered by swallowing, talking, or contact with pharyngeal structures.
  e. Occasionally, glossopharyngeal neuralgia is accompanied by syncope due to associated vagal stimulation.

3. Postherpetic facial pain (postherpetic neuralgia).

   a. Postherpetic neuralgia involving any of the divisions of the trigeminal nerve may follow herpes zoster.

   b. The pain differs from typical neuralgic pain in its tendency to be more constant, its nonparoxysmal quality, and its failure to be triggered by stimuli that ordinarily aggravate conventional neuralgic pain.

   c. Objective sensory loss is usually present, and the skin of the affected area is sensitive to touch.

Atypical Facial Pain

1. The term *atypical facial pain* refers to pain that does not conform to the anatomic distribution of a nerve.

2. The pain is quite variable in character, frequency, and duration.

3. Some authorities think that it may represent a form of migraine.

4. No abnormalities are noted on physical examination. Laboratory and x-ray findings are also negative.

Other Facial Pains

Many facial pains are related to local disease affecting the teeth, nose, paranasal sinuses, mouth, eyes, ears, temporomandibular joints, etc. Careful examination supplemented by appropriate x-ray studies usually establishes the diagnosis in these disorders.

Syncope
H. Harold Friedman

DEFINITION

Syncope, or fainting, is a brief period of unconsciousness caused by reversible disturbances in cerebral function. The most common mechanism is a decrease in cerebral blood flow due to diminished cardiac output, arterial hypotension, or cerebral arterial obstruction. Altered patterns of central nervous system activity or impairment of cerebral metabolism by systemic disorders may be contributory mechanisms in some instances.

ETIOLOGY

1. Vasovagal or vasodepressor syncope (simple faint).

   a. This is the most common form of syncope, accounting for more than 50 percent of cases. Its primary mechanism is a fall in blood pressure. The symptoms and signs of the faint result from vaso-depressor and vagal responses usually initiated by pain, fear, or anxiety. Contributory factors include excessive intake of food or alcohol, close quarters, and excessive heat.

b. Fainting occurs *only* when the patient is sitting or standing.

c. Vasodepressor syncope occurs typically in young people. Fainting that begins in middle age or later in life is usually due to other causes.

d. The clinical picture is well known. The faint is almost always pre-ceded by prodromal symptoms such as a feeling of warmth, nausea, abdominal stress, yawning, or belching. The premonitory symptoms are followed by weakness, lightheadedness or faintness, pallor, sweati-ness, coldness of the hands and feet, and eventually loss of con-sciousness. During the premonitory phase, the heart rate is rapid, but when the systolic pressure falls to a critical level of 55 or 60 mm Hg, the heart rate slows (instead of accelerating) and the radial pulse usually becomes weak. Consciousness is regained rapidly with recumbency. However, symptoms may recur for a brief period after the faint if the patient tries to sit up or stand.

2. Cardiac syncope.

a. Syncope may occur when the heart is beating too fast or too slow, or, obviously, when it is not beating at all. A decreased cardiac out-put is the fundamental mechanism of this type of syncope. Heart block and cardiac arrhythmias are the most common causes.

b. *Heart block*, whether complete or incomplete, may be permanent or intermittent. Unconsciousness usually occurs when the block is complete and the idioventricular pacemaker fails to initiate impulses. However, syncope is not uncommon in second-degree atrioventric-ular block when the ventricular response is slow. The term *Adams-Stokes syndrome* refers to syncope occurring in association with heart block. The mechanism is ventricular tachyarrhythmia or asystole.

c. Fainting may occur at the onset of *paroxysmal tachycardias* because of the sudden fall in cardiac output. It may also occur at the termi-nation of a paroxysm with asystole from overdrive suppression.

d. Syncope may be the result of *sinus arrest* or *sino-atrial block*, and is common in the *"sick sinus" syndrome*. Marked sinus bradycardia, especially in the elderly, may sometimes produce syncope.

e. Fainting is a common occurrence in certain types of *organic heart disease*:

    (1) Severe aortic stenosis, *on exertion* (effort syncope).

    (2) Primary pulmonary hypertension, *on exertion*.

    (3) Idiopathic hypertrophic subaortic stenosis, *after exertion*.

    (4) Mitral valve obstruction due to a left atrial myxoma or ball-valve thrombus, a situation in which embolic phenomena are common.

    (5) Certain congenital or familial syndromes, characterized by syncope due to ventricular fibrillation and sudden death.

(6) Prosthetic mitral or aortic valves that become occluded as a result of malfunction or thrombus formation.

3. Orthostatic hypotensive syncope.

    a. Orthostatic syncope occurs *only* in the upright position (sitting or standing). The faint occurs *without* warning; its mechanism is a precipitous drop in blood pressure.

    b. Orthostatic syncope may occur *physiologically* in some individuals after prolonged standing or upon assumption of an upright position after a long period of recumbency.

    c. Orthostatic syncope may occur after *venous pooling or volume depletion* as a result of factors such as hemorrhage and sodium depletion. It may also occur following the use of drugs such as diuretics, guanethidine, and L-dopa.

    d. Orthostatic syncope may be due to *neurologic disease or disease with neurologic complications,* such as diabetic neuropathy, and tabes dorsalis. The mechanism appears to be a loss of normal sympathetic compensatory mechanisms.

    e. *Idiopathic orthostatic hypotension* may be associated with syncope. The cause of this syndrome is unknown. It is often associated with impotence, anhidrosis, and parkinsonian-like symptoms.

4. Cerebral arterial obstructive syncope. Cerebral vascular disease is one of the less common causes of syncope. It sometimes occurs in basilar artery insufficiency, the subclavian steal syndrome, and the aortic arch syndrome. Unilateral carotid artery insufficiency ordinarily does not cause fainting unless the contralateral artery is compressed. Cerebral arterial obstructive disease may render a patient more susceptible to syncope from other causes.

5. Miscellaneous causes of syncope.

    a. The *carotid sinus syndrome* is an uncommon cause of syncope. The vasodepressor type is characterized by a drop in blood pressure without a change in heart rate; the cardio-inhibitory type, by cardiac standstill; and the cerebral type, by a loss of consciousness without a change in either pulse rate or blood pressure. The diagnosis should be suspected when fainting is induced by turning the head, looking upward, or wearing tight collars.

    b. *Glossopharyngeal neuralgia* is characterized by paroxysmal pain in the throat, bradycardia, hypotension, and syncope.

    c. *Micturition syncope* is not unusual in elderly men. It is usually nocturnal. Syncope occurs during or immediately after urination.

    d. *Cough syncope* is a faint preceded by a violent coughing spell. It usually occurs in overweight men with chronic obstructive pulmonary disease.

    e. *Hysterical fainting* occurs in neurotic young women. The faint characteristically takes place in the presence of other people. Usually there are no premonitory symptoms. The vital signs are unchanged at the time of the syncope episode. Although the fainting is usually involuntary, some individuals can produce a faint at will. Beyond early adult life the diagnosis of hysterical fainting is unlikely and other causes of the fainting should be sought.

f. Syncope may occur during *hypoglycemic episodes.* The diagnosis is established by the clinical picture and low blood sugar values. Injection of glucose intravenously usually leads to a prompt return of consciousness. Although hypoglycemia may be spontaneous, the vast majority of cases occur in diabetics who are receiving insulin or oral hypoglycemic medications.

g. *Hyperventilation* may cause syncope. Paresthesias, numbness, lightheadedness, coldness, and at times tetany are the associated telltale signs of hyperventilation.

DIAGNOSTIC APPROACH

As a first step, conditions such as coma, dizziness and vertigo, seizures, and other neurologic symptoms should be excluded.

History

1. Check for systemic conditions that predispose to volume depletion and venous pooling, or for drugs that have these effects.

2. The age of the patient may be significant. Vasodepressor syncope and hysterical fainting are rare beyond early adult life. Syncope that begins during or after middle age is usually due to other causes.

3. Inquire into the circumstances of the attack.
   a. Symptoms.
     (1) Fainting preceded by pain, fear, or anxiety suggests a vasovagal origin.
     (2) Premonitory symptoms (e.g., weakness, sweating, pallor) are commonly present in vasodepressor and hypoglycemic syncope.
     (3) Associated symptoms of numbness, paresthesias, and coldness of the extremities suggest the diagnosis of hyperventilation.
     (4) Syncope preceded by prolonged standing is probably orthostatic.
     (5) Absence of warning symptoms is typical of cardiac or orthostatic syncope.
   b. Effect of posture.
     (1) In vasovagal syncope, the patient is always upright at the time of the faint.
     (2) In orthostatic hypotensive syncope, fainting occurs after prolonged standing or upon a shift from recumbency to the erect position; it never occurs in recumbency.
     (3) Fainting in the upright position with little or no warning is indicative of cardiac or orthostatic syncope.
     (4) Syncope in recumbency is almost always cardiac.

c. Sleep.   Syncope while the patient is asleep (manifested by inability to arouse the patient) suggests the cause may be cardiac, hypoglycemic, or epileptic.

d. Meals.   Syncope in the fasting state or long after a meal requires investigation for hypoglycemia.

e. Relationship to exercise.   Effort syncope is often due to aortic stenosis or primary pulmonary hypertension; posteffort syncope, to idiopathic hypertrophic subaortic stenosis.

f. Duration of syncope.   Syncope lasts but a few seconds, except in aortic stenosis, hypoglycemia, and hysteria, when it may be of longer duration.

g. Other factors.

(1) Nocturnal fainting in men in relationship to the act of urination suggests micturition syncope.

(2) Fainting following a coughing episode is characteristic of cough syncope.

(3) Fainting that occurs in relationship to head and neck movements or the wearing of tight collars may be indicative of carotid sinus syncope.

(4) Fainting in diabetics receiving insulin or hypoglycemic medications suggests hypoglycemia.

(5) Syncope associated with palpitation suggests a cardiac arrhythmia.

4. Obtain a record, if available, of the blood pressure, heart rate, and associated findings during the attack. Hypotension with a slow rate suggests vasodepressor syncope. Marked bradycardia with normal or elevated pressure implicates atrioventricular block or sino-atrial node dysfunction. Marked hypotension with a normal or rapid heart rate suggests orthostatic syncope.

5. Check for a history of organic heart disease, neurologic disease, diabetes, anemia, or cerebrovascular disease, all of which may predispose to syncope.

Physical Examination and Special Studies

1. Look for diseases or disorders (listed in the preceding paragraph) that predispose to syncope.

2. Listen for carotid bruits, and examine the patient for other evidence of cerebrovascular disease.

3. Search for signs of organic heart disease, particularly for such conditions as aortic and mitral valve disease, primary pulmonary hypertension, and the tetralogy of Fallot.

4. When cardiac arrhythmia is suspected, record an electrocardiogram, and, if necessary, monitor the patient continuously.

5. Determine the heart rate and blood pressure with the patient recumbent and after he has been standing still for at least 1 minute. Since there is normally little change in these parameters on change of position, a significant fall in blood pressure implicates postural hypotension. Orthostatic hypotension is also demonstrable on a tilt table.

6. Have the patient hyperventilate for a 2-minute period while seated to see if the symptoms of hyperventilation are similar to those of spontaneous attacks.

7. When carotid sinus syncope is suspected, massage first the right and then the left carotid bulb with the patient seated. Observe the patient for changes in clinical status, heart rate, and blood pressure. Carotid massage should be employed with great caution in the elderly and is contraindicated in cerebrovascular and some cardiac disorders.

8. When spontaneous hypoglycemia is suspected, blood sugar determinations and 5-hour glucose tolerance tests may be indicated. Specialized procedures may be necessary for the diagnosis of cardiovascular lesions, notably left atrial myxoma. Cerebral arteriography may be indicated for the diagnosis of cerebrovascular disease.

Differential Diagnosis

1. *Coma* is differentiated from syncope by the prolonged duration of the state of unconsciousness.

2. *Dizziness and vertigo* are not associated with unconsciousness, and are characterized by a subjective sensation of motion.

3. The differential diagnosis between *seizures* and *syncope* is summarized in Table 10-1.

TABLE 10-1. Differential Diagnosis of Syncope and Seizures

Parameter	Syncope	Seizures
Onset	Gradual in vasodepressor type; often sudden in other types	Sudden
Warning symptoms	Usual in vasodepressor; absent in other types	Aura common
Duration of unconsciousness	Brief	Prolonged except in petit mal
Position at onset	Usually erect or on change to erect; rarely recumbent	Any
Convulsions	Rare	Common
Incoherence, tongue biting	Rare	Common
Postictal symptoms (headache, drowsiness, confusion)	Usually absent	Usually present

Epilepsy (Seizures)

Sidney Duman
Stanley Ginsburg

DEFINITION

Epilepsy is a paroxysmal disorder of the central nervous system, sudden in onset, usually recurrent, and characterized by one or more of the following manifestations: (1) unconsciousness, (2) localized or generalized tonic spasms or clonic muscle contractions, or both, (3) sensory disturbances, and (4) psychic disturbances. The disorder may be classified into two major categories: (1) idiopathic and (2) symptomatic.

IDIOPATHIC EPILEPSY

Idiopathic epilepsy refers to seizures not directly attributable to demonstrable organic brain disease. The condition usually begins in the first two decades of life and may last well into adult life. A hereditary factor may be present. Idiopathic epilepsy may be manifested as grand mal or petit mal seizures.

Clinical Features

Major Motor Seizures (Grand Mal)

Grand mal seizures are characterized by sudden loss of consciousness, often preceded by a cry, following which the patient falls. Various injuries may occur. Usually a tonic phase, consisting of generalized muscle rigidity, precedes a clonic phase of generalized muscle activity. During this period, the patient may be incontinent of either urine or feces, and he may lacerate his tongue or buccal mucous membranes. Frothing at the mouth may occur. During the tonic phase, respirations often cease and cyanosis may occur. After cessation of the convulsive activity, flaccidity supervenes, but unresponsiveness may persist for a variable period of time. Upon awakening, the patient often is sleepy and confused. He may complain of headache or sore muscles. The postictal symptoms may persist for several hours to several days. The duration of an individual convulsion is variable, lasting from less than a minute to 30 minutes or longer. The frequency of seizures is also extremely variable. They may happen at any time of the night or day. Convulsions may occur only during sleep in some patients.

Minor Motor Seizures (Petit Mal)

1. The petit mal triad consists of:
   a. Myoclonic jerks, which are brief, sudden, involuntary muscle contractions.
   b. Akinetic seizures, in which there is a transitory loss of motor tone sufficient to cause falling without associated clonic muscle activity. Consciousness may be lost briefly.

    c. Brief absences or loss of contact with the environment without a loss of muscle tone.

  2. Classic petit mal is characterized by a blank or vacant expression and momentary cessation of motor activity without loss of muscle tone.

  3. Petit mal seizures are not followed by a postictal state. Consciousness returns promptly. Voluntary motor activity may resume immediately. Petit mal episodes often occur with great frequency. As many as 50 or more attacks in a day may occur. The onset of true petit mal epilepsy is invariably in childhood.

  4. Patients with idiopathic epilepsy often have both major and minor seizures. Although petit mal seizures usually cease spontaneously before the age of 20 years, they occasionally persist into adult life. Idiopathic grand mal seizures, however, frequently continue in adult life.

Physical Examination

Examination of the patient with idiopathic epilepsy demonstrates no localizing neurologic abnormalities. Following a grand mal seizure, bilateral extensor plantar reflexes are often present.

SYMPTOMATIC EPILEPSY

The term *symptomatic epilepsy* refers to seizures attributable to demonstrable organic brain disease. The anatomic localization of the lesion determines the clinical features of the seizure. Symptomatic epilepsy may begin at any age. The various manifestations of symptomatic epilepsy are described below.

Clinical Features

Generalized Convulsions

The generalized convulsions encountered in symptomatic epilepsy do not differ from the grand mal seizures of idiopathic epilepsy. However, unlike the latter, they may be preceded by an aura. The nature of the aura depends upon the focus of origin of the seizures. For example, the aura may be a sensation such as unpleasant odor or paresthesia in a limb. The aura should be regarded as the initial manifestation of the seizure, although it sometimes represents the entire seizure. In some instances, seizures are manifested by unconsciousness without associated involuntary motor activity. It is worth noting that a generalized convulsion may follow any variety of symptomatic epilepsy.

Temporal Lobe Epilepsy

  1. *Absences* found in symptomatic epilepsy are of themselves clinically indistinguishable from those of petit mal epilepsy. However, associated temporal lobe phenomena (e.g., lip smacking) assist in identifying their origin.

2. *Automatisms* ("psychomotor epilepsy") may be defined as repetitive automatic behavior patterns.

3. *Dreamy states,* or feelings of familiarity (*déjà vu*) or unfamiliarity (*jamais vu*) and forced or compulsive thinking.

4. *Auditory, vertiginous, olfactory, or gustatory hallucinations.*

5. *Abdominal sensations,* usually unpleasant or peculiar epigastric feelings that not uncommonly seem to radiate to the head.

6. *Visual hallucinations* are well formed in temporal lobe disturbances but tend to be ill-defined in more posteriorly situated (occipital lobe) lesions.

Focal Motor and Sensory Epilepsy
Focal motor seizures originate in the precentral cortex and are characterized by tonic or clonic muscle activity limited to one extremity, one side of the body, or one side of the face. Focal sensory seizures are similarly localized sensory phenomena that have their origin in the postcentral cortex.

1. Jacksonian seizures are motor or sensory phenomena that spread peripherally in accordance with the anatomic cortical location of the lesion.

2. Epilepsia partialis continua are continuous focal motor seizures of exceptionally prolonged duration, sometimes lasting for months.

Adversive Seizures
Adversive seizures are of frontal lobe origin. They result in deviation of the head and eyes and occasionally the body to the side opposite the lesion.

Reflex Epilepsy
Reflex epilepsy refers to seizures precipitated by some form of external stimulation. Examples are photic stimulation, reading (reading epilepsy), and music (musicogenic epilepsy).

Tonic Postural Seizures
This type of epilepsy refers to the paroxysmal occurrence of generalized muscle rigidity, often with opisthotonos. The limb posture may resemble that observed in decerebrate rigidity. Such seizures are presumed to originate in the brainstem.

Infantile Massive Spasms
This uncommonly occurring syndrome of varied causes is characterized by frequent, abrupt, myoclonic and akinetic seizures. It is often accompanied by mental retardation and a typical electroencephalographic pattern (hypsarrhythmia).

Myoclonus Epilepsy (Unverricht's Epilepsy)
This is a rare familial disorder, beginning in childhood, that is manifested by generalized convulsive and myoclonic seizures and progressive intellectual

deterioration. So-called Lafora bodies are a characteristic pathologic finding in the brain.

Postictal Symptoms

In addition to the general postictal symptoms noted above (p. 390), patients with symptomatic epilepsy may experience focal neurologic symptoms representing dysfunction of that portion of the brain responsible for the seizure. Dysphasia following a generalized convulsion is an example of this type of symptom. The occurrence of such a localized symptom makes it possible to deduce that the seizure is focal in origin, arising from the dominant hemisphere.

Physical Examination

Examination may demonstrate localizing neurologic abnormalities that may be transient (e.g., Todd's postictal paralysis) or permanent. The presence of localizing signs implies a focal lesion and thus rules out the diagnosis of idiopathic epilepsy.

Etiology

The occurrence of symptomatic epilepsy implies a focal lesion in the brain but does not specify its cause. Search for a lesion amenable to specific therapy is imperative. The types of lesions responsible for symptomatic epilepsy are listed below.

1. Localized structural lesions.
    a. Static—local brain atrophy.
    b. Progressive—neoplasms, abscesses, vascular malformations, etc.
    c. Vascular.
        (1) Thrombotic cerebral infarction—seizures uncommon.
        (2) Embolic cerebral infarction and intracerebral hemorrhage—seizures somewhat more common.
        (3) Cortical vein thrombosis—seizures frequent.

2. Diffuse structural lesions.
    a. Infections (e.g., encephalitis).
    b. Metabolic (e.g., uremia, hypoxia, hyponatremia, hypothyroidism).
    c. Degenerative (e.g., Tay-Sachs disease).

3. *Cerebral trauma.* Seizures may occur in cerebral trauma, especially in penetrating brain injuries.

4. Febrile seizures. Seizures may be caused by fever alone in children from 6 months to 3 years of age. Seizures due to focal brain lesions may sometimes be triggered by fever.

DIAGNOSTIC APPROACH TO EPILEPSY

1. All patients with epilepsy should have an EEG, a brain scan, skull films, and determinations of the fasting blood sugar, serum calcium, electrolytes, and BUN or creatinine.

2. If the EEG, skull films, or brain scan demonstrate a localized abnormality, contrast studies may be necessary.

3. Patients with focal epilepsy and those with localized neurologic symptoms or signs or both usually require angiography or pneumoencephalography.

STATUS EPILEPTICUS

Status epilepticus refers to the failure of a patient to recover from one seizure before the next attack occurs. Vigorous attempts to terminate the seizures are mandatory, since death may occur. Petit mal status epilepticus and focal status epilepticus occur occasionally.

Vertigo

Sidney Duman
Stanley Ginsburg

DEFINITION

Vertigo is a subjective sensation of movement. The patient may feel either that he is revolving in space or that the objects in his environment are moving around him. *Dizziness* is the term most commonly used by patients to describe vertigo. However, since this term may have a different meaning to different individuals, the patient should be asked to describe his symptoms in detail. It will then become apparent whether the patient is suffering from vertigo, a sensation of lightheadedness or faintness, unsteadiness of gait, a feeling of fullness in the head, or a visual disturbance (e.g., diplopia).

CLINICAL FEATURES AND ETIOLOGY

Vertigo may result from lesions of the labyrinth, the eighth cranial nerve, the brainstem, or the cerebral cortex.

Labyrinthine Vertigo

Labyrinthine vertigo is generally sudden in onset and of variable duration (several days to several weeks). The vertigo is often aggravated by changes in position. Recurrence is frequent.

Acute Labyrinthine Vertigo
Attacks of acute labyrinthitis are usually self-limiting. The vertigo is not associated with hearing loss, tinnitus, or symptoms of brainstem dysfunction. However, nausea and vomiting occur frequently. Aside from nystagmus and dysequilibrium of gait, no abnormalities are detectable on neurologic examination. It is worth noting, however, that vertical nystagmus is indicative of brainstem rather than labyrinthine disease.

Chronic Labyrinthine Vertigo (Meniere's Syndrome)
Chronic labyrinthitis is characterized by recurrent, acute, usually brief episodes of vertigo associated with tinnitus, hearing loss, nausea, and vomiting. The tinnitus and hearing loss may persist between attacks. No signs of brainstem dysfunction are noted on examination.

Toxic Labyrinthine Vertigo
Many drugs, such as streptomycin, kanamycin, aspirin, and ethacrynic acid, may affect labyrinthine and cochlear function and thereby produce vertigo.

Traumatic Labyrinthine Vertigo
Vertigo may result from relatively mild to severe cranial trauma (e.g., temporal bone fracture). Resolution of the vertigo usually occurs spontaneously.

Labyrinthine Ischemia
The acute vertigo sometimes found in the elderly or in patients with cerebrovascular disease may be the result of interruption of the blood supply to the labyrinth (via the auditory artery). The clinical picture may be similar to or indistinguishable from that which occurs in acute labyrinthitis or brainstem ischemia, but usually there are differences (see Brainstem Lesions, below).

Acoustic Nerve Lesions

Patients with eighth nerve or cerebellopontile angle tumors often complain of dizziness when in fact they mean imbalance or unsteadiness of gait. True vertigo is rare. Involvement of adjacent structures, such as the trigeminal and facial nerves, in association with unilateral ataxia, are clues to the diagnosis of such lesions.

Brainstem Lesions

Vertigo is a common symptom of acute or chronic brainstem dysfunction due, most commonly, to ischemic disease. It may also result from demyelinating diseases, inflammatory and toxic disorders, or, unusually, from destructive intramedullary lesions (e.g., neoplasms, vascular malformations, syringobulbia). The presence or absence of physical signs of brainstem dysfunction permits the differentiation between vertigo due to lesions of the brainstem and labyrinthine disturbances, respectively.

Cerebral Cortex Lesions

Vertigo may in rare instances be the manifestation of a temporal lobe cortical discharge (temporal lobe seizure).

DIAGNOSTIC APPROACH

History and Physical Examination

It is usually possible to determine the anatomic location of the lesion causing vertigo from the history and examination.

1. Labyrinthine vertigo, which is most common, is characterized by nystagmus and dysequilibrium of gait and the absence of other neurologic abnormalities.

2. Acoustic nerve lesions are characterized by evidence of both auditory dysfunction (deafness and tinnitus) and vestibular abnormality (nystagmus and ataxia), as well as by the presence of "neighborhood" neurologic signs.

3. Brainstem lesions are characterized by (1) horizontal or vertical nystagmus, or both, (2) evidence of eye muscle dysfunction or involvement of other cranial nerve nuclei, and (3) abnormalities of long tract motor, sensory, or cerebellar pathways.

4. Cerebral cortical lesions (temporal lobe seizures) are rare causes of vertigo.

5. Ischemic labyrinthine disease can usually be differentiated from ischemic brainstem disease by the absence of the neurologic abnormalities described in paragraph 3 above.

Caloric and Audiometric Testing

These procedures are valuable in suggesting labyrinthine rather than cerebral cortex or brainstem lesions as the cause of vertigo. Electronystagmography, a more sophisticated type of caloric investigation, is employed in some medical centers in place of conventional caloric testing.

X-ray Studies

1. Skull films are of value in viewing the internal auditory meatus and canal.

2. Cervical spine x-rays may be useful in demonstrating vertebral foraminal encroachment, which sometimes causes obstruction of the arterial blood flow to the brainstem and the peripheral auditory apparatus.

Electroencephalogram (EEG)

The EEG may be of help in the identification of irritable cortical foci producing temporal lobe seizures.

Brain Scan

This procedure may be of assistance in the diagnosis of temporal lobe mass lesions and, less commonly, posterior fossa lesions.

Lumbar Puncture

Examination of the spinal fluid is occasionally helpful diagnostically. For example, the protein concentration is typically elevated in acoustic neurinomas, and abnormal protein electrophoretic patterns may be observed in the demyelinating diseases.

Contrast Angiography

Contrast studies may be necessary for the demonstration of specific intracranial lesions.

Weakness of Neuromuscular Origin

Sidney Duman
Stanley Ginsburg

Weakness is one of the most common complaints presented to the physician. This section deals only with weakness produced by neuroanatomic or neurophysiologic lesions. Other causes of weakness are considered elsewhere in the book. Since weakness of neuromuscular origin is manifested by objective evidence of reduced muscle strength, manual testing of muscle function is an important early step in the evaluation of weakness.

ETIOLOGY

The various neuromuscular causes of weakness and paralysis can be divided into five major groups:

1. Disease of the upper motor neurons (the long motor pathways of the brain and spinal cord, consisting of the corticobulbar and corticospinal pathways).

2. Disease of the lower motor neurons (the anterior horn cells of the spinal cord and the motor nuclei of the brainstem).

3. Disease of the nerve roots and the peripheral nerves.

4. Disease of the myoneural junction.

5. Disease of skeletal muscle.

Table 10-2 lists the more common causes of these anatomic lesions.

CLINICAL FEATURES
Upper Motor Neuron Disease
Chronic Lesions
1. The weakness is located below the anatomic level of the lesion.

2. Unilateral lesions situated above the pyramidal decussation in the medulla produce weakness on the contralateral side, whereas those situated below this level produce ipsilateral weakness.

3. The weakness is in "elective distribution," that is, in patients who are not completely paralyzed, the pattern of involvement is selective.

TABLE 10-2.   Common Causes of Neuromuscular Weakness and Paralysis

Anatomic Site of Involvement	Location	Disease State
Upper motor neurons (long motor pathways)	Brain	Infarction Hemorrhage Neoplasm Infection
	Brainstem	Infarction Motor neuron disease (progressive pseudobulbar palsy) Neoplasm
	Spinal cord	Demyelinating diseases Neoplasm Primary lateral sclerosis
Lower motor neurons	Brainstem	Progressive bulbar palsy Syringobulbia Poliomyelitis
	Spinal cord	Progressive muscular atrophy Syringomyelia Poliomyelitis
Nerve roots and peripheral nerves	Nerve roots	Intervertebral disc herniation Metabolic radiculopathies (e.g., diabetic neuropathy)
	Peripheral nerves	Metabolic disorders Inflammatory disorders Trauma
Myoneural junction	. . .	Myasthenia gravis Botulism
Muscle	. . .	Polymyositis Muscular dystrophies

a. In the upper extremity, the muscles that produce abduction, external rotation, and extension of the joints are primarily affected. The antagonistic muscle groups are usually less severely involved.

b. In the lower extremity, the muscles responsible for flexion and internal rotation of the articulations are the ones that are primarily involved. However, with respect to the ankle, it is the dorsiflexors that are weakened and the plantar flexors that are relatively spared.

c. The demonstration of weakness in elective distribution is virtually diagnostic of disease of the long motor tracts.

4. Spasticity of the involved extremities is seen commonly.

5. The deep tendon reflexes are increased and the superficial reflexes are lost on the affected side.

6. Pathologic reflexes, such as the Babinski sign, are noted frequently.

Acute Lesions

1. The onset of weakness is sudden.

2. An elective pattern of weakness is observed, as with chronic lesions.

3. Flaccidity or hypotonia is commonly present during the acute phase.

4. The deep tendon reflexes may be depressed or absent.

Comments

1. Weakness with any of the aforementioned characteristics indicates disease of the central nervous system but does not imply a specific cause. All disease processes involving the long motor pathway produce similar findings.

2. Lesions of the extrapyramidal tracts (e.g., parkinsonism) or cerebellar pathways may also present as weakness but without objective evidence of decreased muscle strength.

Pseudobulbar Palsy

Bilaterally situated corticobulbar lesions, regardless of cause, may produce the syndrome referred to as pseudobulbar palsy. It is characterized by dysphagia, dysarthria associated with clumsy movements of a spastic tongue, loss of emotional control with frequent outbursts of crying or laughter, exaggerated jaw and pharyngeal reflexes, and the appearance of sucking and snout reflexes.

Lower Motor Neuron Disease

1. The motor involvement is segmental in distribution.

2. The affected musculature is flaccid and ultimately becomes atrophic.

3. Fasciculations of the involved muscles are typically observed.

4. Depression or loss of tendon reflexes occurs in the involved segments.

5. Sensory abnormalities do not occur.

6. Bulbar palsy. Lesions of the motor nuclei of the brainstem produce the syndrome of bulbar palsy. The clinical picture is similar to that of pseudobulbar palsy. However, as with other lower motor neuron lesions, the muscles innervated by the motor nuclei of the brainstem (e.g., the tongue) become weak, flaccid, and atrophic, and usually show fasciculations. The jaw jerk and gag reflex are diminished or absent. Loss of emotional control is not a feature of bulbar palsy.

Disease of the Nerve Roots and Peripheral Nerves

Monoradiculopathies and Mononeuropathies

1. Weakness is limited to those muscles innervated by the affected nerve roots or nerves.

2. The weakness produced by these lesions is similar to that found in disease of the lower motor neurons:

a. Hypotonia is commonly present, and the deep tendon reflexes are depressed or absent.

b. Although atrophy often occurs, it is less prominent than that noted with involvement of the anterior horn cells.

c. Fasciculations are a rare occurrence in lesions of the nerve roots or peripheral nerves.

Polyneuropathies

1. The quality of the muscle weakness and the associated phenomena, such as hypotonia and depressed reflexes, are similar to those seen with anterior horn cell disease or lesions of the nerve roots or peripheral nerves.

2. The distinguishing feature of the polyneuropathies is the more widespread distribution of the weakness. It tends to be bilateral, symmetric, and more prominent in the distal than in the proximal portions of the affected extremities. The legs are more likely to be involved than the arms.

3. Sensory changes may or may not accompany the weakness caused by peripheral nerve lesions.

Disease of the Myoneural Junction

Diseases of the myoneural junction resemble the myopathies more than the neuropathies. As a general rule, muscle weakness is more prominent proximally than distally, sensory changes do not occur, and there are no significant early reflex changes.

Myasthenia gravis is a disease of the myoneural junction with very specific clinical characteristics, as listed below.

1. There is undue fatigability of the musculature. The weakness of the muscles is greatest after physical exercise and at the end of the day. Following rest, there is improvement in the muscle strength.

2. Although weakness may be generalized, there is a predilection for involvement of the muscles supplied by the nuclei of the brainstem as well as the proximal limb musculature. Involvement of the ocular muscles is especially frequent.

3. Improvement of muscle strength following the administration of anticholinesterase drugs (neostigmine or edrophonium) is typical and virtually diagnostic.

4. In advanced cases, the muscle weakness may be permanent and may fail to respond either to rest or to drugs.

5. A progressive diminution in the muscle response to repetitive electrical nerve stimulation is typical and often diagnostic.

6. Myasthenic features may occur in patients with myopathy due to various malignancies (Eaton-Lambert syndrome). Electrical studies may help in differentiating this condition from myasthenia gravis. In the Eaton-Lambert syndrome, repetitive electrical nerve stimulation at slow frequencies produces a decreased response, but at higher frequencies there is an augmentation of muscle potentials.

Disease of Skeletal Muscle (Myopathies)

1. Muscle weakness is usually symmetrically distributed but tends to affect the proximal musculature more than the distal musculatures.

2. Sensation is unimpaired.

3. The deep tendon reflexes are preserved.

4. Muscle atrophy is not an early feature.

DIAGNOSTIC APPROACH

1. In the patient with bona fide muscular weakness, it is usually possible to determine clinically whether the lesion is located in the upper motor neurons, the lower motor neurons, the nerve roots or peripheral nerves, the myoneural junction, or the muscles.

2. In the case of suspected central nervous system lesions, it may be advisable to obtain skull films, a brain scan, and an electroencephalogram. When spinal cord involvement is suspected, appropriate x-ray studies of the spine (cervical, dorsal, or lumbar) are indicated. Systemic laboratory studies that may assist in establishing the cause are also warranted.

3. In the case of peripheral lesions, the following routine studies are advisable: CBC, sedimentation rate, muscle enzyme levels, serum protein electrophoresis, immunoglobulins, LE cell preparations, ANA, and serologic test for syphilis. Under some circumstances, investigation for porphyria or heavy-metal poisoning may be indicated.

4. The edrophonium and neostigmine tests and electrical nerve stimulation tests are the procedures of choice for the diagnosis of myasthenia gravis.

5. Electromyography is useful in evaluating suspected lesions affecting the anterior horn cells, muscle, and peripheral nerves.

6. In myopathies, muscle biopsy, with examination of the tissue under both light and electron microscopy, and histochemical studies may be helpful.

Selected Neurogenic Pain Syndromes
Sidney Duman
Stanley Ginsburg

CENTRAL NERVOUS SYSTEM PAIN

Pain arising from disease of the central nervous system is an infrequently diagnosed occurrence clinically. The anatomic structures from which such pain most commonly originates are the thalamus and spinal cord. The causes of painful central lesions are varied.

Pain of central origin is typically constant, intractable, burning in quality, and agonizing. Exacerbations of more severe pain often occur spontaneously or in response to minimal cutaneous stimulation. The associated neurologic findings depend upon the anatomic site of the lesion.

The thalamic syndrome is a classic example of central pain that is cerebral in origin. It is characterized by severe, intractable pain as well as by contralateral hemiparesis and hemihypesthesia, both of which may become permanent. Any lesion of the thalamic structures (e.g., infarction, neoplasm) may produce the thalamic syndrome.

Central pain originating in the spinal cord results from trauma or disease affecting the spinothalamic pathways (e.g., cord injuries, multiple sclerosis). The precise nature of the associated neurologic abnormalities depends on the anatomic site of the lesion.

In the case of cerebral disease, skull films, a brain scan, and an electroencephalogram should be obtained. When the spinal cord appears to be involved, appropriate x-rays of the spine should be done. Lumbar puncture and myelography may also be indicated.

PAINFUL UPPER EXTREMITY

Cervical Radiculopathies

History
The patient usually complains of neck pain that radiates in dermatomal distribution. Suprascapular pain on the affected side is also common. Dysesthesias in the distribution of the involved nerve root may be noted. Both the pain and the dysesthesias are frequently aggravated by neck movements and by the Valsalva maneuver. The nerve roots most commonly involved are C7 and C6. Involvement of C5 and C8 occurs less frequently.

Physical Findings
Tenderness in the cervical and paracervical regions is common. Motor and sensory changes, as well as decreased or absent reflexes, are usually noted. The types of abnormalities that occur are listed in Table 10-3.

Etiology
Of the variety of causes, the most common causes are nerve root compression from foraminal encroachment by bony spurs or intervertebral disc herniation. Less frequent causes are inflammatory masses or neoplasms.

Diagnostic Approach
The level of the lesion can usually be determined clinically. Cervical spine films, including AP, lateral, and oblique views, should be obtained. Other diagnostic studies that may be helpful are electromyography and myelography. In some instances, the correct diagnosis can only be established at the time of surgery.

Brachial Plexus Neuropathy

1. Brachial plexus neuropathy may be idiopathic, or it may follow infectious diseases or inoculations.

TABLE 10-3. Neurologic Signs in the Cervical Radiculopathies

Type of Abnormality	Nerve Root Affected				
	C5	C6	C7	C8	T1
Major sensory abnormality (hypalgesia)	Lateral arm	Lateral forearm and thumb	Middle finger	Little finger	Medial forearm
Major motor abnormality (weakness)	Biceps, supra-spinatus, infraspin-atus, deltoid	Brachio-radialis	Triceps	Wrist and finger flexors	Intrinsic hand muscles
Reflex changes (decreased or absent reflexes)	Biceps	Brachio-radialis	Triceps	None	Finger flexors

2. An acute onset with severe pain, usually located about the shoulder and upper arm, is typical.

3. Muscle weakness usually develops eventually. It has a predilection for the proximal musculature of the arm, but any of the muscles of the upper extremity may be involved. The deltoid, infraspinatus, and supraspinatus muscles are most commonly affected; the trapezius and serratus anterior muscles, somewhat less often.

4. Involvement of the phrenic nerve may cause diaphragmatic paralysis.

5. Physical examination (see above) reveals weakness and often atrophy of the affected musculature. Sensory changes may occur but are less prominent than the motor abnormalities.

6. Spontaneous recovery, which is often complete, generally takes place over a period of several months or years. The recovery time tends to be longer when the distal portion of the limbs is the major site of involvement.

Other Brachial Plexus Lesions

Direct (penetrating injuries) and indirect (torsion, pressure) trauma accounts for about 50 percent of brachial plexus lesions. Pain is usually caused by the musculoskeletal injury rather than by damage to the plexus. Tumors involving the brachial plexus are usually quite painful. Most often these are metastatic (e.g., Pancoast's tumor). In addition to the motor and sensory deficits, Horner's syndrome is a not uncommon finding.

The Thoracic Outlet Syndrome

1. The thoracic outlet syndrome comprises a number of conditions in which the neurovascular bundle is subjected to pressure at the thoracic outlet. The subclavian and axillary vessels as well as the brachial plexus may be compressed.

2. Pain and paresthesias, usually in C8 and T1 distribution, are the most common symptoms. However, sensory disturbances may affect other parts of the extremity. Numbness and clumsiness are also frequent complaints. Ischemic symptoms are present in some cases, but muscle weakness is less common. Positional and postural changes may initiate or aggravate the symptoms.

3. Objective signs of neurologic dysfunction are lacking in most cases, but motor weakness and sensory disturbances in C8 and T1 distribution are observed occasionally.

4. The reproduction of the pain and paresthesias and the diminution or obliteration of the pulse by various maneuvers are considered to have diagnostic significance. The reader is referred to the sections Chest

Pain, Chapter 3, and Painful Shoulder, Chapter 8, for additional information.

5. Plethysmography, nerve conduction studies, and angiography may be helpful diagnostically.

Peripheral Nerve Lesions

Ulnar Neuropathy

Paresthesias involving the little finger and the ulnar side of the ring finger are the major manifestation of ulnar neuropathy. Objective sensory changes occur in similar distribution. Pain is relatively slight. Weakness and atrophy of the intrinsic muscles of the hand, such as the interossei and the two lateral lumbricals, may be noted.

Median Neuropathy (Carpal Tunnel Syndrome)

1. Pain and paresthesias are the most prominent symptoms of the carpal tunnel syndrome. Although these sensations are generally referred to the area of distribution of the median nerve, many patients also complain of discomfort in the forearm. The symptoms are frequently aggravated by inactivity. Nocturnal pain is often quite severe and may awaken the patient from sleep.

2. The syndrome may occur unilaterally or bilaterally. It tends to occur most frequently in individuals whose occupations require repeated wrist movements (e.g., typists). Median neuropathies are also prevalent in such diseases as rheumatoid arthritis, myxedema, and acromegaly.

3. Examination usually discloses tenderness over the transverse carpal ligament. Percussion at this site may reproduce the discomfort (Tinel's sign). Wrist movements may act in a similar fashion. Sensory loss may occur over the palmar surface of the first three fingers, the radial half of the ring finger, and the medial portion of the hand. Weakness, with or without atrophy, of the short abductor of the thumb and the opponens pollicis is observed commonly.

PAINFUL LOWER EXTREMITY

Lumbosacral Radiculopathies

History

The patient typically complains of low back and gluteal pain that radiates to the lower extremity. The distribution of the pain in the lower extremity depends on the nerve root affected. Involvement of the lower nerve roots (L5 and S1) is generally manifested by pain that radiates along the posterior and lateral aspects of the thigh and leg. Lesions of the upper lumbar nerve roots usually produce pain that radiates more anteriorly, especially to the thigh. The pain is characteristically aggravated by back movements and the Valsalva maneuver.

TABLE 10-4. Neurologic Signs in the Lumbosacral Radiculopathies

Type of Abnormality	Nerve Root Affected		
	L4	L5	S1
Major sensory abnormality (hypalgesia)	Medial calf	Lateral calf, dorsomedial aspect of foot and great toe	Posterior calf; sometimes, lateral aspect of the foot
Major motor abnormality (weakness)	Quadriceps, and iliopsoas; sometimes, adductors of the thigh	Extensors of the toes and ankle	May have weakness of the toe extensors
Reflex changes (decreased or absent)	Knee jerk	None	Ankle jerk

Physical Findings
Motor and sensory changes as well as decreased or absent reflexes are usually noted. The types of abnormalities encountered are summarized in Table 10-4.

Etiology
1. Intervertebral disc herniation is the most common cause. The S1 and L5 nerve roots are most frequently affected, although L4 involvement also occurs. Additional information about herniated intervertebral discs may be found in the section Low Back Pain, Chapter 8.

2. Diabetic radiculopathy is also a common cause. The L4 root is most frequently involved in this condition.

3. Primary and metastatic neoplasms may also cause radiculopathies.

Diagnostic Approach
Usually, a fairly accurate diagnosis can be established from the history and physical examination. Lumbosacral spine films should be obtained. Electromyography and myelography may also be helpful diagnostically.

Meralgia Paresthetica (Lateral Femoral Cutaneous Neuralgia)

Meralgia paresthetica is the term applied to the syndrome of entrapment of the lateral femoral cutaneous nerve at the lateral aspect of the inguinal ligament. The primary symptom is a burning, superficial type of discomfort located in the anterior and lateral aspects of the thigh. Complaints of itching and "numbness" may also be noted. Examination usually reveals hypalgesia of the involved area of the thigh. There are no motor or reflex changes.

Spinal Fluid Findings in Disease

Sidney Duman
Stanley Ginsburg

The spinal fluid findings in the more common neurologic abnormalities are shown in Table 10-5.

TABLE 10-5. Spinal Fluid Findings in Disease

Disease	Initial Pressure (mm CSF)	Appearance	Cells (per cubic mm)	Protein (mg/100 ml)
Normal	70 to 150	Clear, colorless	0 to 5; monos	15 to 45
Infections of the Central Nervous System				
Tuberculous meningitis	Often ↑	Opalescent, faintly yellow; fibrin clot	50 to 300; monos	60 to 700
Fungal and yeast meningitis	Often ↑	Opalescent	30 to 500; monos	100 to 700
Acute purulent meningitis	Often ↑	Turbid	Few to 20,000; chiefly polys	100 to 1000
Acute anterior poliomyelitis	N	Clear, colorless	50 to 250; chiefly monos	40 to 100
Viral meningitis and encephalitis	N (rarely elevated)	Clear, colorless	Few to 350; chiefly monos	40 to 100
Brain abscess	May be ↑	Clear, colorless; may be xanthochromic	Few to 100; monos predominate	40 to 140
Landry-Guillain-Barré disease	N	Clear, colorless	N	50 to 1000
Acute syphilitic meningitis	N to slightly ↑	Clear to slightly opalescent	300 to 2000; monos	50 to 400
Meningovascular syphilis	N	Clear, colorless	10 to 50; monos	50 to 100
Parenchymatous syphilis	N	Clear, colorless	10 to 40; monos	50 to 100

N = normal, ↑ = increased, ↓ = decreased, monos = mononuclear leukocytes, polys = polymorphonuclear leukocytes
SOURCE: Modified from R. R. Grinker, P. C. Bucy, and A. L. Sahs, *Neurology*, 6th ed. Springfield, Ill.: Thomas, 1966.

Culture	Sugar (mg/100 ml)	Chlorides	Colloidal Gold Curve	Comments
	40 to 80		0000000000	

		Infections of the Central Nervous System		
Positive for acid-fast bacilli	<20	Diminished	Variable	Polys in acute phase
Positive (smear may demonstrate fungi)	<30	Diminished	Variable	Positive india ink prep in cryptococcosis
Positive (smear often positive)	<20	Often N	Variable	Early, or in partially treated forms, cell count may be low
Negative	N	N	Variable	In preparalytic stage, polys may exceed 80%
Negative	N	N	Variable	Polymorphonuclear reaction early; virus cultures may be positive
Negative	N	N	Variable	
Negative	N	N	Variable	Similar changes in various other polyneuropathies (e.g., diabetes)
Negative	N	N	First or midzone	Serologic tests nearly always positive
Negative	N	N	Usually midzone	Serologic tests positive in 60%
Negative	N	N	First zone in paresis; midzone in tabes	Serologic tests positive in practically all untreated paretics; usually negative in tabes

TABLE 10-5.   (*Continued*)

Disease	Initial Pressure (mm CSF)	Appearance	Cells (per cubic mm)	Protein (mg/100 ml)
Miscellaneous Conditions				
"Bloody tap"	N	Blood-tinged; *supernatant fluid colorless*	RBC; WBC ratio similar to peripheral blood	Slightly ↑ (depends on amount of blood introduced)
Early subarachnoid hemorrhage	Elevated	Bloody; faintly yellow supernatant	Many RBCs	50 to 400
Late subarachnoid hemorrhage	Elevated	Slightly bloody; supernatant deep yellow	Fewer RBCs; WBCs ↑ due to aseptic meningitis	100 to 800
Spinal cord tumor (with "block")	Low	Deep yellow; may coagulate	5 to 50; monos	Up to 6000
Brain tumor	May be ↑	Clear or yellow	Usually normal; may have few monos	N to 150
Meningeal carcinomatosis (carcinomatous meningitis)	May be ↑	Clear to turbid	20 to 300; (may be mixture of malignant and inflammatory cells)	60 to 200
Multiple sclerosis	N	Clear, colorless	5 to 50 monos	N to 80
Cerebral infarction	N (occasionally elevated)	Clear	Usually normal; occasionally a few monos (RBCs frequent in embolic infarction)	N to 80
Cerebral hemorrhage	Often ↑	Blood-tinged (sometimes grossly bloody)	RBCs; varying number WBCs, especially late	50 to 200

Culture	Sugar (mg/100 ml)	Chlorides	Colloidal Gold Curve	Comments
Miscellaneous Conditions				
Negative	N	N	Variable	Progressively less bloody in consecutive tubes
Negative	N	N	Variable	
Negative	May be de-pressed	N	Variable	RBCs disappear in about 2 weeks; xanthochromia may persist for several weeks
Negative	N	N	Variable	No rise of pressure on jugu-lar compression
Negative	N	N	Variable	Occasionally cytologic examination will reveal tumor cells
Negative	Often de-pressed	N	Variable	Cytologic examination often reveals tumor cells
Negative	N	N	First or midzone rise	Gamma globulin fraction may be ↑
Negative	N	N	Variable	Pleocytosis when infarct is in proximity to ven-tricle or subarach-noid space
Negative	N	N	Variable	

Index

Note: To avoid unnecessary repetition within this index, the reader may assume that major discussions of the medical entities indexed include definition and etiology.

Cholinergic drugs, in diagnosis of tachycardia, 130
Cholinergic urticaria, 28, 30
Chordae tendinae, ruptured, as cause of
mitral regurgitation, 102
Christmas disease. *See* Hemophilia, B
Chvostek's sign, and hyperaldosteronism,
60
Chylothorax, pleural effusion in, 175
Cigarette smoking, in chronic cough, 151
Cineradiography
in dysphagia, 182
esophageal, in heartburn, 178, 179
Circulatory disturbances, and pruritus,
25
Cirrhosis of liver
and clubbing, 2
and increased pulse pressure, 51
nonalcoholic etiology, and hepatomegaly, 206
pleural effusion in, 173
Claudication, intermittent, in chronic
arterial occlusion, 134
Clearance, defined, 271
Click, systolic, 79
Clotting, disorders of, 240–251
Clotting factor deficiencies
acquired disorders, 248–249
diagnosis of, 241, 242
hereditary, 243–244
Clotting reaction, 240
Clubbing
bilateral, diagnostic approach to, 2
in bronchiectasis, 155
clinical features of, 1
and cyanosis, 158
defined, 1
as general problem, 1–3
in severe central cyanosis, 160
unilateral, 2
Cluster headaches, 379, 381
Coagulation disorders
diagnosis of, 241, 242
hemoptysis in, 155
physical findings in, 156
roentgenogram in, 156
Coagulation screen, preoperative, 242–
243
Coin lesions. *See* Lung, coin lesions of
Colchicine, in gout, 293
Cold
exposure to, and peripheral cyanosis,
159–160
and urticaria, 28–29
Cold agglutinins, and sputum of dyspnea, 144
"Cold feet," 134

Colic
renal
defined, 256
and ureteral, 256–257
ureteral, defined, 256
Colitis, ulcerative
and basophilia, 236
as cause of FUO, 11, 12
and chronic diarrhea, 192
Colon
disease of
and chronic diarrhea, 191
hematemesis and melena in, 185
proximal, diseases of, and hematemesis and melena, 184
Colonofiberoscopy, in chronic diarrhea,
197
Concentration tests, of kidney function,
270
Congenital heart disease, vs. cardiomyopathy, 118
Congestion, central circulatory, neck vein
distention in, 46
Connective tissue diseases
and clotting factor inhibitors, 244
diagnosis of, 12
dyspnea in, 145
and fever of unknown origin, 10, 11,
12
hemolytic anemia and, 225
kidney involvement in, 254
and myalgia, 305
in painful hip, 317
and peripheral joint arthritis, 292
and proteinuria, 266
Consolidation collapse, of lung. *See*
Atelectasis
Constipation, 197–198
acute, 198
alternating with diarrhea, 193, 197
chronic, etiology of, 197–198
diagnostic approach, 198
Contactants, and urticaria, 30
Contraceptives, oral
and pulmonary embolism, 42
and secondary hypertension, 55
Convulsion(s)
generalized, in symptomatic epilepsy,
391
in grand mal, 390
Coombs' test, in hemolytic anemia, 220,
223
Cor pulmonale, and abnormal jugular
venous pulse, 48
Coronary artery disease, chest pain in,
35

in diagnosis of FUO, 13
in peripheral joint arthritis, 295
regional and generalized, differential diagnosis, 239
Lymphedema
primary, pleural effusion in, 174
unilateral, due to pelvic neoplasm, 4
Lymphocyte count, in lymphocytosis, 234
Lymphocytosis, 234–235
activated, causes of, 235
in chronic dyspnea, 148
drug-induced, 235
infectious, 235
nonactivated, causes of, 235
Lymphoma(s)
fever in, 12
in lymphadenopathy, 240
and pruritus, 22, 23
radiologic signs, 170–171
of spleen, 238
Lymphoproliferative disorders, pleural effusion in, 174

Malabsorption diarrhea, 191, 193, 196
Malabsorptive states, anorexia and weight loss in, 18
Malignancy
anorexia and weight loss in, 18
and ascites, 205
and back pain, severe, 324
of coin lesion of lung, 167–168
evaluation for, as a cause of unexplained pruritus, 26
and goiter, 365
and hematemesis and melena, 186
and hypercalcemia, 373
and mediastinal masses, 169
and myasthenic features, 401
occult, weight loss and, 16
pleural effusion in, 175
and pruritus, 23, 24
and thyroid enlargement, 368
Malingering, and fever of unknown origin, 11, 13
Mallory-Weiss syndrome, and hematemesis and melena, 184, 186
Malnutrition
and edema, 5
in hypoalbuminemia, 7
and hypoglycemia, 335
and weight loss, 17
Mammary souffle
continuous murmurs of, 112
vs. jugular venous hum, 113

Maneuvers, physiologic and pharmacologic, effects on heart murmurs, 84
Manometry, in measurement of venous pressure, 44
Marfan's syndrome, and diastolic murmurs, 107
Massage, carotid sinus. See Carotid sinus massage
Mast cell disease. See Urticaria pigmentosa
Mature, failure to, 339–344
diagnostic approach, 342–344
signs of, 341
symptoms of, 340
with growth retardation, 341
without growth retardation, 341
Mediastinoscopy
in bronchogenic carcinoma, 154
in mediastinal tumors, 172
Mediastinum
location of, 168
masses in, 168–172
diagnostic approach, 169–170
importance of prompt diagnosis, 172
radiologic signs, 170
sites of predeliction of, 169
Mediators, chemical, of pruritus, 21
Medroxyprogesterone acetate, in secondary amenorrhea, 354
Meigs' syndrome
and ascites, 204
pleural effusion in, 173
Melena, 182–188
causes of, 184
diagnostic approach, 186–188
diagnostic studies, 188
Meniere's syndrome. See Vertigo, labyrinthine chronic
Menses, abrupt cessation of, 350
Menstrual bleeding, and anemia, 214, 220
Menstrual history, in hematuria, 268
Menstruation, failure to occur. See amenorrhea
Meralgia paresthetica, 406
Mesantoin, and lymphocytosis, 235
Metabolic disorders
anorexia and weight loss in, 18
kidney involvement in, 253
Metabolic problems, 329–377
Metabolism, accelerated, and weight loss, 16
Metastasis
and marrow failure anemia, 217
and mediastinal mass, 171

Opium derivatives, reactions to, as cause of pruritus, 23, 25
Oral lesions, as cause of weight loss, 18
Osteitis condensans ilii, mimicking sacro-ileitis, 326
Osteitis deformans. *See* Paget's disease
Osteoarthritis
  and chest pain, 36
  clinical features of, 299
  of hip, 318
  and hip pain, 320
  and low back pain, 322
  of lumbar spine, radiologic findings, 325–326
  and peripheral joint arthritis, 292
Osteoarthropathy, hypertrophic
  vs. chronic polyarthritis, 299
  defined, 1
Osteomalacia, and hypocalcemia, 369
Osteoporosis
  and low back pain, 322
  radiologic findings, 325
Ovarian disease, in secondary amenor-rhea, 351
Ovarian dysgenesis, 348
  and amenorrhea, 345
Oxygen saturation, arterial, in polycy-themia, 227

PES. *See* Heart sound(s), systolic, pulmonary ejection
pCO₂. *See under* Blood
pH
  of blood
    abnormalities of, 286–289
    pathophysiology and, 278
  urine, 264
    in nephrolithiasis, 258
PRA. *See* Plasma renin activity
PT. *See* Prothrombin time
PTT. *See* Thromboplastin time, partial
Paget's disease
  and increased pulse pressure, 51
  and myalgia, 306, 307
  radiographic findings in, 326
Pain
  in abdominal distension, 200
  anginal, characteristics of, 34
  central nervous system, 402
  chest. *See* Chest pain
  of chronic arterial occlusion, 134
  of dissecting hematoma, 40
  facial, 383–384
  in gallstones, 208
  of headache, 380
  in hip, 317–319

low back, 311, 321–327, 405
  diagnostic approach, 323
muscle. *See* Myalgia
musculoskeletal, 36–37
of myocardial infarction, 38
neck, 403
in peptic ulcer, 185
in pericarditis, acute, 42–43
pleuritic, in acute pericarditis, 42
psychogenic, 325
  chest pain, 37
in pulmonary embolism, 41
of renal and ureteral colic, 256
sensation to, in arterial occlusion, 133
in shoulder, 312–317
and stimulation of nerve fibers, 21
in thoracic outlet syndrome, 404
in Tietze's syndrome, 36
in thyroid, 364
Pain syndromes, neurogenic, 402
Palpitation, 123–132
  with cardiac arrhythmia, 124–126
  causes of, without arrhythmia, 124
  diagnostic approach, 126–132
Palsy, pseudobulbar, 399
Pancreatic islet cell disease, hypoglycemia in, 335
Pancreatitis
  acute, and prolonged chest pain, 44
  and hypocalcemia, 369
  pleural effusion in, 175
Panhypopituitarism, vs. anorexia nervosa, 17
Papillary muscle, dysfunction of, and mitral regurgitation, 103
Papulosquamous skin disease, as cause of itching, 22
Para-aminosalicylic acid, and lymphocy-tosis, 235
Paracentesis, diagnostic, in ascites, 204
Paralysis, common causes of, 398
Parasitic infestation, and eosinophilia, 236
Parasitosis
  as cause of pruritus, 23, 24
  delusions of, 25
Parasternal pulsations, left, 66
Parathyroid hormone assay, in hyper-calcemia, 378
Parathyroidectomy, and relief of pruritus, 24
Paravertebral ossifications, radiographic findings in, 326
Parenchymal infiltrates, acute, 162
Parkinson's disease, myalgia in, 306

Little, Brown's Paperback Book Series
Little, Brown and Company
34 Beacon Street
Boston, Massachusetts 02106

Basic Medical Sciences

Colton	Statistics in Medicine
Hine & Pfeiffer	Behavioral Science
Kent	General Pathology: A Programmed Text
Levine	Pharmacology
Peery & Miller	Pathology
Richardson	Basic Circulatory Physiology
Selkurt	Physiology
Sidman & Sidman	Neuroanatomy: A Programmed Text
Siegel, Albers, et al.	Basic Neurochemistry
Snell	Clinical Anatomy for Medical Students
Snell	Clinical Embryology for Medical Students
Valtin	Renal Function
Watson	Basic Human Neuroanatomy

Clinical Medical Sciences

Clark & MacMahon	Preventive Medicine
Eckert	Emergency-Room Care
Grabb & Smith	Plastic Surgery
Green	Gynecology
Judge & Zuidema	Methods of Clinical Examination
Keefer & Wilkins	Medicine
MacAusland & Mayo	Orthopedics
Nardi & Zuidema	Surgery
Niswander	Obstetrics
Thompson	Primer of Clinical Radiology
Ziai	Pediatrics

Manuals and Handbooks

Arndt	Manual of Dermatologic Therapeutics
Berk et al.	Handbook of Critical Care
Children's Hospital Medical Center, Boston	Manual of Pediatric Therapeutics
Clawson & Iversen	Manual of Orthopaedic Therapeutics
Condon & Nyhus	Manual of Surgical Therapeutics
Friedman & Papper	Problem-Oriented Medical Diagnosis
Gardner & Provine	Manual of Acute Bacterial Infections
Massachusetts General Hospital	Diet Manual
Massachusetts General Hospital	Manual of Nursing Procedures
Neelon & Ellis	A Syllabus of Problem-Oriented Patient Care
Papper	Manual of Medical Care of the Surgical Patient
Shader	Manual of Psychiatric Therapeutics
Spivak & Barnes	Manual of Clinical Problems in Internal Medicine: Annotated with Key References
Wallach	Interpretation of Diagnostic Tests
Washington University Department of Medicine	Manual of Medical Therapeutics
Zimmerman	Techniques of Patient Care

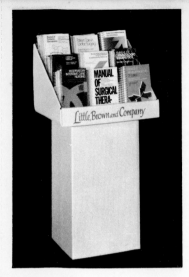

THE LITTLE, BROWN
MANUAL SERIES

Titles in Little, Brown's Manual Series are readily available at all medical bookstores throughout the United States and abroad. You may also order copies directly from Little, Brown and Company, 34 Beacon Street, Boston, Massachusetts 02106, by simply tearing out, filling in, and mailing this postage-free card.

☐ MANUAL OF DERMATOLOGIC THERAPEUTICS — Arndt (#051802-93AD1). $8.95

☐ MANUAL OF PEDIATRIC THERAPEUTICS — Children's Hospital Medical Center, Boston; Graef & Cone, Editors (#139122-88AC1) $8.95

☐ MANUAL OF SURGICAL THERAPEUTICS, 3rd Edition — Condon & Nyhus, Editors (#152838) $8.95

☐ PROBLEM-ORIENTED MEDICAL DIAGNOSIS — Friedman & Papper, Editors, (#293547-88AB1) $8.95

☐ MANUAL OF ACUTE BACTERIAL INFECTIONS: EARLY DIAGNOSIS AND TREATMENT — Gardner & Provine (#303275) $9.95

☐ DIET MANUAL — Massachusetts General Hospital Dietary Department (#549568) .... Due Spring 1976

☐ MASSACHUSETTS GENERAL HOSPITAL MANUAL OF NURSING PROCEDURES — Massachusetts General Hospital Department of Nursing (#549541-88X1) $8.95

☐ A SYLLABUS OF PROBLEM-ORIENTED PATIENT CARE — Neelon & Ellis (#599808-88W1) $4.95

☐ MANUAL OF MEDICAL CARE OF THE SURGICAL PATIENT — Papper, Editor (#690473) $8.95

☐ MANUAL OF PSYCHIATRIC THERAPEUTICS — Shader, Editor (#782203) $8.95

☐ MANUAL OF CLINICAL PROBLEMS IN INTERNAL MEDICINE: ANNOTATED WITH KEY REFERENCES – Spivak & Barnes (#807133-88Y1) $9.95

☐ INTERPRETATION OF DIAGNOSTIC TESTS: A HANDBOOK SYNOPSIS OF LABORATORY MEDICINE, 2nd Edition — Wallach (#920436-88Z1) ... $7.95

☐ MANUAL OF MEDICAL THERAPEUTICS, 21st Edition — Washington University Department of Medicine; Boedeker & Dauber, Editors (#924024-88AD1) $7.95

NAME_____
        (Please print)

STREET_____

CITY_____ STATE _____

        ZIP CODE_____

ORDERS FOR LESS THAN $10.00 MUST BE PREPAID. PUBLISHER PAYS POSTAGE AND HANDLING CHARGES ON ALL ORDERS ACCOMPANIED BY A CHECK. (Please add sales tax if applicable.)

☐ Bill me.
☐ Check enclosed.

The prices listed above are Little, Brown and Company prices as of the printing of this particular book and are subject to change at any time without notice. In no way do they reflect the prices at which books will be sold to you by suppliers other than Little, Brown and Company.

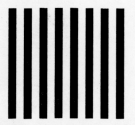